Second Edition

Pocket Guide to

COMMONLY

PRESCRIBED

DRUGS

Glenn N. Levine, MD
Assistant Professor of Medicine
Baylor College of Medicine
Staff Physician, Section of Cardiology
Houston Veterans Affairs Medical Center
Houston, Texas

G7J6VTY- JJJXJG

Ver 1.9 97

7014037

G7QV$Y-TQXJG

APPLETON & LANGE
Stamford, Connecticut

Copyright © 1996 by Appleton & Lange
A Simon & Schuster Company

96 97 98 99 00 / 10 9 8 7 6 5 4 3 2

Prentice Hall International (UK) Limited, *London*
Prentice Hall of Australia Pty. Limited, *Sydney*
Prentice Hall of Canada Inc., *Toronto*
Prentice Hall Hispanoamericana, S.A., *Mexico*
Prentice Hall of India Private Limited, *New Delhi*
Prentice Hall of Japan, Inc., *Tokyo*
Prentice Hall of Southeast Asia Pte. Ltd., *Singapore*
Editora Prentice Hall do Brasil, Ltda., *Rio de Janeiro*
Prentice Hall, *Englewood Cliffs, New Jersey*

ISSN: 1063-7168

Acquisitions Editor: Shelley Reinhardt
Production Service: Rainbow Graphics, Inc.
Cover Designer: Mary Skudlarek

ISBN 0-8385-8099-8

9 780838 0998 90000

PRINTED IN THE UNITED STATES OF AMERICA

Table of Contents

Preface

The *Pocket Guide to Commonly Prescribed Drugs* is a comprehensive, easy-to-use reference to the essential information needed for prescribing medications safely and effectively. Drugs are listed alphabetically, with all information for each drug contained within its individual listing. There is no need to search through a table of contents or index, to turn from chapter to chapter, to consult confusing charts, or to seek cross-referenced information.

Recognizing that medical practitioners are hard pressed for time, each listing has been kept as concise as possible with only the most clinically relevant information included. Comprehensive, easy-to-understand information is included for each drug and presented under clearly labeled subheadings. A quick reading of the introductory pages should better acquaint the reader with how best to use the information contained in the *Pocket Guide*.

Many suggestions by house staff, medical students, and other health care practitioners have been incorporated into the second edition of the *Pocket Guide*. Numerous new drugs are now listed, cost and pregnancy categories have been given their own listings, and the book has been reconfigured to be more compact in order to more easily fit into a lab or other coat pocket.

The *Pocket Guide to Commonly Prescribed Drugs* should prove useful to a wide variety of health care providers, including interns and residents, medical students, primary care physicians, nurses and nurse practitioners, physician assistants, podiatrists, dentists, and other health-related professionals.

I hope that this book will help you, the medical practitioner, to prescribe drugs with confidence and safety, and thus provide your patients with the best medical care.

GNL

Boston
April 1996

Please send comments and suggestions to:

Dr. Glenn N. Levine
Section of Cardiology
VAMC (111B)
2002 Holcombe Blvd.
Houston, TX 77030

Acknowledgments

I wish to express my gratitude to many individuals, including many house staff and medical students, for their suggestions concerning revisions and additions to the second edition of the *Pocket Guide,* to Lori Dawson for her excellent secretarial assistance, and to the many distinguished consultants who have contributed their expertise to the preparation of the *Pocket Guide,* including:

Gary J. Balady, MD, FACC; Director, Preventive Cardiology, Boston University Medical Center Hospital; Associate Professor of Medicine, Boston University School of Medicine

Thomas W. Barber, MD; Associate Director of Housestaff Training, Boston University Residency Program; Assistant Professor of Medicine, Boston University School of Medicine

Dino Beer, MD; Chief, Pulmonary Medicine, Newton-Wellsley Hospital; Medical Director, Intensive Care Unit, Newton-Wellsley Hospital; Associate Professor of Medicine, Tufts University School of Medicine

Sheilah Bernard, MD, FACC; Director, Coronary Care Unit, Boston City Hospital; Director, Heart Station, Boston City Hospital; Director, Clinical Cardiology, Boston City Hospital; Assistant Professor of Medicine, Boston University School of Medicine

Elizabeth Buonepane; Clinical Director, Pharmacy, Boston University Medical Center Hospital

David Cave, MD; Chief, Division of Gastroenterology, St. Elizabeth's Medical Center; Associate Professor of Medicine, Tufts University School of Medicine

Jay D. Coffman, MD, Section Head, Vascular Medicine; Associate Chief, Department of Medicine, Professor of Medicine, Boston University School of Medicine

Robert A. Edelstein, MD; Assistant Professor of Urology, Boston University School of Medicine

Karen M. Freund, MD, MPH; Chief, Women's Health Unit,

Boston University Medical Center Hospital; Associate Professor of Medicine, Boston University School of Medicine

Warren Hershman, MD; Assistant Professor of Medicine, Boston University School of Medicine

Paul J. Hesketh, MD; Codirector, Hematology Oncology Department; St. Elizabeth's Medical Center; Associate Professor of Medicine, Tufts University School of Medicine

James S. Hoffman, MD; Staff Gastroenterologist, St. Elizabeth's Medical Center; Assistant Professor of Medicine, Tufts University School of Medicine

Benton Idelson, MD; Director, Peritoneal Dialysis, Boston University Medical Center Hospital; Professor of Medicine, Boston University School of Medicine

Andra E. Ibrahim, MD; Assistant Professor of Anesthesia, Boston University School of Medicine

Carlos S. Kase, MD; Professor of Neurology, Boston University School of Medicine

Michael D. Klein, MD, FACC; Director, Cardiac Care Unit, Boston University Medical Center Hospital; Associate Professor of Medicine, Boston University School of Medicine

J. Thomas LaMont, MD; Chief, Section of Cardiology, Boston University Medical Center Hospital; Professor of Medicine, Boston University School of Medicine

Joseph Loscalzo, MD, Ph.D., FACC; Chief, Cardiovascular Medicine, Boston University Medical Center Hospital, Boston City Hospital, Boston VA Medical Center; Director, Whitaker Cardiovascular Institute; Vice Chairman, Department of Medicine; Distinguished Professor of Cardiovascular Medicine, Professor of Biochemistry, Boston University School of Medicine

Philip J. Podrid, MD, FACC; Director, Arrhythmia Service, Boston University Medical Center Hospital; Professor of Medicine, Boston University School of Medicine

Neil Ruderman, MD; Director, Diabetes Unit, Boston University Medical Center Hospital; Professor of Medicine, Boston University School of Medicine

Richard Saitz, MD, MPH; Associate Director, Clinical Addiction, Research, and Education Unit, Boston City Hospital; Assistant Professor of Medicine, Boston University School of Medicine

Robert Tarpy, MD; Staff Pulmonologist, Faulkner Hospital;

Assistant Professor of Medicine, Tufts University School of Medicine

Charles P. Tift, MD; Associate Professor of Medicine, Boston University School of Medicine

Sumar Verma, MD; Associate Professor of Psychiatry, Boston University School of Medicine; Lecturer in Psychiatry, Harvard Medical School

Evan Vosberg, MD; Director, Autologous Stem Cell Transplant Service, Boston University Medical Center Hospital; Medical Coordinator, Hematology–Oncology Inpatient Ward, Boston University Medical Center Hospital; Assistant Professor of Medicine, Boston University School of Medicine

Donald A. Weiner, MD, FACC; Director, Exercise Laboratory, Boston University Medical Center Hospital; Professor of Medicine, Boston University School of Medicine

Introduction

This book is designed to be a pocket reference to medications commonly used in clinical medicine. It is not intended to be all inclusive, but rather to list some of the common and clinically important pharmacologic properties of each drug. Information contained in the *Pocket Guide* was compiled from a variety of sources. There is some variation in the literature and among specialists on certain aspects of the clinical profile for many drugs. Listed in this book are what the author considers to be reasonably well accepted and agreed on information for each agent.

Drugs are generally listed by their generic name, in capital letters, and are cross-referenced by trade name; combination drugs are generally listed by trade name. Information included for most drugs consists of dosing schedules; mode of clearance; dosage adjustments necessary in renal failure, liver disease, and following dialysis; side effects; drug interactions; contraindications; pregnancy category; relative cost; therapeutic blood levels; serum values that should be monitored during therapy; and other clinically useful "pearls." The information provided in each section, and how to use it, follows.

The **Dose** section lists the initial, loading, and maintenance or usual dose of each drug, where relevant. For some drugs, the dosing schedule often depends on the route of administration or the specific disease being treated. Doses given are those for adult patients; dosing schedules for children usually differ and are given only for those drugs commonly prescribed for children.

The **Preparations** section lists available forms, sizes, and concentrations of each medication.

The **Actions** section lists the pharmacologic or physiologic action of the drug and what it is used for. Additional information on the mechanism of action is provided where appropriate.

The **Clearance** section describes major modes of elimination for the drug, usually by various degrees of liver metabolism and renal excretion. This section gives general guidelines on dosing changes in patients with renal insufficiency, as listed in the chart below, and whether dosage adjustments are necessary in patients with liver disease. The section also lists whether enough drug is removed by hemodialysis (hemodialysis) or peritoneal dialysis (peritoneal dialysis) to require supplemental doses after dialysis.

Designation	GFR = 10–50 ml/min	GFR < 10 ml/min (ESRD)
"no change"	No adjustment necessary	No adjustment necessary
"slight"	Give 75–100% the usual dose or increase the dosing interval up to 1½ times the normal interval	Up to 2 times the normal interval
"moderate"	Give 50–75% the usual dose or increase the dosing interval to ≈ ½–2 times the normal interval	Give only 25–50% the usual dose or increase the dosing interval to ≈2–4 times the normal interval
"marked"	Give ≤50% the usual dose or increase the dosing interval to ≈2–4 times the normal interval	Give <25% the usual dose or increase the dosing interval to 2–4 times the normal interval

The **Selected Side Effects** section lists several of the more common or more clinically important side effects associated with each drug, particularly those side effects that one should learn to associate with each respective drug. *This section is NOT designed to list every reported side effect of each medication.* Reported side effects that occurred with similar frequency in control groups, and thus did not appear to be causally related to the medication, are usually not included. For a full listing of reported side effects for each drug, the *Physicians Desk Reference (PDR)* should be consulted.

The **Selected Drug Interactions** section lists several selected important interactions that the listed drug has with other medications, particularly those drug interactions that one should learn to associate with each respective drug. *This section is NOT designed to list every reported drug interaction for each medication.* For a full listing of reported drug interactions for each drug, the *Physicians Desk Reference (PDR)* should be consulted. Interactions include reciprocal effects on serum level of the listed drug or drugs taken with it; increased metabolism of the listed drug through induction of hepatic enzymes by other drugs; and effects of the listed drug on prothrombin time (PT) in patients taking warfarin.

The **Cautions** section lists some of the clinically important contraindications and relative contraindications to the use of each drug.

The **Pregnancy Category** listing gives the Food and Drug Administration (FDA) categorization of the drug with respect to potential effects on the embryo or fetus of pregnant patients. Brief summaries of each pregnancy category are listed below. For medications that do not have an FDA-established pregnancy category, important information may nevertheless be available to guide prescribing decisions, and *PDR* or other sources should be consulted.

Category A: Controlled studies in women have failed to demonstrate a risk to the first-trimester fetus, and the possibility of fetal harm appears remote.

Category B: (1) Animal studies have not shown a fetal risk but there are no controlled studies in pregnant women, *or* (2) animal studies have shown an adverse effect that was not confirmed in controlled studies of women.

Category C: (1) Studies in animals have revealed adverse effects on the fetus but there are no controlled studies in women, *or* (2) studies in women and animals are not available. Drugs in this category should be given only if the potential benefit justifies the potential risk to the fetus.

Category D: There is positive evidence of human fetal risk, but the benefits from use in pregnant women may be acceptable despite the risk.

Category X: Studies in animals, humans, or both have demonstrated fetal abnormalities, and the risk of using the

drug in pregnant women clearly outweighs any possible benefit. The drug is contraindicated in women who are pregnant or
potentially pregnant.

The **Cost** section gives a relative cost for each drug. The
relative cost of each drug is denoted with one ($) to four
($$$$) dollar signs, with each drug somewhat arbitrarily rated
into one of the four categories that best describes its cost. Average retail costs for many drugs are also given. Cost rating
criteria are as follows:

$ Inexpensive
   Affordable to patients on even a limited income; inex-
   pensive compared with other drugs with similar functions.

$$ Should be affordable to most patients.
   Cost should generally not be a significant concern when
   using or prescribing this drug.

$$$ Somewhat or relatively expensive.
   May be difficult for many patients to afford (if not ade-
   quately covered by insurance); cost may be a considera-
   tion when using or prescribing this drug; consider using
   less expensive drugs with similar actions or functions.

$$$$ Expensive in both relative and absolute terms.
   Cost should be considered when using or prescribing
   this drug; consider using (substantially) less expensive
   drugs with similar actions or functions.

The **Pearls** section lists any other clinically useful information concerning the drug, including, when appropriate, blood
levels to monitor, onset and duration of action, and therapeutic
drug levels.

Commonly Used Drugs by Category

ACNE TREATMENT
Benzamycin (BENZOYL PEROXIDE + ERYTHROMYCIN)
BENZOYL PEROXIDE (Benoxyl, Benzac, Benzagel, Clearasil, Fostex, Oxy Lotion, etc)
CLINDAMYCIN PHOSPHATE topical solution, lotion, and gel (Cleocin T)
ERYTHROMYCIN topical solution and gel (Erycette, Ery-Derm, Erygel, Erymax)
ISOTRETINOIN (Accutane)
TRETINOIN topical cream, gel, and liquid (Retin-A)

AIDS: *see* HIV INFECTIONS

ALCOHOL WITHDRAWAL (Prophylaxis and Acute Treatment)
CHLORDIAZEPOXIDE (Librium)
DIAZEPAM (Valium)

ANALGESICS
ACETAMINOPHEN (Tylenol)
ACETYLSALICYLIC ACID (aspirin, ASA, enteric-coated aspirin, Ecotrin, ZORprin)
CODEINE
Tylenol with Codeine
Darvocet
Darvon
DIFLUNISAL (Dolobid)
Esgic (BUTALBITAL + ACETAMINOPHEN + CAFFEINE)
ETODOLAC (Lodine)
FENTANYL transdermal system (Duragesic)
FENTANYL CITRATE injection (Sublimaze)
Fioricet (BUTALBITAL, ACETAMINOPHEN + CAFFEINE)
Fiorinal (BUTALBITAL, ASA + CAFFEINE)
HYDROMORPHONE (Dilaudid)

IBUPROFEN (Advil, IBU, IBU-Tabs, Medipren, Motrin, Motrin IB, Nuprin, Rufen)
INDOMETHACIN (Indocin, Indocin SR)
KETOROLAC (Toradol)
Lorcet 10/650 (HYDROCODONE + ACETAMINOPHEN)
MEPERIDINE (Demerol)
METHADONE
MORPHINE (*long-acting preparation:* MS Contin)
NABUMETONE (Relafen)
NAPROXEN (Naprosyn)
Percocet (OXYCODONE + ACETAMINOPHEN)
Percodan (OXYCODONE HCl, OXYCODONE TEREPH-THALATE + ASA)
PIROXICAM (Feldene)
PROPOXYPHENE (Darvon, Darvon-N; *see also* Darvocet)
SALSALATE (Disalcid)
SULINDAC (Clinoril)
Tylenol with Codeine
Vicodin, Vicodin ES (ACETAMINOPHEN + HYDROCO-DONE)

ANESTHETIC AND PARALYTIC AGENTS
DIPRIVAN (Propofol)
FENTANYL CITRATE (Sublimaze)
MIDAZOLAM (Versed)
PANCURONIUM (Pavulon)
PENTOBARBITAL (Nembutal)
SECOBARBITAL (Seconal)
SUCCINYLCHOLINE
VECURONIUM (Norcuron)

ANTACIDS/ULCER TREATMENTS
BISMUTH SUBSALICYLATE (Pepto-Bismol)
CIMETIDINE (Tagamet)
CISAPRIDE (Propulsid)
FAMOTIDINE (Pepcid)
LANSOPRAZOLE (Prevacid)
Maalox (MAGNESIUM HYDROXIDE + ALUMINUM HYDROXIDE)
NIZATIDINE (Axid)

OMEPRAZOLE (Prilosec; formerly Losec)
RANITIDINE (Zantac)
Rolaids (DIHYDROXYALUMINUM SODIUM CARBONATE)
SUCRALFATE (Carafate)

ANTIANGINALS
ATENOLOL (Tenormin)
DILTIAZEM (Cardizem)
ESMOLOL (Brevibloc)
ISOSORBIDE DINITRATE (Isordil, Isordil Tembids)
ISOSORBIDE MONONITRATE (Imdur, Ismo, Monoket)
LABETALOL (Normodyne, Trandate)
METOPROLOL (Lopressor, Toprol XL)
NADOLOL (Corgard)
NICARDIPINE (Cardene)
NIFEDIPINE (Procardia, Procardia XL)
NITROGLYCERIN
PINDOLOL (Visken)
PROPRANOLOL (Inderal, Inderal LA)
TIMOLOL (Blocadren)
VERAPAMIL (Calan, Calan SR, Isoptin, Isoptin SR, Verelan)
Zestoretic (LISINOPRIL + HYDROCHLOROTHIAZIDE)

ANTIARRHYTHMICS
ADENOSINE
AMIODARONE (Cordarone)
BRETYLIUM (Bretylol)
DILTIAZEM (Cardizem)
DISOPYRAMIDE (Norpace)
ESMOLOL (Brevibloc)
FLECAINIDE (Tambocor)
LIDOCAINE (Xylocaine)
MEXILETINE (Mexitil)
MORICIZINE (Ethmozine)
PROCAINAMIDE (Procan SR, Pronestyl)
PROPAFENONE (Rythmol)
QUINIDINE (QUINIDINE SULFATE, Quinaglute, Quinidex
    Extentabs)

SOTALOL (Betapace)
TOCAINIDE (Tonocard)
VERAPAMIL (Calan, Calan SR, Isoptin, Isoptin SR, Verelan)

ANTIBIOTICS
AMIKACIN
AMOXICILLIN
AMPICILLIN
AUGMENTIN
AZITHROMYCIN (Zithromax)
AZTREONAM
BACTRIM
CEFACLOR (Ceclor)
CEFADROXIL (Duricef)
CEFAZOLIN (Ancef, Kefzol)
CEFIXIME (Suprax)
CEFOPERAZONE (Cefobid)
CEFOTAXIME (Claforan)
CEFOTETAN (Cefotan)
CEFOXITIN (Mefoxin)
CEFTAZIDIME (Fortaz, Tazicef, Tazidime)
CEFTIZOXIME (Cefizox)
CEFTRIAXONE (Rocephin)
CEFUROXIME (Ceftin, Kefurox, Zinacef)
CEPHALEXIN (Keflex, Keftab)
CHLORAMPHENICOL (Chloromycetin)
CIPROFLOXACIN (Cipro)
CLARITHROMYCIN (Biaxin)
CLINDAMYCIN (Cleocin)
DICLOXACILLIN
DOXYCYCLINE (Vibramycin, Vibra-Tabs)
ERYTHROMYCIN (E-Mycin, Ery-Tab, Erythrocin, PCE 333, PCE 500)
GENTAMICIN (Garamycin)
LOMEFLOXACIN (Maxaquin)
METRONIDAZOLE (Flagyl)
MEZLOCILLIN (Mezlin)
NITROFURANTOIN (Macrodantin)
NORFLOXACIN (Noroxin)

OFLOXACIN (Floxin)
OXACILLIN
PENICILLIN (Pen-Vee K)
PENTAMIDINE (NebuPent, Pentam)
PIPERACILLIN
Primaxin (IMIPENEM + CILASTATIN)
SEPTRA
TETRACYCLINE
TICARCILLIN
Timentin (TICARCILLIN + CLAVULANATE)
TOBRAMYCIN
Unasyn (AMPICILLIN + SULBACTAM)
VANCOMYCIN

ANTICONVULSANTS
CARBAMAZEPINE (Tegretol)
CLONAZEPAM (Klonopin)
DIAZEPAM (Valium)
ETHOSUXIMIDE (Zarontin)
GABAPENTIN (Neurontin)
LAMOTRIGINE (Lamictal)
PENTOBARBITAL (Nembutal)
PHENOBARBITAL
PHENYTOIN (Dilantin)
VALPROIC ACID (DIVALPROEX SODIUM, VPA, Depakene, Depakote)

ANTIDEPRESSANTS
AMITRIPTYLINE (Elavil)
AMOXAPINE (Asendin)
BUPROPION (Wellbutrin)
CLOMIPRAMINE (Anafranil)
DESIPRAMINE (Norpramin)
FLUOXETINE (Prozac)
IMIPRAMINE (Tofranil)
NORTRIPTYLINE (Pamelor)
PAROXETINE (Paxil)
SERTRALINE (Zoloft)
TRAZODONE (Desyrel)

ANTIDIARRHEAL AGENTS (*see also* TRAVELERS' DIARRHEA)
Deodorized Tincture of Opium (DTO)
Kaopectate liquid (KAOLIN + PECTIN)
Lomotil (DIPHENOXYLATE + ATROPINE)
LOPERAMIDE (Imodium)

ANTIEMETICS
CHLORPROMAZINE (Thorazine)
HYDROXYZINE (Atarax, Vistaril)
MECLIZINE (Antivert)
METOCLOPRAMIDE (Reglan)
ONDANSETRON (Zofran)
PERPHENAZINE (Trilafon, etc)
PROCHLORPERAZINE (Compazine)
PROMETHAZINE (Phenergan)
SCOPOLAMINE
TRIMETHOBENZAMIDE (Tigan)

ANTIEPILEPTIC AGENTS (*see* ANTICONVULSANTS)

ANTIFUNGAL AGENTS
Topical
CLOTRIMAZOLE (Lotrimin, Mycelex)
Cortisporin Cream (POLYMYXIN B + NEOMYCIN + HYDROCORTISONE)
Cortisporin Ointment (POLYMYXIN B + BACITRACIN + NEOMYCIN + HYDROCORTISONE)
KETOCONAZOLE topical (Nizoral topical)
Lotrisone topical cream (CLOTRIMAZOLE + BETAMETHASONE)
NYSTATIN (Mycostatin cream and ointment)
TERCONAZOLE vaginal cream and suppositories
Systemic
FLUCONAZOLE (Diflucan)
ITRACONAZOLE (Sporanox)
KETOCONAZOLE (Nizoral)

ANTIHISTAMINES
ASTEMIZOLE (Hismanal)
CHLORPHENIRAMINE (Chlor-Trimeton)
Contac (CHLORPHENIRAMINE + PHENYLPROPANOL-AMINE)
DIPHENHYDRAMINE (Benadryl)
LORATADINE (Claritin)
HYDROXYZINE (Atarax, Vistaril)
TERFENADINE (Seldane)

ANTIHYPERTENSIVE AGENTS
Intravenous Agents
ESMOLOL (Brevibloc)
DIAZOXIDE (Hyperstat)
HYDRALAZINE (Apresoline)
LABETALOL (Normodyne, Trandate)
METHYLDOPATE (Aldomet)
NITROGLYCERIN
NITROPRUSSIDE (Nipride)
Oral Agents
Aldactazide
ATENOLOL (Tenormin)
BENAZEPRIL (Lotensin)
Capozide (CAPTOPRIL + HCTZ)
CAPTOPRIL (Capoten)
CHLOROTHIAZIDE (Diuril)
CLONIDINE (Catapres)
DILTIAZEM (Cardizem)
DOXAZOSIN (Cardura)
Dyazide (HYDROCHLOROTHIAZIDE + TRIAMTERENE)
ENALAPRIL (Vasotec)
ESMOLOL (Brevibloc)
FELODIPINE (Plendil)
FOSINOPRIL (Monopril)
GUANABENZ (Wytensin)
GUANETHIDINE (Ismelin)
HYDRALAZINE (Apresoline)
HYDROCHLOROTHIAZIDE (HCTZ, HydroDIURIL, etc.)
Hyzaar (LOSARTAN + HYDROCHLOROTHIAZIDE)

INDAPAMIDE (Lozol)
ISRADIPINE (DynaCirc)
LABETALOL (Normodyne, Trandate)
LISINOPRIL (Prinivil, Zestril)
LOSARTAN (Cozaar)
Lotensin HCT (BENAZEPRIL + HYDROCHLOROTHIA-
    ZIDE)
Maxzide, Maxzide-25 (TRIAMTERENE + HYDROCHLO-
    ROTHIAZIDE)
METHYLDOPA (Aldomet)
METOPROLOL (Lopressor, Toprol XL)
MODURETIC (AMILORIDE + HYDROCHLOROTHI-
    AZIDE)
NADOLOL (Corgard)
NICARDIPINE (Cardene)
NIFEDIPINE (Procardia, Procardia XL)
PINDOLOL (Visken)
PRAZOSIN (Minipress)
Prinzide (LISINOPRIL + HYDROCHLOROTHIAZIDE)
PROPRANOLOL (Inderal, Inderal LA)
QUINAPRIL (Accupril)
RAMIPRIL (Altace)
RESERPINE (Serpasil)
TERAZOSIN (Hytrin)
TIMOLOL (Blocadren)
TRIAMTERENE (Dyrenium)
VERAPAMIL (Calan, Calan SR, Isoptin, Isoptin SR, Verelan)
Ziac (BISOPROLOL + HYDROCHLOROTHIAZIDE)
Topical Agents
CLONIDINE (Catapres)
NITROGLYCERIN

ANTIPARASITIC AGENTS
LINDANE cream and lotion (Kwell)

ANTIPARKINSONIAN AGENTS
AMANTADINE (Symmetrel)
BENZTROPINE (Cogentin)
BROMOCRIPTINE (Parlodel)
PERGOLIDE MESYLATE (Permax)

SELEGILINE (Eldepryl)
Sinemet (CARBIDOPA + LEVODOPA)
TRIHEXYPHENIDYL (Artane)

ANTIPLATELET AGENTS
ACETYLSALICYLIC ACID (aspirin, ASA, enteric-coated
   aspirin, Ecotrin, ZORprin)
DIPYRIDAMOLE (Persantine)
TICLOPIDINE (Ticlid)

ANTIPSYCHOTIC AGENTS
CHLORPROMAZINE (Thorazine)
HALOPERIDOL (Haldol)
PERPHENAZINE (Trilafon, etc)
THIORIDAZINE (Mellaril)
TRIFLUOPERAZINE (Stelazine)

ANTIPYRETIC AGENTS
ACETAMINOPHEN (Tylenol)
ACETYLSALICYLIC ACID (aspirin, ASA, enteric-coated
   aspirin, Ecotrin, ZORprin)

ANTISPASMODICS
BACLOFEN (LIORESAL)
CYCLOBENZAPRINE (Flexeril)
DANTROLENE (Dantrium)
QUININE (QUININE SULFATE, Quinamm)

ANTITUSSIVE AGENTS
CODEINE
Robitussin A-C
Robitussin DM
DEXTROMETHORPHAN (Delsym)
HYDROMORPHONE (Dilaudid, Hydrostat IR)

ANXIOLYTIC AGENTS
ALPRAZOLAM (Xanax)
BUSPIRONE (BuSpar)

CHLORDIAZEPOXIDE (Librium)
CLONAZEPAM (Klonopin)
DIAZEPAM (Valium)
HYDROXYZINE (Atarax, Vistaril)
LORAZEPAM (Ativan)
MIDAZOLAM (Versed)
OXAZEPAM (Serax)

BRONCHITIS (Outpatient)
AMOXICILLIN
AUGMENTIN
AZITHROMYCIN (Zithromax)
Bactrim (TRIMETHOPRIM + SULFAMETHOXAZOLE)
Septra (TRIMETHOPRIM + SULFAMETHOXAZOLE)
CEFACLOR (Ceclor)
CEFUROXIME (Ceftin)
CLARITHROMYCIN (Biaxin)
ERYTHROMYCIN
OFLOXACIN (Floxin)

BRONCHODILATORS
ALBUTEROL (Proventil, Ventolin)
AMINOPHYLLINE
IPRATROPIUM (Atrovent)
ISOETHARINE (Bronkometer, Bronkosol)
METAPROTERENOL (Alupent, Metaprel)
TERBUTALINE inhaler (Brethaire)
THEOPHYLLINE (Slo-bid, Slo-Phyllin, Theo-24, Theo-Dur,
   Theolair)

CATHARTICS: *see* LAXATIVES

CELLULITIS (Outpatient)
AZITHROMYCIN (Zithromax)
CEFACLOR (Ceclor)
CLARITHROMYCIN (Biaxin)
DICLOXACILLIN
ERYTHROMYCIN

CHOLESTEROL LOWERING AGENTS
CHOLESTYRAMINE (Cholybar, Questran)
COLESTIPOL (Colestid)
FLUVASTATIN (Lescol)
GEMFIBROZIL (Lopid)
LOVASTATIN (Mevacor)
NICOTINIC ACID (Lipo-Nicin, Niacin, Nicobid, Nicolar, Slo-Niacin)
PRAVASTATIN (Pravachol)
PROBUCOL (Lorelco)
SIMVASTATIN (Zocor)

CONJUNCTIVITIS
ERYTHROMYCIN ophthalmic ointment (Ilotycin)
GENTAMICIN SULFATE eye drops (Garamycin Ophthalmic, Genoptic)

CONTRACEPTIVES
Desogen contraceptive pills (DESOGESTREL + ETHINYL ESTRADIOL
MEDROXYPROGESTERONE (Depo-Provera)
Levlen oral contraceptive (LEVONORGESTREL + ETHINYL ESTRADIOL
LEVONORGESTREL (Norplant)
Norinyl oral contraceptive pills (NORETHINDRONE + ETHINYL ESTRADIOL or NORETHINDRONE + MESTRANOL)
Ortho-Cyclen contraceptive pills (NORGESTIMATE + ETHINYL ESTRADIOL)
Ortho-Novum contraceptive pills (NORETHINDRONE + ETHINYL ESTRADIOL or NORETHINDRONE + MESTRANOL)
Ortho Tri-Cyclen contraceptive pills (NORGESTIMATE + ETHINYL ESTRADIOL)
Tri-Levlen (LEVONORGESTREL + ETHINYL ESTRADIOL)
Tri-Norinyl (NORETHINDRONE + ETHINYL ESTRADIOL)
Triphasil (LEVONORGESTREL + ETHINYL ESTRADIOL)

CORTICOSTEROIDS
Systemic
CORTISONE
DEXAMETHASONE (Decadron)
FLUDROCORTISONE (Florinef)
HYDROCORTISONE (Solu-Cortef)
METHYLPREDNISOLONE (Solu-Medrol)
PREDNISOLONE (Delta-Cortef, Hydeltrasol, Hydeltra-TBA)
PREDNISONE
Topical
FLUOCINONIDE cream, gel, ointment, and solution (Lidex)
Cortisporin Cream (POLYMYXIN B + NEOMYCIN + HYDROCORTISONE)
Cortisporin Ointment (POLYMYXIN B + BACITRACIN + NEOMYCIN + HYDROCORTISONE)
HYDROCORTISONE (Anusol-HC and many other brands)
TRIAMCINOLONE ACETONIDE cream, lotion, and ointment (Aristocort A, Kenalog)

COUGH SUPPRESSANTS (*see* ANTITUSSIVE AGENTS)

DECONGESTANTS
Contac (CHLORPHENIRAMINE + PHENYLPROPANOL-AMINE)
PSEUDOEPHEDRINE (Sudafed)

CYSTITIS (Outpatient, uncomplicated)
Bactrim (TRIMETHOPRIM + ULFAMETHOXAZOLE)
CEPHALEXIN (Keflex, Keftab)
CIPROFLOXACIN (Cipro)
DOXYCYCLINE (Doryx, Vibramycin, Vibra-Tabs)
NORFLOXACIN (Noroxin)
OFLOXACIN (Floxin)
NITROFURANTOIN (Macrobid, Macrodantin)
PHENAZOPYRIDINE (Pyridium—as an analgesic)
Septra (TRIMETHOPRIM + SULFAMETHOXAZOLE)

DIARRHEA: *see* ANTIDIARRHEAL AGENTS and TRAVELERS' DIARRHEA

DIURETICS
ACETAZOLAMIDE (Diamox)
Aldactazide
AMILORIDE (Midamor)
BUMETANIDE (Bumex)
CHLOROTHIAZIDE (Diuril)
Dyazide (HYDROCHLOROTHIAZIDE + TRIAMTERENE)
FUROSEMIDE (Lasix)
HYDROCHLOROTHIAZIDE (HCTZ, HydroDIURIL, etc.)
INDAPAMIDE (Lozol)
Maxzide, Maxzide-25 (TRIAMTERENE + HYDROCHLO-ROTHIAZIDE)
METOLAZONE (Zaroxolyn)
MODURETIC (AMILORIDE + HYDROCHLOROTHIA-ZIDE)
SPIRONOLACTONE (Aldactone)
TORSEMIDE (Demadex)
TRIAMTERENE (Dyrenium)

EAR INFECTIONS: *see* ANTIBIOTICS/otitis externa or otitis media

EAR WAX BUILD-UP
TRIETHANOLAMINE otic solution (Cerumenex)

EMETICS
IPECAC syrup

EXPECTORANTS
GUAIFENESIN expectorant (Robitussin)

EYE INFECTIONS: *see also* CONJUNCTIVITIS
Cortisporin Ophthalmic Suspension (HYDROCORTISONE + NEOMYCIN + POLYMYXIN B)

FLATULENCE
SIMETHICONE (Gas-X, Mylicon, Phazyme)

GOUT TREATMENT/PREVENTION
ALLOPURINOL (Zyloprim)
COLCHICINE
INDOMETHACIN (Indocin); *see also* other NONSTER-
OIDAL ANTI-INFLAMMATORY AGENTS

H$_2$-BLOCKERS
CIMETIDINE (Tagamet)
FAMOTIDINE (Pepcid)
NIZATIDINE (Axid)
RANITIDINE (Zantac)

HEMORRHOIDS
Anusol suppositories and ointment
Preparation H ointment, cream, and suppositories

HERPES ZOSTER INFECTIONS
ACYCLOVIR (Zovirax)
FAMCICLOVIR (Famvir)

HIV INFECTION
DIDANOSINE (DDI, Videx)
ZALCITABINE (ddc, DIDEOXYCYTIDINE, Hivid)
ZIDOVUDINE (AZT, Retrovir, ZDV)

HYPERKALEMIA
SODIUM POLYSTYRENE SULFONATE (Kayexalate)

HYPERPHOSPHATEMIA
ALUMINUM CARBONATE (Basaljel)
ALUMINUM HYDROXIDE (Amphojel)

HYPERTHYROIDISM
METHIMAZOLE (Tapazole)

HYPNOTIC AGENTS
DIPHENHYDRAMINE (Benadryl)
ESTAZOLAM (ProSom)
FLURAZEPAM (Dalmane)
LORAZEPAM (Ativan)
TEMAZEPAM (Restoril)
TRIAZOLAM (Halcion)

HYPOCALCEMIA
CALCIUM CARBONATE (Os-Cal–PO)
CALCIUM CHLORIDE (IV)
CALCIUM GLUCONATE (IV)

HYPOGLYCEMIC AGENTS
CHLORPROPAMIDE (Diabinese)
GLIPIZIDE (Glucotrol)
GLYBURIDE (DiaBeta, Micronase)
METFORMIN (Glucophage)
TOLAZAMIDE (Tolinase)
TOLBUTAMIDE (Orinase)

HYPOKALEMIA
POTASSIUM CHLORIDE (K-Dur, K-Tab, Micro-K, Slow-K)

HYPOMAGNESEMIA
MAGNESIUM OXIDE (Mag-Ox 400)
MAGNESIUM SULFATE

HYPOPHOSPHATEMIA
PHOSPHORUS (K-Phos, Neutra-Phos)

HYPOTHYROIDISM
L-THYROXINE (LEVOTHYROXINE, T, Levoxine, Synthroid)

INOTROPIC AGENTS
AMRINONE (Inocor)
DIGOXIN (Lanoxin)
DOBUTAMINE (Dobutrex)

DOPAMINE (Intropin)
EPINEPHRINE

LAXATIVES
BISACODYL (Dulcolax)
Ex-Lax (unflavored), Ex-Lax Chocolate laxative, Extra Gentle Ex-Lax
MAGNESIUM HYDROXIDE (MILK OF MAGNESIA, M.O.M.)
Peri-Colace (CASANTHRANOL + DOCUSATE)

LICE: *see* ANTIPARASITIC AGENTS

MUSCLE RELAXANTS (*see* ANTISPASMODICS)

NEUROMUSCULAR BLOCKERS (*see* PARALYTIC AGENTS)

NONSTEROIDAL ANTI-INFLAMMATORY AGENTS (NSAIDs)
DIFLUNISAL (Dolobid)
ETODOLAC (Lodine)
IBUPROFEN (Advil, IBU, IBU-Tabs, Medipren, Motrin, Motrin IB, Nuprin, Rufen)
INDOMETHACIN (Indocin, Indocin SR)
KETOROLAC (Toradol)
NABUMETONE (Relafen)
NAPROXEN (Naprosyn)
PIROXICAM (Feldene)
SALSALATE (Disalcid)
SULINDAC (Clinoril)

OCULAR INFLAMMATION: *see also* CONJUNCTIVITIS
Cortisporin Ophthalmic Ointment (POLYMYXIN B + BACI-TRACIN + NEOMYCIN + HYDROCORTISONE)
FLUOROMETHOLONE ophthalmic ointment and suspension (FML, FML Forte)

Naphcon-A ophthalmic solution (NAPHAZOLINE + PHENI-
RAMINE)

ORAL HYPOGLYCEMIC AGENTS (*see* HYPOGLYCEMIC AGENTS)

OTITIS EXTERNA
Cortisporin Otic Solution (POLYMYXIN B + NEOMYCIN +
HYDROCORTISONE)

OTITIS MEDIA (Outpatient)
AMOXICILLIN
AUGMENTIN
Bactrim (TRIMETHOPRIM + SULFAMETHOXAZOLE)
Septra (TRIMETHOPRIM + SULFAMETHOXAZOLE)
CEFACLOR (Ceclor)
CEFUROXIME (Ceftin)
CLARITHROMYCIN (Biaxin)

PARALYTIC AGENTS
PANCURONIUM (Pavulon)
SUCCINYLCHOLINE
VECURONIUM (Norcuron)

PNEUMOCYSTIS CARINII PNEUMONIA (PCP)
BACTRIM
DAPSONE
PENTAMIDINE (NebuPent, Pentam)
SEPTRA

PNEUMONIA (Outpatient, uncomplicated)
AMOXICILLIN
AUGMENTIN
AZITHROMYCIN (Zithromax)
Bactrim (TRIMETHOPRIM + SULFAMETHOXAZOLE)
Septra (TRIMETHOPRIM + SULFAMETHOXAZOLE)
CEFACLOR (Ceclor)
CEFUROXIME (Ceftin)

CLARITHROMYCIN (Biaxin)
ERYTHROMYCIN

PRESSORS
AMRINONE (Inocor)
DOPAMINE (Intropin)
EPINEPHRINE
NOREPINEPHRINE (Levophed)
PHENYLEPHRINE (Neo-Synephrine)

POTASSIUM SUPPLEMENTS
POTASSIUM CHLORIDE (K-Dur, K-Tab, Micro-K, Slow-K)

RESPIRATORY AGENTS
ACETYLCYSTEINE (*N*-ACETYLCYSTEINE, Mucomyst)
ALBUTEROL (Proventil, Ventolin)
BECLOMETHASONE nasal inhaler and spray (Beconase, Vancenase)
BECLOMETHASONE oral inhaler (Beclovent, Vanceril)
BUDESONIDE Nasal Inhaler (Rhinocort)
GUAIFENESIN expectorant (Robitussin)
IPRATROPIUM (Atrovent)
ISOETHARINE (Bronkometer, Bronkosol)
METAPROTERENOL (Alupent, Metaprel)
Organidin (IODINATED GLYCEROL)
SALMETEROL (Serevent)
TERBUTALINE inhaler (Brethaire)
TRIAMCINOLONE (Azmacort)

SCABIES: *see* ANTIPARASITIC AGENTS

SEDATIVES (*see* ANXIOLYTIC AGENTS)

SEIZURE TREATMENTS (*see* ANTIEPILEPTIC AGENTS)

SINUSITIS (Outpatient)
AMOXICILLIN
AUGMENTIN

Bactrim (TRIMETHOPRIM + SULFAMETHOXAZOLE)
Septra (TRIMETHOPRIM + SULFAMETHOXAZOLE)
CEFACLOR (Ceclor)
CEFUROXIME (Ceftin)
CLARITHROMYCIN (Biaxin)

SKIN INFECTIONS (Superficial); *see also* CELLULITIS
CLINDAMYCIN PHOSPHATE topical solution, lotion, and gel (Cleocin T)
ERYTHROMYCIN topical solution and gel (Erycette, Ery-Derm, Erygel, Erymax)

SUBARACHNOID HEMORRHAGE
NIMODIPINE (Nimotop)

STEROIDS: *see* CORTICOSTEROIDS

STOOL SOFTENERS
DOCUSATE SODIUM (Colace)
Metamucil (PSYLLIUM)

THROMBOLYTIC AGENTS
ANISTREPLASE (APSAC, Eminase)
STREPTOKINASE (Kabikinase, Streptase)
TISSUE PLASMINOGEN ACTIVATOR (ALTEPLASE, t-PA, Activase)
UROKINASE (Abbokinase Open-Cath)

TRANSIENT ISCHEMIC ATTACKS (TIAs)
ACETYLSALICYLIC ACID (aspirin, ASA, enteric-coated aspirin, Ecotrin, ZORprin)
TICLOPIDINE (Ticlid)

TRAVELERS' DIARRHEA (Antibiotic treatment; *see also* DIARRHEA)
Bactrim (TRIMETHOPRIM + SULFAMETHOXAZOLE)
CIPROFLOXACIN (Cipro)

NORFLOXACIN (Noroxin)
Septra (TRIMETHOPRIM + SULFAMETHOXAZOLE)

TUBERCULOSIS
ETHAMBUTOL
ISONIAZID (INH, Nydrazid)
PYRAZINAMIDE (PZA)
RIFAMPIN (Rifadin, Rimactane)
STREPTOMYCIN

ULCER TREATMENTS (*see* ANTACIDS, H_2 BLOCKERS)

URINARY TRACT INFECTION: *see* CYSTITIS

VASOCONSTRICTORS: *see* PRESSORS

URINARY TRACT INFECTIONS: *see* CYSTITIS

VITAMINS AND COFACTORS
COBALAMIN (Vitamin B)
PYRIDOXINE (Vitamin B_6)
THIAMINE (VITAMIN B_1)
Vitamin K

COMMONLY USED DRUGS

Accupril: *see* QUINAPRIL

Accutane: *see* ISOTRETINOIN

ACEBUTOLOL (Sectral)
Dose:
- Initial: 200 mg PO bid.
- Can increase to 600–1200 mg PO daily, given in divided doses.
- Maximum daily dose in elderly patients is 800 mg.

Preparations: 200 and 400 mg capsules.

Actions: β_1-selective β-blocker with intrinsic sympathomimetic activity (ISA); used in the treatment of ventricular arrhythmias.

Clearance: Acebutolol is excreted via the GI tract; its active metabolite, diacetolol, is excreted mainly by the kidney.
- Markedly reduce the dose in patients with decreased renal function.
- Use with caution in patients with liver disease.

Selected Side Effects: Bradycardia, hypotension, heart failure, asthma exacerbation and other side effects associated with β-blockers.

Cautions:
- *Contraindicated in patients with severe bradycardia, overt congestive heart failure or cardiogenic shock, or second- or third-degree AV block.*
- Use with caution in patients with reactive airway disease.

Pregnancy Category: B.

Pearls: Withdraw dose gradually to avoid β-blocker withdrawal.

ACETAMINOPHEN (Tylenol; *see also* Darvocet, Fioricet, Percocet, Tylenol with Codeine, Vicodin, Vicodin ES)
Adult Dose: Preparation dependent:
- Regular-strength: One or two 325 mg tablets PO q4–6h; maximum, 12 tablets in 24 h.

- Extra-strength: Two 500 mg tablets PO q6–8h; maximum, 8 tablets in 24 h.
- Liquid: 30 mL (2 tbsp) of Extra-Strength Tylenol liquid q4–6h prn; maximum, 4000 mg (4 doses) in 24 h.

Children's Dose:

- 2–3 years: 2 Children's Tylenol Chewable Tablets (ie, 160 mg dose) or 1 tsp Children's Tylenol Elixir or Suspension q4h prn (up to a maximum of 5 doses over 24 h).
- 4–5 years: 3 Children's Tylenol Chewable Tablets (ie, 240 mg dose) or 1.5 tsp Children's Tylenol Elixir or Suspension q4h prn (up to a maximum of 5 doses over 24 h).
- 6–8 years: 4 Children's Tylenol Chewable Tablets (ie, 320 mg dose) or 2 tsp Children's Tylenol Elixir or Suspension q4h prn (up to a maximum of 5 doses over 24 h).
- 9–10 years: 5 Children's Tylenol Chewable Tablets (ie, 400 mg dose) or 2.5 tsp Children's Tylenol Elixir or Suspension q4h prn (up to a maximum of 5 doses over 24 h).
- 11–12 years: 6 Children's Tylenol Chewable Tablets (ie, 480 mg dose) or 3 tsp Children's Tylenol Elixir or Suspension q4h prn (up to a maximum of 5 doses over 24 h).

Adult PO Preparations:

- 325 caplets.
- 8 oz bottles of Extra-Strength Tylenol liquid containing 500 mg/15 mL (1 tbsp).

Children's PO Preparations:

- 80 mg Children's Tylenol Chewable Tablets.
- 2 and 4 oz Children's Tylenol Elixir containing 160 mg/5 mL (1 tsp).
- 2 and 4 oz Children's Tylenol Suspension containing 160 mg/5 mL (1 tsp).

Actions: Analgesic and antipyretic agent; used to treat pain and fever.

- Produces analgesia by elevation of the pain threshold.
- Antipyretic effect mediated through action on the hypothalamic heat-regulating center.
- The analgesic and antipyretic effects of acetaminophen are comparable to those of aspirin.

Clearance: Metabolized via liver.

- Slightly increase dosing interval in patients with impaired renal function (metabolites can accumulate).

- Avoid in patients with significant liver disease.
- Supplemental dose suggested after hemodialysis but not after peritoneal dialysis.

Selected Side Effects: *Hepatotoxicity* (at "overdose" levels and with chronic use of 4–8 g daily).

Cautions: *Avoid in patients with liver disease and heavy alcohol users.*

Cost: $.

Pearls:

- Hepatotoxicity is rare if <10 g is ingested (unless patient has history of alcohol abuse); fatalities rare if <15 g is ingested.
- Early symptoms of overdose include nausea and vomiting, diaphoresis, anorexia, and general malaise.
- Clinical and laboratory evidence of hepatotoxicity may not become apparent until 48–72 h after ingestion.
- Marked "synergistic" liver toxicity with alcohol.

ACETAZOLAMIDE (Diamox)

Dose: (for metabolic alkalosis): 500 mg PO or IV q8h.

PO Preparations:

- 125 and 250 mg tablets.
- 500 mg sustained-release capsules.

Actions:

- Carbonic anhydrase inhibitor with mild diuretic properties; used primarily to treat glaucoma; occasionally used to treat metabolic alkalosis.
- In the kidney, causes loss of HCO_3^- ion (which carries off Na^+, K^+, and H_2O), resulting in alkalization of the urine.

Clearance: Primarily renally excreted.

- Slightly increase dosing interval in patients with impaired renal function; avoid in patients with end-stage renal disease.
- Clearance is reduced in elderly patients.

Selected Side Effects: Paresthesias (especially tingling), hearing dysfunction, changes in appetite, GI disturbances, electrolyte abnormalities, sulfonamide-derivative adverse/allergic reactions (fever, rash, anaphylaxis, bone marrow depression, hemolytic anemia, decreased WBC and platelets, Stevens–Johnson syndrome).

Cautions:
- *Contraindicated in patients with cirrhosis (increases risk of hepatic encephalopathy), decreased serum levels of Na^+ or K^+, marked liver or kidney dysfunction, hyperchloremic acidosis, or adrenal insufficiency.*
- Patients allergic to sulfonamides can have cross-sensitivity allergic reactions to acetazolamide.

Pregnancy Category: C.

Cost: \$\$ ($\approx$ \$0.50 each 250 mg tablet).

Pearls:
- Use with caution in COPD (can aggravate acidosis).
- Periodically check CBC.
- Alternate-day therapy may increase response by allowing the kidney to recover.

ACETYLCYSTEINE (*N*-ACETYLCYSTEINE, Mucomyst)

As Mucolytic Agent:

Dose: 3–5 mL of 20% solution in nebulizer (or 6–10 mL of 10% solution) tid–qid or prn.

Actions: Mucolytic agent that decreases viscosity by theoretically "opening" disulfide linkages.

Selected Side Effects: Bronchospasm, stomatitis, nausea, rhinorrhea.

Pregnancy Category: B.

Cost: \$\$.

Pearls: Actual clinical role, if any, is controversial.

ACETYLCYSTEINE (*N*-ACETYLCYSTEINE, Mucomyst)

For Acetaminophen Overdose:

Dose: 140 mg/kg loading dose PO or via NG tube, then 17 doses of 70 mg/kg PO or via NG tube q4h.

Actions: Prevents liver injury in acetaminophen overdose (most likely by restoring glutathione levels).

Selected Side Effects: Rare urticaria. The nitrogen load in *N*-acetylcysteine can exacerbate hepatic encephalopathy and necessitate dosage reduction.

Pregnancy Category: B.

Cost: $$.
Pearls:

- *In suspected overdose do not wait for serum level determinations or signs of clinical hepatotoxicity before starting therapy.*
- Do not give concurrently with activated charcoal (which absorbs it).
- Repeat any dose that is vomited within 1 h of administration.
- May be administered by duodenal intubation if necessary.
- Is a potent emetic; therefore, give diluted in fruit juice or soda, in a 3:1 concentration (3 parts soda or juice for every 1 part of acetylcysteine).
- Is available for IV administration in Canada and Europe.
- Dosing regimens vary, but one suggested regimen is a total dose of 30 mg/kg administered over 20 h.

ACETYLSALICYLIC ACID (ASPIRIN, ASA, ENTERIC-COATED ASPIRIN, Ecotrin, ZORprin)

Dose: Disease dependent:

- Acute MI: Single dose of 160 mg of nonenteric-coated ASA (usually two 80 mg baby aspirin tablets) **chewed** (for quicker absorption), then 325 mg PO qd of enteric-coated aspirin.
- Primary and secondary MI prevention: 325 mg of enteric-coated aspirin qod–qd.
- TIA treatment/stroke prevention: 325 PO mg qd–qid (dependent on response).
- Rheumatologic disease: Up to 1 g PO qid.

PO Preparations:

- 80 mg ("baby aspirin"), 325 and 500 mg tablets.
- Ecotrin is an enteric-coated aspirin available in 325 mg tablets.
- ZORprin is controlled-release aspirin.

Actions: Antipyretic, anti-inflammatory, analgesic, antiplatelet, and antithrombotic agent that irreversibly inhibits platelet aggregation, used to treat fever, pain, cardiovascular disease, and cerebrovascular disease.

Clearance: Metabolized via liver; excreted through the kidneys.

- Avoid in patients with end-stage renal disease.
- Modify dosing regimen when used for chronic therapy in patients with liver disease.
- Supplemental dose suggested after hemodialysis or peritoneal dialysis.

Selected Side Effects: GI irritation and bleeding, nausea and vomiting, tinnitus, metabolic acidosis, respiratory alkalosis, ARDS.

Cautions:

- Use with caution, if at all, in patients with liver dysfunction, impaired renal function, elevated uric acid, history of salicylate sensitivity or asthma, or nasal polyps.
- Use with caution in patients taking warfarin or nonsteroidal anti-inflammatory agents (NSAIDs), or with prior upper GI bleeding.
- Avoid in children or teenagers with varicella or other viral infections.

Pregnancy Category: D; *should not be taken during the third trimester.*

Cost: Generic $, Brand names $$.

Pearls:

- Regular use is frequently associated with heme (+) stools without a significant lesion in the GI tract; however, overt ulceration without symptoms can also occur.
- Signs and symptoms of overdose (salicylism) include tinnitus, vertigo, headache, confusion, drowsiness, sweating, hyperventilation, diarrhea, and vomiting.

Achromycin: *see* TETRACYCLINE

Activase: *see* TISSUE PLASMINOGEN ACTIVATOR

ACTIVATED CHARCOAL: *see* CHARCOAL

Acutrim: *see* PHENYLPROPANOLAMINE

ACYCLOVIR (Zovirax)

Dose: Disease dependent.
- Mucocutaneous lesion: 5% ointment q3h 6 times daily.
- Genital herpes: (1) 200 mg PO q4h 5 times daily or (2) 400 mg PO tid.
- Herpes zoster (shingles): 800 mg PO q4h 5 times daily.
- Severe genital herpes: 5 mg/kg IV q8h.
- Herpes simplex encephalitis: 10 mg/kg IV q8h.
- Herpes zoster (shingles) in immunocompromised host:
  - ▶ mild cases: 800 mg PO q4h 5 times daily.
  - ▶ severe cases: 10-12 mg/kg IV q8h.
- Secondary prevention of recurrent genital herpes (especially in immunocompromised patients): 200–400 mg PO bid.

Preparations:
- 200 capsules, and 400 & 800 mg tablets.
- 1 pint bottle of suspension containing 200 mg/5 mL (1 tsp).
- 3 and 15 g containers of 5% ointment.

Actions: Antiviral agent that inhibits DNA synthesis; used to treat HSV-I, HSV-II, varicella-zoster virus, and Herpes simplex infection.

Clearance: Predominantly renally excreted.
- Moderately increase dosing interval in patients with impaired renal function.
- No change in dosage needed for patients with liver disease.
- Supplemental dose suggested after hemodialysis.

Selected Side Effects: Route dependent:
- PO: Nausea and vomiting.
- IV: Local phlebitis, rash, transient rise in serum creatinine, rare CNS changes (1%).

Pregnancy Category: C.

Cost: $$$$ (≈ $1 each 200 mg tablet; ≈ $3.50 each 800 mg tablet).

Pearls:
- Patients should be well hydrated to avoid renal tubule crystallization.
- Can be taken without regard to meals.

Adalat, Adalat CC: *see* NIFEDIPINE

ADENOSINE

Dose:
- Initial: 6 mg IV.
- If no response, may give 12 mg IV.
- This 12 mg dose may be repeated one additional time.

Actions: Slows conduction through the AV node, and thus can terminate supraventricular tachycardias (SVT) involving the AV node (including those caused by Wolf–Parkinson–White [WPW] syndrome)
- Has -dromotropic (reduces conduction) but not -inotropic action.

Clearance: $t_{1/2}$ is 30 s; extensively degraded in the body.

Selected Side Effects: Facial flushing, frequent transient chest pain or pressure, dyspnea, transient AV block (including complete heart block).

Selected Drug Interactions:
- Dipyridamole decreases its uptake and markedly delays its clearance.
- Methylxanthines, theophylline, and caffeine all block adenosine receptors and reduce its effectiveness.

Pregnancy Category: C.

Cost: $$ ($15–30; IV verapamil is much less expensive).

Pearls:
- Does not terminate atrial fibrillation, atrial flutter, or ventricular tachycardia, as these arrhythmias do not directly involve the AV node.
- Works within 30 s.
- Inject *quickly* (within 1–2 s), preferably through a large-bore or central IV catheter.

ADH: *see* VASOPRESSIN

Adriamycin: *see* DOXORUBICIN

Advil: *see* IBUPROFEN

ALBUMIN

Dose: 25 g IV initially, then as indicated by clinical situation.

Actions: Albumin preparation that increases plasma osmotic pressure; used (1) to treat peripheral or pulmonary edema,

(2) in certain cases of shock, and (3) by some physicians during paracentesis.

Selected Side Effects: Febrile reactions, nausea and vomiting, increased salivation.

Cautions: Contraindicated in patients with severe anemia or CHF.

Pearls:
- If patient is anemic, packed red blood cells are preferred.
- Use in subjects with hypoalbuminemia and "third-spacing" is very controversial.

ALBUTEROL [SALBUTAMOL] (Proventil, Ventolin, Volmax)

Dose: Route dependent:
- Nebulizer: 0.25–0.5 mL of 0.5% solution in 3 mL NS.
- Metered-dose inhaler: 2 inhalations q4–6h.
- Regular-acting PO: 2–4 mg tid–qid; maximum 8 mg daily.
- Long-acting PO: 4–8 mg of long-acting tablets (Proventil Repetabs, Volmax) q12h.

Preparations:
- 2 and 4 mg regular tablets.
- 4 mg long-acting tablets (Proventil Repetabs, Volmax).
- 16 oz bottles of syrup containing 2 mg/5 mL (1 tsp).
- 17 g inhaler canisters.

Actions: β_2 receptor-selective stimulant used to treat reactive airway disease.

Selected Side Effects: Tachycardia, palpitations, tremor, restlessness and anxiety, rare cough or bronchospasm.

Selected Drug Interactions: MAOI and tricyclics increase its vascular effects (use with caution).

Cautions: Use with caution in patients with CAD, hypertension, or tachyarrhythmias.

Pregnancy Category: C.

Cost: $$$ ($\approx$ $23 each inhaler).

Aldactazide (HYDROCHLOROTHIAZIDE + SPIRONOLACTONE)

Dose: 25–200 mg PO daily of each component, given either qd or in divided doses.

PO Preparations:
- Tablets containing 25 mg hydrochlorothiazide and 25 mg spironolactone.
- Tablets containing 50 mg hydrochlorothiazide and 50 mg spironolactone.

Actions: Combination diuretic with K^+-sparing properties; used to treat hypertension.

Pregnancy Category: Not established.

Cost: Generic \$, Aldactazide \$\$\$ ($\approx$ \$0.15 each 25 mg/25 mg generic tablet; $\approx$ \$0.45 each 25 mg/25 mg Aldactazide tablet).

Aldactone: *see* SPIRONOLACTONE

Aldomet: *see* METHYLDOPA

Aleve: *see* NAPROXEN

Alkeran: *see* MELPHALAN

ALLOPURINOL (Zyloprim)
Dose:
- Initial, 100 mg PO qd.
- May increase by 100 mg at weekly intervals until serum uric acid reaches < 6 mg/dL.
- Usual, 200–300 mg PO qd.

PO Preparations: 100 and 300 mg tablets.

Actions: Xanthine oxidase inhibitor that decreases uric acid production, used to treat gout.

Clearance: Allopurinol and its oxidized metabolite oxypurinol are excreted by the kidneys.
- Moderately to markedly reduced dosage or increased dosing interval in patients with impaired renal function.
- No change in dosage needed for patients with liver disease.

Selected Side Effects: Precipitation of acute gout attack, drowsiness, nausea and vomiting, elevated LFTs, *aller-*

gic reactions (which may begin as a skin rash and progress to Stevens–Johnson syndrome or toxic epidermal necrosis).

Selected Drug Interactions:
- Dramatically reduce dosage of mercaptopurine or azathioprine (Imuran) when given concurrently. Decreases renal excretion of chlorpropamide.

Pregnancy Category: C.

Cost: $.

Pearls:
- Give colchicine when allopurinol is started (to decrease likelihood of precipitating gout attacks).
- *Warn patients to discontinue use immediately if the following symptoms appear (which may signify severe systemic or allergic reaction and may be followed by the development of Stevens–Johnson syndrome or toxic epidermal necrosis): fever, chills, nausea and vomiting, skin rash, itching, painful urination, hematuria, eye irritation, or swelling of lips or mouth.*

ALPHA INTERFERON: *see* INTERFERON

ALPRAZOLAM (Xanax)

Dose:
- Initial: 0.25–0.50 mg PO tid.
- maximum: 4–6 mg PO daily.

PO Preparations: 0.25, 0.5, 1.0, and 2.0 mg tablets.

Actions: Benzodiazepine analog; used to treat anxiety and panic attacks.

Clearance: Metabolized via liver; renally excreted.
- No change in dosage needed in patients with impaired renal function; use with caution in patients with end-stage renal disease (can cause sedation and encephalopathy).

Selected Side Effects: Drowsiness.

Selected Drug Interactions:
- Raises serum levels of tricyclics.
- Potentiates CNS-depressant effects of other CNS depressants.

Pregnancy Category: D.

Cost: Generic $$, Xanax $$$$ (≈ $0.30 each 1 mg generic tablet; ≈ $0.85 each 1 mg Xanax tablet)
Pearls:
- Withdrawal seizures can occur with abrupt discontinuance after even relatively brief use.
- Prolonged use is associated with physical dependence.

Altace: *see* RAMIPRIL

ALTEPLASE: *see* TISSUE PLASMINOGEN ACTIVATOR

ALternaGEL: *see* ALUMINUM HYDROXIDE

ALUMINUM CARBONATE (Basaljel)
Dose:
- 15–30 mL or 2–4 tablets with or after meals and qhs.
- Maximum: 24 capsules, 24 tablets, or 24 tsp in 24 h.
PO Preparations:
- Standard-dose scored tablets.
- 12 oz bottle of standardized suspension.
Actions: Antacid that reduces intestinal absorption of phosphorus; usually used to treat hyperphosphatemia in patients with end-stage renal disease.
Selected Side Effects: Constipation.
Pregnancy Category: C.
Cost: $.

ALUMINUM HYDROXIDE (ALternaGEL)
Dose: 1–2 tsp prn, taken between meals and qhs.
PO Preparations: 5 and 12 oz bottles.
Actions: Antacid that lacks laxative properties of magnesium-containing antacids.
Selected Side Effects: Constipation.
Cost: $$.

ALUMINUM HYDROXIDE (Amphojel)
Dose: 30–60 mL, two 300 mg tablets, or one 600 mg tablet PO tid with meals.

Preparations:
- 300 and 600 mg tablets.
- 12 oz bottles of 320 mg/5 mL (1 tsp) unflavored and peppermint-flavored suspension.

Actions: Antacid that reduces intestinal absorption of phosphorous; usually used to treat hyperphosphatemia in patients with end-stage renal disease.

Selected Side Effects: Constipation.

Cost: $$.

ALUMINUM PHOSPHATE (Phosphaljel)

Dose: 15–30 mL PO q2h between meals and qhs.

Selected Side Effects: Constipation.

Selected Drug Interactions: Reduces effectiveness of tetracyclines.

Cost: $$.

Pregnancy Category: C.

Alupent: *see* METAPROTERENOL

AMANTADINE (Symmetrel)

Dose: Disease dependent:
- Parkinsonian and extrapyramidal symptoms: 100 mg PO bid initially; may increase dose slowly to 300–400 mg daily, given in divided doses.
- Influenza A virus infection: 200 mg PO qd; if CNS side effects develop, may give 100 mg PO bid instead.

PO Preparations:
- 100 mg capsules and tablets.
- 16 oz bottles containing 50 mg/5 mL (1 tsp) syrup.

Actions:
- Antiparkinsonian agent that increases neuronal release of dopamine and other catecholamines and delays presynaptic reuptake of these neurotransmitters; used to treat parkinsonism.
- Antiviral agent used in prevention and treatment of influenza A.

Clearance: Renally excreted.
- *Markedly increase dosing interval and reduce dosage in patients with impaired renal function.*

- No change in dosage needed in patients with liver disease.
- Supplemental dose not required after hemodialysis.
- Significantly decrease dosage in elderly patients.

Selected Side Effects: Multiple CNS effects (dizziness, light-headedness, blurred vision, anxiety, irritability, hallucinations, confusion, depression, ataxia, increased seizure activity), anorexia, constipation, orthostatic hypotension, peripheral edema, reversible livedo reticularis, dry mouth.

Selected Drug Interactions:
- Potentiates CNS depressant effects of other CNS depressants.
- Produces increased atropine-like effects when used with anticholinergic agents.

Cautions: Use with caution in patients with history of seizures or liver disease.

Pregnancy Category: C.

Cost: Generic $$, Symmetrel $$$ (≈ $0.30/generic tablet; ≈ $1/Symmetrel tablet).

Pearls:
- Onset of action is within 48 h.
- Discontinue gradually to prevent withdrawal reactions.
- Signs and symptoms of overdose include urinary retention, hyperactivity, convulsions, arrhythmias, hypotension, acid–base disturbances, and acute toxic psychosis.
- Sometimes used to treat fatigue in patients with multiple sclerosis.

Ambien: *see* ZOLPIDEM

AMIKACIN
Dose:
- Loading: 7.5 mg/kg IV.
- Maintenance: 5 mg/kg q8h or 7.5–10 mg/kg q12h IM or IV.

Actions: Bactericidal aminoglycoside antibiotic that irreversibly inhibits protein synthesis.
- Excellent aerobic gram (≈) coverage, including *Pseudomonas*.
- Not effective against anaerobes.
- *NOTE:* The above-mentioned antimicrobial coverage summary should be used as a guideline only; treatment deci-

sions should take into account not only local epidemiologic patterns of antibiotic susceptibility but also, when available, culture susceptibility results.

Clearance: Renally excreted.

- Markedly decrease dosage or increase dosing interval in patients with impaired renal function.
- No change in dosage needed in patients with liver disease.
- Supplemental dose suggested after hemodialysis or peritoneal dialysis.

Selected Side Effects: Nephrotoxicity, ototoxicity, rare increased neuromuscular blockade.

Selected Drug Interactions:

- Concomitant use with cephalothin, vancomycin, cisplatin, amphotericin B, nitrogen mustard compounds, loop diuretics, and cyclosporin all increase risk of nephrotoxicity or ototoxicity.
- Can inactivate mezlocillin, azlocillin, and piperacillin if given concurrently.

Pregnancy Category: D.

Cost: $$$$ ($2000/week wholesale); consider using significantly less expensive gentamicin.

Pearls:

- Used primarily in patients with gentamicin- and tobramycin-resistant organisms.
- (+) CSF penetration in patients with meningeal inflammation.
- Follow peak and trough levels.

AMILORIDE (Midamor; *see also* Moduretic)

Dose: 5–10 mg PO qd–bid.

PO Preparations: 5 mg tablets.

Actions: K+-sparing diuretic, used to treat hypertension.

Clearance: Metabolized via liver; renally excreted.

- Avoid if creatinine clearance <50 mL/min.
- May need to adjust dosage in patients with liver disease.

Cautions:

- *Avoid in patients with diabetes 2° increased risk of hyperkalemia.*
- Use with caution with ACE inhibitors, the angiotensin II antagonist losartan, and with other potassium-sparing diuretics

(triamterene, spironolactone, etc.), due to an increased risk of hyperkalemia.
Cost: $$$ ($\approx$ $0.55/tablet).

AMINOPHYLLINE (*see also* THEOPHYLLINE for PO preparations)
Dose:
- Loading: 5–6 mg/kg (ideal weight) IV over 30 min.
- Maintenance: 0.5–0.6 mg/kg/h (ideal weight).

Actions: Respiratory agent with bronchodilating, diaphragmatic stimulating, and probably other actions, which is used to treat reactive airway disease.

Clearance: Metabolized via liver in cytochrome 450 system.
- No change in dosage needed in patients with impaired renal function.
- Significantly increase dosing interval or significantly reduce dose in patients with liver dysfunction or significant systolic heart dysfunction (due to decreased blood flow to the liver).
- Supplemental dose suggested after hemodialysis or peritoneal dialysis.

Selected Side Effects: Tachycardia, palpitations, arrhythmias, headache, seizures, coma, nervousness, irritability, nausea and vomiting, diarrhea, esophageal reflux (because of decreased lower esophageal sphincter tone), tachypnea, rash.

Selected Drug Interactions:
- Drugs that lead to elevated theophylline levels: cimetidine, propranolol, fluoroquinolones (Cipro, Floxin, etc), macrolide antibiotics (erythromycin, Biaxin, etc), isoniazid (INH), oral contraceptives.
- Drugs that lead to lower theophylline levels: phenytoin (Dilantin), phenobarbital, rifampin, ketoconazole, carbamazepine, furosemide.

Pregnancy Category: C.
Cost: $.
Pearls:
- IV dose (in mg/h) can be calculated by dividing total daily PO dose by 20 (eg, 300 mg PO bid = 600 mg PO daily; 600 divided by 20 yields an IV dose of 30 mg/h).

- The definition of a "therapeutic range" varies greatly with each practitioner and hospital; therapeutic ranges may include levels between 5–20 μg/mL.
- Risk of toxicity is increased when serum level > 20 μg/mL.
- $t_{1/2}$ is decreased in smokers and in patients taking phenytoin (Dilantin).
- $t_{1/2}$ is increased in the elderly and in patients with liver disease, CHF (due to decreased blood flow to the liver), COPD, viral infection, or high fever.
- Methods of giving additional aminophylline to raise a subtherapeutic level are highly variable. One method is to anticipate that every 1 mg/kg bolus will raise the serum level by approximately 2 mg/mL.

AMIODARONE (Cordarone)
IV Preparation (*see also* the following entry for the PO preparation):
Dose: *Amiodarone shows considerable interindividual variation in response. Close monitoring with adjustment of dose as needed is necessary.*

- Loading: 150 mg over 10 minutes (15 mg/min) then 360 mg over the next 6 hours (1 mg/min).
- Maintenance: 540 mg over the next 24 hours (0.5 mg/min).
- Treatment of breakthrough VT/VF: 150 mg administered over 10 minutes (15 mg/min).
- Maintenance infusions of up to 0.5 mg/min may be cautiously continued for up to 2–3 weeks.

Actions: Class III antiarrhythmic; IV preparations at present are currently approved only for the treatment of life-threatening ventricular arrhythmias not responsive to other standard medications.

- The primary electrophysiologic effects of IV administration of amiodarone are prolongation of intranodal conduction and increased refractoriness of the AV node; it has little or no effect on sinus node rate, intraventricular conduction, infranodal conduction (His-Purkinje system) and ventricular refractoriness.

Clearance:
- Due to rapid distribution, serum concentrations decline to 10% of peak values within 30–45 minutes after the end of infusion.
- Elimination is primarily via hepatic metabolism and biliary excretion; there is negligible renal excretion.
- Neither amiodarone nor the main active metabolite are dialyzable.
- Age, renal disease, and hepatic disease do not have marked effects of clearance of amiodarone or its main active metabolite.

Selected Side Effects: *Hypotension,* bradycardia, proarrhythmic effects, *asystole* cardiac arrest/EMD.

Selected Drug Interactions: Available information is based on drug interactions with the PO preparation of amiodarone.
- Raises serum levels of digoxin and antiarrhythmics.
- Can potentiate β-blocker- and calcium-antagonist-mediated bradycardia, sinus arrest, or AV block.
- Prolongs PT in patients taking warfarin.

Cautions: *Contraindicated in patients with cardiogenic shock, marked sinus bradycardia, and second- or third-degree AV block (unless a functioning pacemaker is present).*

Pregnancy Category: D.

Cost: $$$$.

Pearls:
- Correct hypokalemia or hypomagnesemia when possible prior to treatment.
- Should be administered when possible through a central venous catheter dedicated to that purpose.
- Multiple cautions exist about how IV amiodarone should be administered; nursing staff should review these before administering.
- Changing from IV amiodarone to PO amiodarone (assuming maintenance IV infusion of 0.5 mg/min):

Duration of IV Amiodarone Infusion	Initial Daily Dose of PO Amiodarone
< 1 week	800–1600 mg
1–3 weeks	600–800 mg

AMIODARONE (Cordarone)
<u>PO Preparation</u> (*see also* the previous entry for the IV preparation):
Dose: Disease dependent.

- *NOTE: Amiodarone required a prolonged and variable period of "loading"; the following are only suggested guidelines.*
- Life-threatening ventricular arrhythmias: 800–1600 mg PO daily for 1–3 weeks, then 400–800 mg PO daily for 1–3 weeks, then 200–400 mg daily (some patients require higher maintenance doses).
- Atrial fibrillation and other supraventricular arrhythmias (not FDA approved for this at present): 600 mg PO daily for 1–3 weeks, then 400 mg daily for up to 3 weeks (consider electrical cardioversion at this point if necessary); maintenance dose once normal sinus rhythm is restored: 200 mg PO qd.

PO Preparations: 200 mg tablets.

Actions: Class III antiarrhythmic used to treat VT and VF; is also effective for atrial and supraventricular arrhythmias (though not FDA approved for this use).

- Blocks the potassium channels, prolonging membrane repolarization and the QT interval.

Clearance: Metabolized via liver.

- Metabolites are active.
- Significant enterohepatic recirculation and hepatobiliary excretion occur.
- No change in dosage needed in patients with impaired renal function.
- There are no studies examining the need to reduce dosage in patients with liver dysfunction.
- Supplemental dose not required after hemodialysis.

Selected Side Effects: Bradycardia, conduction abnormalities, arrhythmias, CNS symptoms (especially ataxia, neuropathy), GI symptoms (nausea and vomiting, constipation, anorexia), elevated LFTs and hepatitis, pulmonary fibrosis, corneal microdeposits, hypothyroidism or hyperthyroidism, elevated thyroid function tests, photodermatitis.

Selected Drug Interactions:

- Raises serum levels of digoxin and antiarrhythmics.

- Can potentiate β-blocker- and calcium-antagonist-mediated bradycardia, sinus arrest, or AV block.
- Prolongs PT in patients taking warfarin.

Cautions: Use with caution with β-blockers and general anesthetics (can cause decreased BP and HR, conduction abnormalities, and CHF).

Pregnancy Category: D.

Cost: $$$$ (≈ $2.80/tablet).

Pearls:

- Obtain chest x-ray and liver and thyroid function tests every 6 months.
- Loading dose is often limited by GI or CNS side effects, and may require a reduction in loading dose.
- Monitor for bradycardia and conduction abnormalities during loading.
- QT prolongation with PO amiodarone is not considered by some to predict the occurrence of torsade de pointes.
- Changing from IV amiodarone to PO amiodarone (assuming maintenance IV infusion of 0.5 mg/min):

Duration of IV Amiodarone Infusion	Initial Daily Dose of PO Amiodarone
< 1 week	800–1600 mg
1–3 weeks	600–800 mg

AMITRIPTYLINE (Elavil)

Dose: (for depression):

- Initial: 75 mg daily in divided doses or 50–100 mg qhs
- Maintenance: 40–150 mg qhs.

PO Preparations: 10, 25, 50, 75, 100, and 150 mg tablets.

Actions: Tricyclic antidepressant with sedative effects used to treat depression and other disorders, including painful neuropathies and chronic fatigue syndrome.

Clearance: Metabolized via liver.

- No change in dosage needed in patients with impaired renal function.
- Substantially reduce dosage in elderly patients.

- Supplemental dose not required after hemodialysis or peritoneal dialysis.

Selected Side Effects: Multiple CNS effects, multiple cardiovascular effects (including effects on the conduction system, including QT interval prolongation, similar to type Ia antiarrhythmics such as quinidine), atropine-like effects, multiple other effects (see *PDR*).

Selected Drug Interactions:

- *Hyperpyrexia when used with MAOI, anticholinergic agents, or neuroleptics.*
- Paralytic ileus when used with anticholinergic agents.

Cautions:

- *Contraindicated in patients who have taken MAOI within 2 weeks.*
- Use with caution, if at all, in elderly patients and in patients with history of seizures, cardiovascular disease, hyperthyroidism, urine retention, angle-closure glaucoma, or increased intraocular pressure.

Pregnancy Category: Not established.

Cost: Generic $, Elavil $$$$ ($\approx$ $0.20 each 150 mg generic tablet; $\approx$ $1.60 each 150 mg Elavil tablet).

Pearls:

- Signs and symptoms of overdose include confusion, seizure, coma, visual hallucinations, dilated pupils and ocular dysmotility, hypothermia or hyperpyrexia, arrhythmias, decreased conduction and bundle-branch block, CHF, hypotension, muscle rigidity, and hyperreflexia.
- Patients with drug overdose must be monitored for arrhythmias and conduction abnormalities, with regular checks of the QRS and QT intervals, since amitriptyline has type Ia antiarrhythmic effects.

AMLODIPINE (Norvasc)
Dose:

- Initial: 5 mg PO qd.
- Consider an initial dose of 2.5 mg in small, fragile, or elderly patients, and those with hepatic disease or taking other antihypertensive agents.
- Maximum: 10 mg PO qd.

Preparations: 2.5, 5, and 10 mg tablets.

Actions: Calcium channel blocker used to treat hypertension and angina (including vasospastic angina).

Clearance: Metabolized via liver; no significant renal clearance.

- No change in dosage needed in patients with impaired renal function.
- Decrease starting dose (to 2.5 mg qd) in patients with significant liver disease.

Selected Side Effects: peripheral edema (especially in women), dizziness, hypotension.

Cautions:

- *Contraindicated in patients with severe aortic stenosis.*
- Use with caution in patients with severe hepatic insufficiency and severe heart failure.

Pregnancy Category: C.

Cost: $$$ (≈ $0.50 each 5 mg tablet).

Pearls:

- Appears not to lead to any worsening of heart failure in patients with compensated heart failure.
- Does not have any significant effects on the cardiac conduction system.

AMOXAPINE (Asendin)

Dose:

- Initial: 50 mg PO tid or 150 mg PO qhs.
- May gradually increase to maximum of 400–600 mg daily in patients without history of seizures.
- Usual: 200–300 mg daily.

PO Preparations: 25, 50, 100, and 150 mg tablets.

Actions: Antidepressant used to treat depression.

Clearance: Metabolized via liver to a dopamine receptor antagonist neuroleptic.

- No change in dosage needed in patients with impaired renal function.
- Reduce dosage in elderly patients.

Selected Side Effects:

- Sedation, postural hypotension, anticholinergic effects.
- In theory, tardive dyskinesia and neuroleptic malignant syndrome can develop.

Cautions:
- *Contraindicated in patients taking MAOI.*
- Use with caution in patients with history of seizures.

Pregnancy Category: C.

Cost: $$$$ (≈ $1.50 each 100 mg tablet).

Pearls:
- Taper dose when discontinuing.
- Signs and symptoms of overdose are predominantly neurologic, including seizures.
- A small percentage of patients may develop renal failure, particularly acute tubular necrosis (ATN) secondary to myoglobinuria, 2–5 days after an overdose.

AMOXICILLIN (Amoxil; *see also* Augmentin)

Dose:
- 250–500 mg PO tid without regard to meals.
- For uncomplicated cystitis, may give high-dose therapy (3 g PO qd for 1–3 days).
- Pediatric dose:
  - ▶ For otitis, sinusitis, pharyngitis, or GU infection: children weighing 8–20, kg 20 mg/kg daily in 3 divided doses given q8h; children > 20 kg (44 lb), 250 mg PO q8h.
  - ▶ For lower respiratory tract infection: children weighing 8–20 kg, 40 mg/kg daily in 3 divided doses given q8h; children > 20 kg (44 lb), 500 mg PO q8h.

PO Preparations:
- 125 and 250 mg chewable tablets.
- 5, 80, 100, and 150 mL bottles containing 125 mg/5 mL (1 tsp) suspension.
- 5, 80, 100, and 150 mL bottles containing 250 mg/5 mL (1 tsp) suspension.

Actions: Bactericidal β-lactam antibiotic that inhibits cell wall synthesis.
- Some gram (+) coverage, including strep and most enterococci (but *not* most staph).
- Some gram (−) coverage, including *Escherichia coli, Salmonella,* most *Haemophilus influenzae,* some *Proteus,* and some *Klebsiella* but *not Shigella* or β-lactamase-producing organisms (including some *H influenzae*).

- Some anaerobic coverage.
- *NOTE:* The above-mentioned antimicrobial coverage summary should be used as a guideline only; treatment decisions should take into account not only local epidemiologic patterns of antibiotic susceptibility but also, when available, culture susceptibility results.

Clearance: Primarily renally excreted.

- Increase dosing interval slightly to moderately in patients with impaired renal function.
- No change in dosage needed in patients with liver disease.
- Supplemental dose suggested after hemodialysis but not after peritoneal dialysis.

Selected Side Effects: GI discomfort, diarrhea, abdominal cramps, rash, anaphylactic reaction, allergic interstitial nephritis.

Cautions: *Contraindicated in patients with penicillin allergy.*

Pregnancy category: B.

Cost: $ (≈ $10 for 250 mg tid for 10 days).

Pearls:

- Tolerated better than oral ampicillin and only needs to be taken tid (vs. qid for ampicillin).
- With the emergence of resistant *Haemophilus influenzae,* most sources no longer consider amoxicillin adequate therapy for sinusitis and instead recommend Augmentin, Bactrim, or Ceclor.
- Increases risk of rash in patients with mononucleosis or taking allopurinol.

Amphojel: *see* ALUMINUM HYDROXIDE

AMPHOTERICIN B

Dose: Disease dependent:

- Systemic illness: Give 1 mg IV test dose (after patient has received premedication) over 30 min, then 0.20–0.25 mg/kg on the first day; may increase by 0.1–0.2 mg/kg daily to a maximum of 0.5–1.0 mg/kg/day.
- Bladder irrigation: Sources vary; regimens include: (1) 15–50 mg in 1 L sterile water as continuous irrigation over

24 h; (2) 50 mg daily in 1 L sterile water as continuous irrigation for 3–5 days; (3) 5–15 mg in sterile water q6–8h for 3–5 days.

Actions: Polyene antibiotic that alters membrane permeability; used to treat fungal infections.

Clearance: Metabolic pathways unclear but presumed hepatic metabolism; 2–5% excreted unchanged in urine.

- Slightly increase dosing interval in patients with end-stage renal disease; no change needed in milder renal dysfunction.
- May need to reduce dosage in patients with liver disease.
- Supplemental dose not required after hemodialysis or peritoneal dialysis.

Selected Side Effects: Nephrotoxicity, electrolyte wasting (especially K^+ and Mg^{2+}), fever and shaking chills (usually 15 min after injection), nausea and vomiting.

Selected Drug Interactions:
- Corticosteroids can exacerbate K^+ wasting.
- Other nephrotoxic agents and nitrogen mustard can increase its nephrotoxicity.

Pregnancy Category: B.

Cost: $.

Pearls:
- In critically ill patients, some sources recommend proceeding directly to maximum dose after initial test dose.
- Give slowly IV over 4–6 h.
- *Carefully* follow K^+, Mg^{2+}, renal function, CBC, and LFTs.
- Premedicate with acetaminophen (Tylenol) or ASA, diphenhydramine 25–50 mg PO or IV, and hydrocortisone 25–50 mg IV (to reduce side effects). Over time, may be able to give without premedication.
- Nephrotoxicity may be reduced by prehydration, salt loading, and keeping the patient well hydrated.
- Meperidine 50 mg IV is useful if chills develop.

AMPICILLIN (*see also* Unasyn)

Dose: Route dependent:
- PO: 250–1000 mg qid 30 min before or 2 h after meals.
- IM or IV: 0.5–2 g q6h.

- May give high-dose therapy (3.5 g PO qd for 1–3 days) for uncomplicated cystitis.
- Oral absorption can be affected by food.

PO Preparations:
- 250 and 500 mg tablets.
- Multiple suspensions at various concentrations.

Actions: Bactericidal β-lactam antibiotic that inhibits cell wall synthesis.

- Some gram (+) coverage, including strep and enterococci (but *not* most staph).
- Some gram (−) coverage, including *Escherichia coli,* most *Haemophilus influenzae, Shigella,* and *Salmonella* (but *not* β-lactamase-producing bacteria, including some *H influenzae*).
- Some anaerobic coverage.
- Also effective against *Listeria,* an important (although uncommon) cause of meningitis in elderly and immunocompromised patients, which cephalosporins do not cover.
- *NOTE:* The above-mentioned antimicrobial coverage summary should be used as a guideline only; treatment decisions should take into account not only local epidemiologic patterns of antibiotic susceptibility but also, when available, culture susceptibility results.

Clearance: Some liver metabolism; primarily renally excreted.

- Increase dosing interval slightly to moderately in patients with impaired renal function.
- No change in dosage needed in patients with liver disease.
- Supplemental dose suggested after hemodialysis but not after peritoneal dialysis.

Selected Side Effects: GI discomfort, rash, anaphylactic reaction, allergic interstitial nephritis.

Cautions: *Contraindicated in patients with penicillin allergy.*

Pregnancy Category: B.

Cost: $ (≈ $10 for 250 mg qid for 10 days).

Pearls:
- Amoxicillin is often preferred over ampicillin for oral use (because of its tid dosing schedule and because its absorption is not affected by food).

- Increases risk of rash in patients with mononucleosis or those taking allopurinol.

AMRINONE (Inocor)
Dose:
- Initial: 0.75 µg/kg bolus over 2–3 min; a second loading dose may be repeated 30 min later if clinically indicated.
- Maintenance: 5–10 µg/kg/min.
- Doses up to 40 µg/kg/min may be used for refractory CHF.

Actions:
- Phosphodiesterase inhibitor with positive inotropic and direct vasodilator effects used to treat CHF.
- Hemodynamic effects include increases in cardiac index and BP, and decreases in pulmonary vascular resistance, pulmonary capillary wedge pressure, and HR.

Clearance: Metabolized via liver; renally excreted.
- Slightly decrease dosage in patients with end-stage renal disease; no change needed in patients with milder renal impairment.
- Reduce dosage in patients with liver disease.

Selected Side Effects: Increased PVCs and occasional arrhythmias, hypotension, mild reduction in platelets (secondary to reduced $t_{1/2}$ of platelets), rare hepatotoxicity.

Selected Drug Interactions: Can produce hypotension when used with disopyramide.

Pregnancy Category: C.

Cost: $$$$ ($\geq$$600/day wholesale).

Pearls:
- Inotropic effects are additive with digoxin.
- Generally does not produce any increase in myocardial oxygen demand.
- May lead to slight enhancement of AV conduction and possible increased ventricular response rate in patients in atrial fibrillation or atrial flutter.
- Should not be diluted with solutions containing dextrose or administered through IV tubing in which dextrose is running because this can lead to drug precipitation.

Anafranil: *see* CLOMIPRAMINE

Anaprox: *see* NAPROXEN

Ancef: *see* CEFAZOLIN

ANISTREPLASE (APSAC, Eminase)

Dose: 30 unit IV bolus over 2–5 min.

Actions:

- Thrombolytic agent used to treat acute MI.
- Enzyme is activated after deacylation of the protective anisole group, leading to both clot-specific and nonclot-specific conversion of plasminogen to plasmin with resulting thrombolysis.

Selected Side Effects: *Bleeding and rare intracranial bleeding, arrhythmias, hypotension, and anaphylactic reactions.*

Pregnancy Category: C.

Pearls: *The lists of what constitutes absolute contraindications to thrombolytic therapy and what other factors should be considered as increasing the risks of adverse events have been evolving and are being updated as new data become available.* The following should serve as guidelines only; *in decisions regarding thrombolytic therapy, the risks of administering thrombolytic agents must be weighed against the potential benefit.*

- Generally accepted absolute contraindications:
  - ▶ History of hemorrhagic strokes (regardless of when the bleed occurred); thromboembolic stroke within the past 1 year.
  - ▶ Active or recent (within 2 weeks) internal bleeding (*not* including menses).
  - ▶ Recent CNS surgery or trauma; known CNS (or spinal cord) tumor, or AV malformation.
  - ▶ Severe hypertension on presentation (> 180/110), which increases the risk for hemorrhagic stroke.
  - ▶ Major recent (within 2 weeks) surgery.
  - ▶ CPR that is prolonged (> 10 min) or suspected to have been traumatic (ie, suspected multiple rib fractures).
  - ▶ Suspected aortic dissection.
  - ▶ Pregnancy.

- Other factors that should be considered when the potential risks and benefits of thrombolytic therapy are considered:
  - ▶ Thromboembolic strokes greater than 1 year old; TIA within the prior 6 months *may* increase the risk of CNS adverse events.
  - ▶ Known bleeding diathesis or significantly elevated INR (≥ 2–3) from warfarin therapy.
  - ▶ Active peptic ulcer disease or recent significant GI bleeding (a distant history of a GI bleed may not be a significant risk factor with thrombolytic therapy).
  - ▶ Hemorrhagic retinopathy was in the past regarded as a relative contraindication to therapy; some sources no longer regard it as a contraindication; vitreous hemorrhage may, however, be a contraindication to treatment.
  - ▶ Older age was in the past considered a relative contraindication to therapy; however, although the risk of CNS bleeding in elderly patients is greater, the benefits in terms of mortality reduction are also greater, thus age *per se* is now not generally regarded as a contraindication to thrombolytic therapy. The greater risks and benefits with thrombolytic therapy in elderly patients should be weighed when considering such therapy in these patients.
  - ▶ Patients with cardiogenic shock on presentation do not generally derive significant benefit from thrombolytic therapy, and primary angioplasty, when available, should be considered.

Antabuse: *see* DISULFIRAM

Antivert: *see* MECLIZINE

Anusol suppositories and ointment
Dose: Route dependent:
- Rectal suppository: 1 bid and after each evacuation.
- Ointment: Apply and rub into cleansed and dried anal tissue q3–4h.
PO Preparations:
- 1 and 2 oz tubes.
- Boxes of 12, 24, and 48 suppositories.

Actions:
- Suppositories contain phenylephrine and "hard fat"; temporarily relieves the swelling associated with hemorrhoids and helps to relieve hemorrhoidal burning, itching, and discomfort.
- Ointment contains pramoxine (a local anesthetic), mineral oil, and zinc oxide; forms a temporary protective coating over inflamed tissues and helps to relieve hemorrhoidal burning, itching, and discomfort.

Anusol-HC: *see* **HYDROCORTISONE SUPPOSITORIES**

Apresoline: *see* **HYDRALAZINE**

APSAC: *see* **ANISTREPLASE**

ARA-C: *see* **CYTOSINE ARABINOSIDE**

Aristocort A: *see* **TRIAMCINOLONE ACETONIDE cream, lotion, and ointment**

Artane: *see* **TRIHEXYPHENIDYL**

ASA: *see* **ACETYLSALICYLIC ACID**

Asendin: *see* **AMOXAPINE**

ASPIRIN: *see* **ACETYLSALICYLIC ACID**

ASTEMIZOLE (Hismanal)
Dose: 10 mg PO qd.
PO Preparations: 10 mg scored tablets.
Actions: Long-acting antihistamine that blocks H_1 receptors; used to treat allergic conditions.
Clearance: Metabolized via liver; excreted primarily in feces.

Selected Side Effects: Fatigue, initial increase in appetite and weight gain, dry mouth, QT interval prolongation and rare ventricular arrhythmias.

Drug Interactions: Increased risk of ventricular arrhythmias with erythromycin, ketoconazole, and itraconazole.

Cautions:

- *Do not exceed daily dose of 10 mg (increased risk of ventricular arrhythmias).*
- Concurrent use of astemizole with erythromycin and ketoconazole have been associated with ventricular arrhythmias and death, and hepatic dysfunction has been associated with ventricular arrhythmias in the related drug terfenadine (Seldane). Therefore, astemizole should not be prescribed in patients taking erythromycin and the related drugs clarithromycin and troleandomycin, ketoconazole and the related drugs itraconazole, fluconazole, metronidazole, and miconazole, and in patients with hepatic dysfunction.
- Avoid in patients taking medications that can prolong the QT interval, in patients with congenital QT prolongation, patients with electrolyte abnormalities, or those on diuretics with the potential to induce electrolyte abnormalities (secondary concerns about ventricular arrhythmias).

Pregnancy Category: C.

Cost: $$$ (≈ $2/tablet); similar to daily cost of Seldane.

Pearls:

- *Warn patients that if they experience syncope they should discontinue the medicine and consult their physician.*
- Should be taken on an empty stomach to increase bioavailability.
- Does not generally have the sedative/drowsiness effects of many other antihistamines.

Atarax: *see* HYDROXYZINE

ATENOLOL (Tenormin)

Dose: Route dependent:

- PO: 50–200 mg qd.
- IV in acute MI: 5 mg over 5 min; repeat dose 10 min later, then begin PO therapy.

PO Preparations: 25, 50, and 100 mg tablets.

Actions: β_1-selective β-blocker used to treat angina and hypertension.

Clearance: Renally excreted; no liver metabolism.

- Moderately reduce dosage in patients with impaired renal function.
- No change in dosage needed in patients with liver disease.
- Supplemental dose suggested after hemodialysis but not peritoneal dialysis.

Selected Side Effects: Cardiovascular (CHF, bradycardia, AV block, postural hypotension), CNS (vertigo, fatigue, depression, lethargy), bronchospasm, impotence.

Cautions:

- Relatively contraindicated in patients with greater than first-degree AV block, CHF, or reactive airway disease.

Pregnancy Category: D.

Cost: Generic $$, Tenormin $$$ (generic ≈ $0.35 each 100 mg tablet, Tenormin ≈ $0.65 each 100 mg tablet).

Pearls: Taper when discontinuing (abrupt discontinuance can cause rebound reactions).

Ativan: *see* LORAZEPAM

ATROPINE

Dose: Situation dependent:

- Situations other than cardiac arrest: 0.5–1.0 mg IV; may repeat q5 min as clinically indicated (maximum total dose of 2–3 mg in patients with coronary artery disease).
- Cardiac arrest (extreme bradycardia or asystole):
  - ▶ 1 mg IV q3–5 min to a maximum total dose of 3 mg.
  - ▶ If IV access is not available, can give 1–2 mg of atropine, diluted in several mL of water or normal saline, down the endotracheal tube.

Actions: Antimuscarinic agent that enhances sinus node automaticity and AV node conduction; used primarily to treat symptomatic bradycardia, heart block, and in certain situations, cardiac arrest.

- Also used in therapy for insecticide poisoning.

Side Effects: Excess tachycardia, myocardial ischemia, ventricular tachycardia or fibrillation, "anticholinergic syndrome" (delirium, tachycardia, coma, flushed and hot skin, ataxia, blurred vision).

Pearls:

- Administration of atropine in doses of less than 0.5 mg can produce paradoxical bradycardia due to parasympathomimetic effects at low doses.
- After peripheral administration of atropine in a code situation, give a 20–30 mL bolus of intravenous fluid and immediately elevate the extremity. This enhances delivery of the drug to the central circulation, which can take 1–2 minutes (AHA, Advanced Cardiac Life Support, 1994).
- The administration of a total dose of 3 mg produces full vagolytic effect in most patients.
- Can be given via endotracheal tube if no IV access available.

Atrovent: *see* IPRATROPIUM

Augmentin (AMOXICILLIN + CLAVULANATE)
Dose:

- Adults: 250–500 mg PO q8h.
- Pediatric: (for otitis media, sinusitis, lower respiratory tract infection): Children weighing < 40 kg, 40 mg/kg daily (of amoxicillin component) given in 3 divided doses q8h; for children ≥ 40 kg, give usual adult dosage.

Preparations: Quantity of amoxicillin (A) and clavulanate (C) components.

- "250" tablets containing 250 mg A and 125 mg C; "500" tablets containing 500 mg A and 125 mg C; "125" chewable tablets containing 125 mg A and 31.25 mg C; "250" chewable tablets containing 250 mg A and 62.5 mg C.
- 75 and 150 mL bottles of banana-flavored suspension containing 125 mg A and 31.25 mg C per 5 mL (1 tsp); 75 and 150 mL bottles of orange-flavored suspension containing 250 mg A and 62.5 mg C per 5 mL (1 tsp).

Actions: Semisynthetic bactericidal β-lactam antibiotic that inhibits cell wall synthesis, combined with clavulanate, a β-lactamase inhibitor.

- Good gram (+) coverage, including enterococci, strep, and most staph (*not* MRSA).

- Good gram (–) coverage and good anaerobic coverage, including *Bacteroides fragilis.*
- *NOTE:* The above-mentioned antimicrobial coverage summary should be used as a guideline only; treatment decisions should take into account not only local epidemiologic patterns of antibiotic susceptibility but also, when available, culture susceptibility results.

Clearance: Some renal excretion of amoxicillin and clavulanate.

- Moderately increase dosing interval in patients with impaired renal function.
- Supplemental dose suggested after hemodialysis.

Selected Side Effects: Allergic and anaphylactic reactions, diarrhea, nausea, elevated LFTs.

Cautions: *Contraindicated in patients with penicillin allergy.*

Pregnancy Category: B.

Cost: $$$ (≈ $65 for 250 mg tid for 10 days).

Pearls:

- Can produce false (+) result on dipstick test for urine glucose.
- Increases risk of rash in patients with mononucleosis or those taking allopurinol.
- May be taken without regard to meals.

Axid: *see* NIZATIDINE

Axsain: *see* CAPSAICIN cream

AZATHIOPRINE (Imuran)

Dose: Disease dependent:

- Renal transplant patients: Usually 3–5 mg/kg PO or IV qd initially; maintenance, 1–3 mg/kg daily.
- Rheumatoid arthritis: often 1.0 mg/kg PO or IV qd initially, given in 1 or 2 divided doses; may gradually increase to maximum of 2.5 mg/kg daily.

PO Preparations: 50 mg tablets.

Actions: Immunosuppressive antimetabolite, used in patients who have received homograft transplants and to treat autoimmune diseases.

Clearance: Cleaved in vivo to mercaptopurine. Both it and mercaptopurine are metabolized in the liver and in RBCs; there is little renal excretion.

- Slightly decrease dosage in patients with impaired renal function.
- One source suggests avoiding azathioprine in patients with liver disease.
- Supplemental dose suggested after hemodialysis.

Selected Side Effects: *Severe leukopenia* (dose limiting), macrocytic anemia, decreased platelets, nausea and vomiting, elevated LFTs, hepatitis with biliary stasis, cholestatic hepatotoxicity, pancreatitis, mucositis, restrictive lung disease.

Selected Drug Interactions: Allopurinol markedly reduces its metabolism (substantially decrease the dosage).

Cautions: *Contraindicated in pregnant or potentially pregnant patients.*

Pregnancy Category: X.

Cost: $$$$ (PO ≥ $2.50/day wholesale).

Pearls:

- Should be taken on an empty stomach to enhance absorption.
- Usually takes 6–8 weeks for response in rheumatoid arthritis; patients not responding within 12 weeks are considered treatment failures.

AZITHROMYCIN (Zithromax)

Dose: Disease dependent:

- COPD exacerbation, uncomplicated pneumonia, pharyngitis, uncomplicated skin infection: Single dose of 500 mg PO on day 1, then 250 mg PO qd for days 2–5 (longer courses of therapy may be necessary in some cases).
- Nongonococcal urethritis or cervicitis from *Chlamydia:* Single dose of 1000 mg PO.

PO Preparations: 250 mg capsules.

Actions: Macrolide antibiotic that inhibits protein synthesis. Has been shown to have *in vitro* activity against the following organisms, although the clinical significance of this activity for some listed organisms is not established:

- Gram (+) coverage, including *Staphylococcus aureus, S pyogenes,* and *Viridans* group strep (but *not* MRSA or en terococci).
- Gram (−) coverage, including *Haemophilus influenzae* and *H ducreyi, Moraxella catarrhalis (Branhamella catarrhalis), Campylobacter jejuni,* and *Legionella pneumophila* (but *not Escherichia coli, Klebsiella,* or *Proteus*).
- Anaerobic coverage, including *Bacteroides bivius, Clostridium perfringens,* and peptostreptococci.
- Other coverage includes *Mycoplasma pneumoniae, Treponema pallidum,* and *Ureaplasma urealyticum.*
- *NOTE:* The above-mentioned antimicrobial coverage summary should be used as a guideline only; treatment decisions should take into account not only local epidemiologic patterns of antibiotic susceptibility but also, when available, culture susceptibility results.

Clearance: Metabolized and excreted primarily via liver.
- Little data are available on its use in liver or kidney disease, so use with caution in these patients.

Selected Side Effects: Diarrhea, nausea, abdominal pain.

Selected Drug Interactions:
- Little data are currently available.
- Other macrolide antibiotics have been shown to raise serum levels of theophylline, digoxin, carbamazepine, phenytoin, and cyclosporine to decrease clearance of triazolam (Halcion), and to prolong PT in patients taking warfarin. These effects should be borne in mind when using azithromycin.

Cautions: *Contraindicated in patients with history of allergic reaction to any macrolide antibiotic.*

Pregnancy Category: B.

Cost: $$$ ($40 for a 6-day course of treatment).

Pearls:
- Should be taken at least 1 h before or 2 h after meals.
- Should not be used for treatment of infections in patients < 16 years old.

Azmacort: *see* TRIAMCINOLONE

AZT: *see* ZIDOVUDINE

AZTREONAM
Dose:
- 500 mg–2 gram IV q8h.
- Usual dose: 1 g IV q8h.
- May give IM up to 1 g q8h.

Actions: Monobactam bactericidal antibiotic that inhibits cell wall synthesis.
- Excellent aerobic gram (−) coverage (variable, hospital-dependent *Pseudomonas aeruginosa* coverage).
- Not active against gram (+) organisms or anaerobes.
- *NOTE:* The above-mentioned antimicrobial coverage summary should be used as a guideline only; treatment decisions should take into account not only local epidemiologic patterns of antibiotic susceptibility but also, when available, culture susceptibility results.

Clearance: Primarily renally excreted.
- Moderately decrease dosage in patients with impaired renal function.
- No change in dosage needed in patients with liver disease.
- Supplemental dose suggested after hemodialysis.

Selected Side Effects: Eosinophilia (8%).
Selected Drug Interactions: β-lactam antibiotics may decrease the antibiotic effect of aztreonam and thus should not be used at the same time.
Pregnancy Category: B.
Cost: $$$; consider using less expensive gentamicin.

Azulfidine: *see* SULFASALAZINE

BACITRACIN (Baciguent, Bacitrin; *see also* Cortisporin)
Dose: Apply thin film to skin bid–qid.
Preparations: 15 and 30 g tubes.
Actions: Topical antibiotic that inhibits cell wall synthesis.
- Good gram (+) coverage (bacteriocidal against strep, staph and pneumococci).
- Poor gram (−) coverage.

Selected Side Effects: Skin rashes, itching, burning, tingling.
Cost: $.

BACLOFEN (Lioresal)
Dose: 40–80 mg daily in divided doses.
PO Preparations: 10 and 20 mg tablets.
Actions: Muscle relaxant used to treat spasticity (usually due to multiple sclerosis).
Clearance:
• Renally excreted.
• Reduce dose in patients with impaired renal function.
Selected Side Effects: Drowsiness, dizziness, weakness, fatigue, confusion, headache, insomnia, urinary frequency, hypotension.
Pregnancy Category: Not established.
Cost: Generic $$, Lioresal $$$$ (≈ $0.35 each 20 mg generic tablet; ≈ $0.95 each 20 mg Lioresal tablet).
Pearls:
• Abrupt withdrawal may cause seizures and hallucinations.
• Patients fully dependent on leg spasticity for sustaining upright posture and gait may lose functional abilities after reduction of spasticity.

Bactrim, Septra (TRIMETHOPRIM + SULFAMETHOXAZOLE)
Dose: Disease dependent:
• Outpatient bronchitis: 1 double-strength (DS) tablet PO bid for 14 days.
• Outpatient urinary tract infection: 1 double-strength (DS) tablet PO bid for 3 days.
• Inpatient urinary tract infection: 5 mg/kg/day trimethoprim (with 25 mg/kg/day of sulfamethoxazole) IV in 2 or 3 divided doses.
• Inpatient nonurinary-tract infection: 8–10 mg/kg/day trimethoprim (with 40–50 mg/kg/day of sulfamethoxazole) IV in 3 divided doses.
• PCP: 20 mg/kg/day trimethoprim (with 100 mg/kg/day sulfamethoxazole) IV in 4 divided doses.

- PCP prophylaxis: 1 single-strength tablet qd or 1 double-strength tablet qod–qd

PO Preparations: Regular- and double-strength tablets; each regular-strength tablet contains 80 mg trimethoprim and 400 mg sulfamethoxazole.

Actions: Antibiotic that blocks the folic acid synthesis pathway.

- Good gram (+) coverage, including strep and staph (but *not* enterococci).
- Good gram (−) coverage, including ampicillin-resistant *Haemophilus influenzae* (but *not Pseudomonas aeruginosa*).
- *NOTE:* The above-mentioned antimicrobial coverage summary should be used as a guideline only; treatment decisions should take into account not only local epidemiologic patterns of antibiotic susceptibility but also, when available, culture susceptibility results.

Clearance: Some systemic metabolism; renally excreted.

- Decrease dosage in patients with impaired renal function.
- Reduce dosage in patients with severe liver disease; no change needed for patients with milder liver dysfunction.
- Supplemental dose suggested after hemodialysis.

Selected Side Effects: GI disturbances (nausea and vomiting, anorexia, cholestasis and hepatitis, pancreatitis), common allergic reactions, multiple hematologic abnormalities, hallucinations, depression, and seizure.

Selected Drug Interactions: Can inhibit phenytoin and warfarin (Coumadin) metabolism.

Cautions: *Contraindicated in sulfa allergy or G6PD deficiency.*

Pregnancy Category: C.

Cost: Generic $, Bactrim $$ (≈ $11 for 1 generic DS tab bid x 10 days; ≈ $35 for 1 Bactrim DS tab bid x 10 days).

Pearls:

- G6PD-deficient patients can develop hemolysis.
- May cause *falsely* elevated creatinine measurements.
- Check CBC frequently.
- PO dose (in mg) is equivalent to IV dose (in mg).
- Patients with AIDS undergoing treatment for PCP have an increased frequency of side effects.

Basaljel: *see* ALUMINUM CARBONATE

BECLOMETHASONE nasal inhaler and spray (Beconase, Beconase AQ, Vancenase, Vancenase AQ)

Dose: Delivery dependent:
- Beconase and Vancenase: 1–2 inhalations in each nostril bid.
- Beconase AQ and Vancenase AQ: 1 or 2 inhalations in each nostril bid.

Preparations:
- Beconase and Vancenase: 6.7 and 7.0 g canisters, respectively containing approximately 80 metered doses.
- Beconase AQ and Vancenase AQ: 25 g bottle with fitted metering atomizing pump and nasal adaptor.

Actions: Topical steroid; used to treat allergic rhinitis and "NARES."

Selected Side Effects: Local irritation and burning, sneezing attacks, rare *Candida* infections, systemic absorption, and steroid-mediated side effects.

Pregnancy Category: C.

Cost: $$$ (≈ $35 each inhaler).

BECLOMETHASONE oral inhaler (Beclovent, Vanceril)

Dose: 2–4 inhalations PO qid.

PO Preparations: 16.8 g canister containing 200 metered doses.

Actions: Inhaled steroid used to treat reversible airway disease.

Selected Side Effects: Oral candidiasis, suppression of adrenal axis, dysphonia (hoarse voice), osteoporosis (after chronic high-dose therapy).

Pregnancy Category: C.

Cost: $$$ (≈ $35 each inhaler).

Pearls:
- Rinsing the mouth after use and using a "spacer" may decrease local side effects.
- Is considered a first-line treatment for asthma.

Beclovent: *see* **BECLOMETHASONE oral inhaler**

Beconase, Beconase AQ: *see* **BECLOMETHASONE nasal inhaler and spray**

Benadryl: *see* **DIPHENHYDRAMINE**

BENAZEPRIL (Lotensin); *see also* **Lotensin HCT**
Dose:
- Initial: 10 mg PO qd (5 mg PO qd if patient is currently taking a diuretic).
- After 2 weeks may increase to 20 mg PO qd.
- Maximum: 20 mg PO bid.

PO Preparations: 5, 10, 20 and 40 mg tablets.

Actions: ACE inhibitor that causes vasodilation and is used to treat hypertension and CHF 2° systolic dysfunction.

Clearance: Predominantly removed by renal clearance in healthy patients.
- Liver metabolism appears to compensate in patients with renal insufficiency.
- No change in dosage needed in patients with mild to moderate renal impairment.
- For GFR < 30 mL/min, begin with 5 mg PO bid.
- No change in dosage needed for patients with liver disease.

Selected Side Effects: Hypotension and dizziness, hyperkalemia (especially in patients with impaired renal function or taking K^+-sparing drugs or K^+ supplements), nonproductive cough, impairment of renal function, angioedema, rare neutropenia.

Cautions:
- *Contraindicated during second and third trimesters of pregnancy and in patients with significant aortic stenosis or hyperkalemia.*
- Patients should not be given both an ACE inhibitor and a K^+ supplement, unless clearly indicated by serial serum K^+ testing.

Pregnancy Category: D.
Cost: $$$ ($0.80 each 20 mg tablet).
Pearls:

• Diuretics potentiate its antihypertensive effects; the risk of hypotension is increased in volume-depleted and elderly patients.
• Follow BUN, creatinine, and K when beginning therapy.
• Patients should be instructed not to use potassium supplements or salt substitutes containing potassium.
• Patients should be made aware of the possibility of developing a nonproductive cough and of developing angioedema.
• The nonproductive cough with ACE inhibitors is presumed to be due to the inhibition of the degradation of endogenous bradykinin.
• Patients who develop a cough with one ACE inhibitor will usually also develop such a cough with other ACE inhibitors.

Benzac: *see* BENZOYL PEROXIDE

Benzagel: *see* BENZOYL PEROXIDE

Benzamycin (BENZOYL PEROXIDE + ERYTHROMYCIN)

Dose: Apply to cleansed, dried skin bid.
Preparations: Supplied as a package containing 20 g of benzoyl peroxide gel and a plastic vial containing 0.8 g of erythromycin powder (which is mixed with 3 mL of ethyl alcohol).
Actions: Combination antibacterial used to treat acne vulgaris.
Selected Side Effects: Dry skin, pruritus, allergic reactions, erythema.
Pregnancy Category: C.
Cost: $$$ (tube: ≥ $24 retail).
Pearls:

• Avoid contact with mucous membranes or inflamed, denuded skin.
• Needs to be stored in the refrigerator.

BENZOYL PEROXIDE (Benoxyl, Benzac, Benzagel, Clearasil, Fostex, Oxy Lotion, etc; *see also* Benzamycin)

Dose: Apply to skin 1–3 times daily.
Preparations: Tubes containing 2.5, 5, and 10% preparations.
Actions: Topical antibacterial used to treat acne vulgaris.
Pearls:
- Bleaches hair and clothing.
- Patients allergic to benzoic acid derivatives may show cross-sensitivity.
- Most preparations now available without prescription.

BENZTROPINE (Cogentin)

Dose: Disease dependent:
- Idiopathic parkinsonism (adjunctive therapy): Initial 0.5–1.0 mg PO or IM qhs; usual 1–2 mg PO tid.
- Drug-induced extrapyramidal disorder: 1–2 mg PO or IM daily, given qd–tid.
PO Preparations: 0.5, 1.0, and 2.0 mg tablets.
Actions: Synthetic competitive anticholinergic agent that also has antihistaminic and atropine-like effects, used to treat Parkinson's disease and other extrapyramidal disorders.
Clearance: Metabolized primarily via liver.
Selected Side Effects: Numerous CNS effects (psychosis, nervousness, depression, etc), atropine-like effects (tachycardia, constipation, dry mouth, blurred vision, dilated pupils, urine retention, anhidrosis, and hyperthermia).
Selected Drug Interactions:
- Can cause paralytic ileus or exacerbate psychotic behavior in patients taking phenothiazines or tricyclics.
- Potentiates CNS-depressant effects of other CNS depressants.
Cautions: Use with caution in patients with arrhythmias, prostate hypertrophy, or wide-angle glaucoma.
Pregnancy Category: Not established.
Cost: Generic $$, Cogentin $$$ ($\approx$ $0.10 each 1 mg generic tablet; $\approx$ $0.25 each 1 mg Cogentin tablet).
Pearls:
- Is equally effective IM or IV; may give IV if IM is contraindicated.

- Is more effective in treating tremor and rigidity than for bradykinesia.

BEPRIDIL (Vascor)
Dose: 200–400 mg PO qd.
- Allow 10 days between dosing changes.

Actions: Calcium channel blocker used in the treatment of refractory angina.
- Also blocks the fast sodium channel.
- Has class III (potassium channel blocking) antiarrhythmic actions.

Clearance: Primarily metabolized in liver, negligible amount excreted unchanged in urine.

Selected Side Effects: Negative inotropy, QT prolongation (dose related).

Selected Drug Interactions: Increases serum level of digoxin.

Cautions: *Contraindicated in patients with history of ventricular arrhythmias, sick sinus syndrome, second- or third-degree heart block, or cardiogenic shock.*

Pregnancy Category: C

Cost: $$$.

Pearls: It is prudent to follow corrected QT interval.

BETAMETHASONE cream and lotion (many brands including Diprolene cream, lotion, ointment and gel; *see also* Lotrisone topical cream)
Dose: Apply to skin qd–tid.

Preparations: All contain 0.05% betamethasone.
- Diprolene AF Cream: 15 and 45 g tubes.
- Diprolene Lotion: 30 and 60 mL squeeze bottles.
- Diprolene Ointment: 15 and 45 g tubes.
- Diprolene Gel: 15 and 45 g tubes.

Actions: Potent topical corticosteroid used to treat many dermatologic conditions.

Pregnancy Category: C.

Cost: Generic $, Diprolene $$$; 45 g tube: generic ≈ $10, Diprolene ≈ $45.
Cautions:
- Extensive use over prolonged periods, especially with occlusive dressings, may lead to systemic absorption and related side effects of systemic steroids; treatment for more than 2 weeks and treatment with more than 50 g/week should be avoided because this may lead to suppression of the hypothalamic–pituitary axis (ie, adrenal suppression).
- Avoid use on face, breasts, axilla, and groin.
- Prolonged use of such class I steroids can lead to skin atrophy, telangiectasias, and pigmentary changes

Betapace: *see* SOTALOL

BETHANECHOL (Urecholine)
Dose: Route dependent:
- PO: Initial 5–10 mg/h until satisfactory response or maximum dose of 50 mg is reached; for maintenance dose give minimum effective dose (as determined by cumulative initial dose) tid–qid; usual dose 10–50 mg tid–qid.
- SQ: Initial 0.5 mL (2.5 mg); repeat every 15–30 min until satisfactory response or maximum of 2.0 mL (10 mg) is reached; for maintenance dose give minimum effective dose (as determined by cumulative initial dose) tid–qid; usual dose 1 mL (5 mg) tid–qid.
PO Preparations: 5, 10, 25, and 50 mg tablets.
Actions: Parasympathomimetic (cholinergic) agent that increases detrusor muscle contraction and stimulates micturition, used to treat nonobstructive urine retention.
Selected Side Effects: Increased gastric motility and tone, abdominal discomfort, diarrhea, hypotension and reflex tachycardia, flushing, bronchial constriction, lacrimation, miosis, salivation, urinary urgency.
Cautions: Must never be used when urinary tract obstruction is present.
Pregnancy Category: C

Cost: Generic $$, Urecholine $$$$ (25 mg generic ~ $0.30/ day, 25 mg Urecholine ≈ $2.70/day).

Pearls:

- Tablets should be taken 1–2 h after meals to avoid GI distress.
- Warn patients about possible orthostatic hypotension-like effects.
- Bethanechol is used now only rarely by many urologists.

Biaxin: *see* CLARITHROMYCIN

BICARBONATE (SODIUM BICARBONATE)

Dose: Route dependent:

- PO: 300–600 mg bid–tid.
- IV drip: Mix 2 ampules (88 mEq) in 1 L 0.45% NS (approximately equal to 0.9% solution) at IV rate appropriate for clinical setting.
- IV bolus: 1 mEq/kg; may give additional 0.5 mg/kg q10–12 min as indicated.

Pearls:

- Use with caution in patients with CHF (carries significant Na^+ load).
- During a code situation, can usually call for administration of "one amp" of a standard premixed solution.

BISACODYL (Dulcolax)

Dose: Route dependent:

- PO: 5–10 mg taken on an empty stomach with water.
- PR: 10 mg.
- Enema: 37.5 mL.

Preparations:

- 5 mg enteric-coated tablets.
- 10 mg suppositories.
- Liquid enema preparations.

Actions: Nondiarrheogenic cathartic that stimulates smooth muscle contractions, used to treat constipation.

Pearls: Onset of action 6–10 h PO, 15–60 min PR, immediate when given as enema.

BISMUTH SUBSALICYLATE (Pepto-Bismol)
Dose:
- Ulcers believed due to *Helicobacter pylori:* Usual dose is 2 tablets or 2 tbsp of regular-strength liquid preparation PO qid.

Preparations:
- Caplets containing 262 mg subsalicylate (99 mg salicylate).
- 4, 8, 12, and 16 oz bottles of regular-strength liquid containing 262 mg bismuth subsalicylate (102 mg salicylate)/ 16 mL (1 Tbsp).
- 4, 8, and 12 oz bottles of maximum strength liquid containing 525 mg bismuth subsalicylate (236 mg salicylate)/ 15 mL (1 Tbsp).

Actions: Used in the treatment of ulcer disease believed to be due, in part, to *H pylori* infections.
- Binds bacteria toxins and has antimicrobial effects on *H pylori*.

Selected Side Effects: Tinnitus.

Cautions:
- *Should not be given to children with chicken pox or the flu (since medication contains salicylates and the potential of causing Reye's syndrome exists).*
- Should not be taken by patients allergic to aspirin (since medication contains salicylates).

Cost: $.

Pearls: Warn patients that medication may darken tongue and stools.

BLEOMYCIN (Blenoxane)
Dose: Tumor dependent.
- Usually first give a "test dose" (to assess for anaphylactoid reaction).
- One regimen for many malignancies is 0.25–0.50 units/kg (10–20 units/m^2) IV, IM, or SQ weekly or twice weekly.

Actions: Antineoplastic agent that inhibits DNA synthesis, and possibly RNA and protein synthesis, used to treat many malignancies.

Clearance: 60–70% renally excreted.
- Slightly to moderately reduce dosage in patients with impaired renal function.

- For patients with serum creatinine of 2.5–4.0 mg/L, give 1/4 the normal dose; 4.0–6.0 mg/L, 1/5 the normal dose; 6.0–10.0 mg/L, 5–10% of the normal dose.
- No change in dosage needed for patients with liver disease.
- Supplemental dose not required after hemodialysis.

Selected Side Effects: *Pneumonitis and pulmonary fibrosis,* skin toxicity (erythema, rash, hyperpigmentation, vesiculations, tenderness, etc, usually occurring 2–3 weeks after therapy), rare renal or hepatic toxicity, *severe idiosyncratic reaction* in 1% of lymphoma patients (hypotension, mental status changes, fever and chills, wheezing).

Pregnancy Category: Not established.

Cost: $$$.

Pearls:

- Pulmonary fibrosis is the most severe toxicity usually associated with therapy; earliest symptoms and signs are dyspnea and fine rales.
- Decreased total lung volume and vital capacity are the most common abnormalities on pulmonary function tests but do not predict development of pulmonary fibrosis.
- DL_{CO} (diffusing capacity) may be a sensitive measure of subclinical pulmonary toxicity; *PDR* recommends checking it monthly.
- Pulmonary toxicity increases when cumulative dose exceeds 400 units.

Blocadren: *see* TIMOLOL

Brethaire: *see* TERBUTALINE inhaler

Brethine: *see* TERBUTALINE

BRETYLIUM (Bretylol)

Dose: Situation dependent (dosing regimens based on AHA 1994 ACLS guidelines).

- Ventricular fibrillation: Initial rapid injection of 5 mg/kg IV; if defibrillation fails and VF persists, after 5 min a dose of 10 mg/kg can be given; the 10 mg/kg dose can be repeated twice at q5–30 min up to a maximum total dose of 35 mg/kg.

- Refractory or recurrent ventricular tachycardia: 5–10 mg/kg injected IV over a period of 8–10 min; if VT persists, can give second dose of 5–10 mg/kg in 10–30 min.
- Maintenance: 1–2 mg/min IV.

Actions: Class III antiarrhythmic used to treat ventricular tachyarrhythmias.

Clearance: Renally excreted.

- Moderately to markedly reduce dosage in patients with impaired renal function; avoid in patients with end-stage renal disease.
- Dosage change probably unnecessary in patients with liver disease.

Selected Side Effects:
- Hypotension, orthostatic hypotension.
- Causes initial rise in norepinephrine levels, which may lead to initial increases in blood pressure, heart rate and arrhythmias.

Selected Drug Interactions:
- Increases risk of digoxin toxicity.
- Concomitant use with other antiarrhythmics increases risk of inducing hypotension.
- Augments pressor effects.

Pregnancy Category: C.

Cost: $$.

Pearls:
- After peripheral administration in a code situation, give a 20–30 mL bolus of intravenous fluid and immediately elevate the extremity. This enhances delivery of the drug to the central circulation, which can take 1–2 minutes.
- In non-code situations should be administered slowly.
- Onset of action in VF usually within a few minutes; onset of action in VT may be 20 minutes or more.
- Is more effective for VF and rapid VT (> 220 bpm); less effective for slower VT (< 220 bpm).

Brevibloc: *see* **ESMOLOL**

Bricanyl: *see* **TERBUTALINE**

BROMOCRIPTINE MESYLATE (Parlodel)
Dose (for Parkinson's disease):
- Initial: 1.25 mg (half of a 2.5 mg "SnapTab") PO bid with meals.
- May increase total daily dose by 2.5 mg (ie, bid dose by 1.25 mg) every 14–28 days.
- Maximum: 50 mg bid given with meals.

PO Preparations: 2.5 mg scored "SnapTabs" and 5 mg capsules.

Actions:
- Ergot derivative with potent agonistic activity against postsynaptic dopamine receptors, used to treat Parkinson's disease and other disorders (including pituitary adenoma, neuroleptic malignant syndrome, amenorrhea, galactorrhea, and female infertility).
- Like dopamine, inhibits pituitary secretion of prolactin.

Clearance: Metabolized via liver.
- No change in dosage needed in patients with impaired renal function.

Selected Side Effects: GI symptoms (nausea and vomiting, abdominal discomfort), CNS effects (abnormal involuntary movements, hallucinations, confusion, drowsiness, "on–off" phenomenon, ataxia, insomnia, depression), first-dose hypotensive effect, dizziness, or orthostatic hypotension.

Selected Drug Interactions:
- Concomitant use with antihypertensive agents increases risk of hypotension.
- Dopamine antagonists (phenothiazines, haloperidol, etc) decrease its therapeutic effect.

Cautions:
- *Contraindicated in uncontrolled hypertension (occasionally substantially increases BP), in toxemia of pregnancy, and in patients sensitive to ergot alkaloids.*
- Should not be used by nursing mothers (prevents lactation).

Pregnancy Category: B.

Cost: $$$$ (≥$2 per 5 mg tablet).

Bronkometer: *see* ISOETHARINE

Bronkosol: *see* ISOETHARINE

BUDESONIDE Nasal Inhaler (Rhinocort)

Dose: Two possible regimens: (1) two sprays in each nostril in the morning and evening *or* (2) four sprays in each nostril in the morning.

Preparations: 7.0 g cannister that delivers 200 metered doses.

Actions: Potent anti-inflammatory glucocorticoid; used in the treatment of allergic seasonal or perennial allergic rhinitis and nonallergic perennial rhinitis.

Selected Side Effects: Irritation of nasal mucous membranes, possible adrenal suppression with long-term use.

Pregnancy Category: C.

Pearls: Onset of action may be within 24 h; maximum benefit usually takes 3–7 days.

BUMETANIDE (Bumex)

Dose: Route dependent:
- PO: 0.5–2.0 mg qd.
- IV: 0.5–1.0 mg over 1–2 min; may repeat dose q2–3h.
- Maximum: 10 mg daily.

PO Preparations: 0.5, 1.0, and 2.0 mg tablets.

Actions: Potent loop diuretic that inhibits sodium reabsorption in the ascending loop of Henle, used as a diuretic, often in patients responsive only to high-dose furosemide (Lasix).

Clearance: 81% excreted in urine, 45% in unchanged form.
- No change in dosage needed in patients with impaired renal function.

Selected Side Effects: Profound water loss and electrolyte depletion, reductions in PO_4^{2-}, K^+, and Cl^-, ototoxicity (but less than with the equally effective amount of furosemide).

Cautions:
- Contraindicated in anuria, hepatic coma, severe electrolyte depletion, and in patients taking aminoglycosides (increases risk of ototoxicity).
- Patients allergic to sulfonamides may show cross-hypersensitivity.

Pregnancy Category: C.

Cost: $$$ ($\approx$ $0.85 each 2 mg tablet).

Pearls:
- 1 mg bumetanide is approximately as effective as 40 mg furosemide (Lasix).
- Can be given IM if necessary.
- Patients allergic to furosemide may exhibit cross-sensitivity.

Bumex: *see* BUMETANIDE

BUPROPION (Wellbutrin)
Dose:
- Initial: 100 mg PO bid.
- After 3 days may increase to 100 mg PO tid.
- If needed, may increase after several weeks to 100–150 mg PO tid (allow at least 4–5 h between doses).
- Maximum single dose: 150 mg.

PO Preparations: 75 and 100 mg tablets.

Actions:
- Monocyclic agent, unrelated to other antidepressants, that may act by D_2 receptor blockade (inhibits dopamine uptake), used to treat depression.
- Unlike tricyclics, minimally inhibits norepinephrine and serotonin reuptake.

Clearance:
- Extensively metabolized; some metabolites are active; renal excretion may play an important role in their clearance.
- Studies in patients with cirrhosis show that metabolites accumulate at 2–3 times the levels in normal patients, so reducing the dosage in patients with liver disease is probably advisable.

Selected Side Effects: CNS symptoms (*agitation,* tremor, confusion, blurred vision, auditory and taste disturbances, etc), dizziness, constipation, menstrual complaints.

Selected Drug Interactions: L-Dopa increases its side effects.

Cautions:
- *Use with extreme caution in patients predisposed to seizures or taking medications that lower the seizure threshold.*
- Use with great caution in patients who are being withdrawn from benzodiazepines or those who had them discontinued recently.

Pregnancy Category: B.
Cost: $$$$ (≈ $0.90 each 100 mg tablet).
Pearls:
- Risk of seizures is approximately 0.4% at doses up to 450 mg daily and increases substantially at higher dosages.
- Its potential advantages over other antidepressants include lack of autonomic and cardiovascular effects, sedation, or weight gain.

BuSpar: *see* BUSPIRONE

BUSPIRONE (BuSpar)
Dose:
- Initial: 5 mg PO q8h.
- May increase total daily dose (*not* tid dose) by 5 mg every 2–3 days.
- Maximum: 20 mg PO q8h.

PO Preparations: 5 and 10 mg tablets.
Actions: Anxiolytic, unrelated to benzodiazepines or barbiturates, that may act on 5-hydroxytryptophan, used to treat anxiety disorders.
Clearance: Metabolized primarily via liver.
- One source recommends against giving to patients with renal impairment, but others claim no change in dosage is necessary.

Selected Side Effects: Dizziness, nervousness, occasional other CNS or neuropsychiatric symptoms
Selected Drug Interactions:
- Raises serum level of haloperidol.
- *Greatly increases BP when given with MAOI.*

Cautions: *Contraindicated in patients receiving MAOI.*
Pregnancy Category: B.
Cost: $$$$ (≈ $1 each 10 mg tablet).
Pearls:
- Should not be taken "prn."
- Is less sedating than other anxiolytics.
- More effective in patients who have not previously taken benzodiazepines.
- Maximum effect may take weeks to achieve.
- Signs and symptoms of overdose include nausea and vomiting, dizziness, drowsiness, miosis, and GI distress.

BUSULFAN (Myleran)
Dose:
- Induction: 4–8 mg PO daily.
- After induction, a maintenance dose of 1–3 mg PO daily is sometimes used.

PO Preparations: 2 mg scored tablets.

Actions: Alkylating agent, nonspecific for cell cycle phase, used to treat neoplastic disease, primarily myeloproliferative disorders.

Clearance: Metabolized via liver.
- Reduce dosage in patients with end-stage renal disease (give 50% of normal dose); no change in dosage needed for milder renal impairment.
- Supplemental dose not required after hemodialysis.

Selected Side Effects:
- *Myelosuppression,* hyperpigmentation, hyperuricemia, rare pulmonary fibrosis.
- Prolonged use can cause adrenal insufficiency and suppression of testicular and ovarian function.

Pregnancy Category: D.

Cost: $$$.

Pearls:
- Myelosuppression is the dose-limiting toxicity; may be cumulative and irreversible with prolonged use.
- WBC and platelet nadirs occur 14–21 days after pulse dosing.
- Follow CBC.
- Pulmonary fibrosis ("busulfan lung") is a rare but important side effect that usually occurs after months to years of prolonged treatment.
- Leukemogenic with prolonged use in hematologic disorders.

Calan: *see* VERAPAMIL

CALCIUM CARBONATE (Os-Cal; *see also* Rolaids, Tums)
Dose: 250–500 mg PO tid.
PO Preparations: 250 and 500 mg tablets.
Cost: $

CALCIUM CHLORIDE
Dose: 1 amp (13.6 mEq) of a premixed 10% solution IV.
Actions: Calcium supplement that can be used during cardiac arrests or to reverse the peripheral-dilating properties of the calcium antagonists.
Pearls:
- In emergency situations, the use of calcium chloride is preferred over other calcium supplements (such as calcium gluconate).
- During a code situation, can usually call for administration of "1 amp" of a standard premixed solution.

Capoten: *see* CAPTOPRIL

Capozide (CAPTOPRIL + HYDROCHLOROTHIAZIDE)
Dose: 1 tablet PO bid–tid 1 h before meals.
PO Preparations:
- Tablets containing 25 mg captopril with 15 or 25 mg hydrochlorothiazide.
- Tablets containing 50 mg captopril with 15 or 25 mg hydrochlorothiazide.

Actions: Drug that combines vasodilating and K^+-sparing properties of the ACE inhibitor captopril with diuretic action of hydrochlorothiazide, used to treat hypertension.
Cautions: *Contraindicated during second and third trimesters of pregnancy (because of captopril component).*
Pregnancy Category: D.
Cost: $$$$.
Pearls: BP-lowering action of ACE inhibitors is often strongly enhanced in fluid-depleted patients, which may increase risk of a hypotensive response.

CAPSAICIN cream (Axsain, Zostrix)
Dose: Apply to affected areas tid–qid.
PO Preparations:
- Axsain: 1.0 and 2.0 oz tubes containing 0.075% capsaicin.
- Zostrix: 1.5 and 3.0 oz tubes containing 0.025% capsaicin.

Actions: Topical analgesic that may inhibit synthesis, transport, and release of substance P, a neurotransmitter of pain; used to treat pain associated with arthritis and neuralgias.

Selected Side Effects: Transient burning sensation at application site (caused by initial release of substance P).

Cost: $$$–$$$$.

Pearls:

- Inform patients that they may experience a burning sensation for the first several days of use.
- Warn patients to wash hands immediately after applying cream, not to apply cream to wounds or damaged skin, and to avoid contact with eyes.
- Manufacturer states that optimal benefit may take 4–6 weeks to achieve, but most patients should notice some relief of symptoms by 1–2 weeks.
- Preparations of this type have a substantial placebo effect, but there appears to be at least some additional benefit from using capsaicin.

CAPTOPRIL (Capoten; *also* Capozide)

Dose:

- Initial test dose: 6.25 mg.
- Usual: 25–50 mg bid–tid (increase stepwise).

PO Preparations: 12.5, 25, 50, and 100 mg tablets.

Actions: ACE inhibitor that promotes peripheral dilatation, used to treat hypertension and CHF secondary to systolic dysfunction.

- Is also now approved for the prevention of renal insufficiency progression in diabetic patients.

Clearance: Metabolized via liver; renally excreted.

- Either slightly decrease dosage or moderately increase dosing interval in patients with impaired renal function.
- One source suggests that dosage should probably be reduced in patients with liver disease.
- Supplemental dose suggested after hemodialysis.

Selected Side Effects: Hypotension and dizziness, hyperkalemia (especially in patients with impaired renal function or taking K^+-sparing drugs or K^+ supplements), nonproductive cough, impairment of renal function, angioedema, rare neutropenia.

Cautions:
- *Contraindicated during second and third trimesters of pregnancy and in patients with significant aortic stenosis or hyperkalemia.*
- Patients should almost never be given both an ACE inhibitor and a K⁺ supplement, unless clearly indicated by serial serum K⁺ testing.

Pregnancy Category: D.
Cost: $$$$ (≈ $0.70 each 25 mg tablet).
Pearls:
- Diuretics potentiate its antihypertensive effects; the risk of hypotension is increased in volume-depleted and elderly patients.
- Follow BUN, creatinine, and K when beginning therapy.
- Patients should be instructed not to use potassium supplements or salt substitutes containing potassium.
- Patients should be made aware of the possibility of developing a nonproductive cough and of developing angioedema.
- The nonproductive cough with ACE inhibitors is presumed to be due to the inhibition of the degradation of endogenous bradykinin.
- Patients who develop a cough with one ACE inhibitor usually also develop such a cough with other ACE inhibitors.

Carafate: *see* SUCRALFATE

CARBAMAZEPINE (Tegretol)
Dose:
- Initial: 200 mg PO bid.
- May increase up to 400 mg tid–qid.
- Usual maintenance: 400 mg PO bid–tid.

PO Preparations:
- 100 mg chewable tablets; 200 mg adult tablets.
- 450 mL bottle of suspension containing 100 mg/5 mL (1 tsp).

Actions: Anticonvulsant that probably acts by reducing polysynaptic responses and blocking posttetanic potentiation, used to treat seizure disorders.

Clearance: Metabolized via liver; metabolites are active.
- Slightly reduce dosage in patients with end-stage renal disease; no change needed for milder renal impairment.
- Decrease in dosage (or at least *careful* blood level monitoring) may be needed in patients with liver disease.
- Supplemental dose not required after hemodialysis.

Selected Side Effects: Numerous CNS effects, including drowsiness and dizziness, rare hemopoietic suppression (WBCs, RBCs and/or platelets), rare severe dermatologic reactions (toxic epidermal necrolysis, Stevens–Johnson syndrome).

Selected Drug Interactions:
- *Concomitant use with MAOI causes hyperpyrexia and seizures.*
- Phenytoin and phenobarbital decrease its serum level.
- Erythromycin, cimetidine, isoniazid, and calcium channel blockers raise its serum level, increasing its potential toxicity.

Cautions: *Contraindicated in patients taking MAOI or with history of hypersensitivity to any tricyclic.*

Pregnancy Category: C.

Cost: $$ (≈ $0.20 each 200 mg tablet).

Pearls:
- Abrupt discontinuance may precipitate seizures.
- Not indicated for the treatment of *petit mal* ("absence") seizures; treatment with carbamazepine may precipitate "absence status."
- Usual therapeutic level is 4–12 mg/mL.
- Signs and symptoms of overdose include respiratory depression, convulsions, coma, tremor, arrhythmia, marked fluctuations in BP, and marked tachycardia.

CARBIDOPA: *see* Sinemet

CARBOPLATIN (Paraplatin)
Dose: Disease dependent.

Actions: Platinum analog that cross-links DNA molecules, used to treat malignancies, most commonly of the lung, ovary, and breast.

Clearance: Significant renal excretion because of low protein binding.
- Reduce dosage in patients with impaired renal function.
- No change in dosage needed in patients with liver disease.

Selected Side Effects: *Myelosuppression,* rare anaphylactic reaction, dose-related nausea and vomiting.

Pregnancy Category: D.

Cost: $$$.

Pearls:
- A new agent with several advantages over the similar cisplatin: less nephrotoxicity, nausea and vomiting; minimal ototoxicity, neurotoxicity, and magnesium wasting.
- Has greater myelosuppression, principally of platelets, than cisplatin.

Cardene: *see* **NICARDIPINE**

Cardizem: *see* **DILTIAZEM**

Cardura: *see* **DOXAZOSIN**

CASANTHRANOL: *see* **Peri-Colace**

Catapres: *see* **CLONIDINE**

Ceclor: *see* **CEFACLOR**

CEFACLOR (Ceclor)

Dose: 250–500 mg PO q8h.

PO Preparations:
- 250 and 500 mg capsules.
- 75 mL suspension containing 125 mg/5 mL (1 tsp).
- 50 mL suspension containing 187 mg/5 mL (1 tsp).
- 75 mL suspension containing 250 mg/5 mL (1 tsp).
- 50 mL suspension containing 375 mg/5 mL (1 tsp).

Actions: Bactericidal second-generation cephalosporin that inhibits cell wall synthesis.
- Good gram (+) coverage, including strep and most staph (but *not* enterococci or MRSA).
- Some gram (−) coverage, including *Escherichia coli, Klebsiella, Proteus,* and β-lactamase-producing *Haemophilus influenzae* (though nosocomial gram (−) organisms are usually resistant).
- Poor anaerobic coverage.
- *NOTE:* The above-mentioned antimicrobial coverage summary should be used as a guideline only; treatment decisions should take into account not only local epidemiologic patterns of antibiotic susceptibility but also, when available, culture susceptibility results.

Clearance: Primarily renally excreted.
- Slightly reduce dosage in patients with impaired renal function.
- No change in dosage needed in patients with liver disease.
- Supplemental dose suggested after hemodialysis or peritoneal dialysis.

Selected Side Effects: Hypersensitivity reactions, rare anaphylactic reactions.

Cautions:
- *Contraindicated in patients with cephalosporin allergy.*
- Use with caution in patients with penicillin allergy.

Pregnancy Category: B.

Cost: $$$ (≈ $65 for 250 mg tid for 10 days).

Pearls: Can be taken without regard to meals.

CEFADROXIL (Duricef)

Dose: 1–2 g PO daily given in 1 or 2 divided doses.

PO Preparations:
- 500 mg capsules and 1 g tablets.
- 50 and 100 mL bottles of orange–pineapple-flavored suspension containing 125 mg/mL (1 tsp) or 250 mg/mL.
- 50, 75, and 100 mL bottles of orange–pineapple-flavored suspension containing 500 mg/mL (1 tsp).

Actions: Semisynthetic bactericidal cephalosporin that inhibits cell wall synthesis.

- Good gram (+) coverage, including strep and many staph (but *not* enterococci or MRSA).
- Some gram (−) coverage (but not *Pseudomonas aeruginosa,* β-lactamase-producing *Haemophilus influenzae,* or nosocomial organisms).
- Poor anaerobic coverage.
- *NOTE:* The above-mentioned antimicrobial coverage summary should be used as a guideline only; treatment decisions should take into account not only local epidemiologic patterns of antibiotic susceptibility but also, when available, culture susceptibility results.

Clearance:
- Excreted unchanged in urine.
- Slightly to moderately increase dosing interval in patients with impaired renal function.

Selected Side Effects: Allergic reactions, rare anaphylactic reactions.

Cautions:
- *Contraindicated in patients with cephalosporin allergy.*
- Use with caution in penicillin allergy.

Pregnancy Category: B.

Cost: $$$ (≈ $75 for 500 mg bid for 10 days).

Pearls: Should be taken with meals to decrease GI side effects.

CEFAZOLIN (Ancef, Kefzol)

Dose: Infection dependent:
- Mild infection: 250–500 mg IM or IV q8h.
- Moderate to severe infection: 500–1000 mg IM or IV q6–8h.
- Life-threatening infection: 1–2 g IV q8h.

Actions: Bactericidal first-generation cephalosporin that inhibits cell wall synthesis.
- Good gram (+) coverage, including *Staphylococcus aureus* and strep (but *not* MRSA or enterococci).
- Some gram (−) coverage, including *Escherichia coli, Klebsiella,* and *Proteus* (nosocomial gram [−] organisms are usually resistant).
- Poor anaerobic coverage.

- *NOTE:* The above-mentioned antimicrobial coverage summary should be used as a guideline only; treatment decisions should take into account not only local epidemiologic patterns of antibiotic susceptibility but also, when available, culture susceptibility results.

Clearance: Primarily renally excreted.
- Moderately reduce dosage in patients with impaired renal function.
- No change in dosage needed in patients with liver disease.
- Supplemental dose suggested after hemodialysis but not after peritoneal dialysis.

Selected Side Effects: Allergic reactions, rare anaphylactic reactions.

Selected Drug Interactions: Concomitant use with aminoglycosides increases risk of nephrotoxicity.

Cautions:
- *Contraindicated in patients with cephalosporin allergy.*
- Use with caution in patients with penicillin allergy.

Pregnancy Category: B.

Cost: $.

Pearls: Well-tolerated IM.

CEFIXIME (Suprax)

Dose: 200 mg PO q12h or 400 mg PO qd.

PO Preparations:
- 200 and 400 mg scored tablets.
- 50, 75, and 100 mL bottles containing powder for strawberry-flavored oral suspension that contains 100 mg/5 mL (1 tsp) when reconstituted.

Actions: Semisynthetic bactericidal cephalosporin that inhibits cell wall synthesis.
- Poor gram (+) coverage with variable coverage for strep (but *not* staph or enterococci).
- Good gram (−) coverage, including *Haemophilus influenza* (but *not Pseudomonas aeruginosa*).
- Poor anaerobic coverage.
- *NOTE:* The above-mentioned antimicrobial coverage summary should be used as a guideline only; treatment deci-

sions should take into account not only local epidemiologic patterns of antibiotic susceptibility but also, when available, culture susceptibility results.

Clearance: 50% of absorbed dose is excreted unchanged in the urine.

- Slightly reduce dosage in patients with impaired renal function.
- Is not significantly removed by hemodialysis or peritoneal dialysis.

Selected Side Effects: Frequent GI symptoms (diarrhea, nausea, dyspepsia, abdominal pain, flatulence), hypersensitivity reactions, rare anaphylactic reactions.

Cautions:

- *Contraindicated in patients with cephalosporin allergy.*
- Use with caution in patients with penicillin allergy.

Pregnancy Category: B.

Cost: $$$$ (≈ $85 for 200 mg bid for 10 days).

Pearls: Can be given without regard to meals.

Cefizox: *see* CEFTIZOXIME

Cefobid: *see* CEFOPERAZONE

CEFOPERAZONE (Cefobid)
Dose:

- Many infections: 2 g IV q12h to 4 g IV q6h (higher dose and more frequent dosing interval required for *Pseudomonas aeruginosa).*

Actions: Bactericidal third-generation cephalosporin that inhibits cell wall synthesis.

- Excellent gram (−) coverage, including *P aeruginosa;* some gram (+) coverage.
- Variable *Bacteroides fragilis* coverage.
- *NOTE:* The above-mentioned antimicrobial coverage summary should be used as a guideline only; treatment decisions should take into account not only local epidemiologic patterns of antibiotic susceptibility but also, when available, culture susceptibility results.

Clearance: Excreted in bile.
- No change in dosage needed in patients with impaired renal function.
- Serum $t_{1/2}$ is increased 2–4 times in patients with significant liver disease.

Pregnancy Category: B.

Cost: $$.

Pearls:
- Poor CNS penetration.
- Can cause disulfiram (Antabuse)-like reactions with alcohol.

Cefotan: *see* CEFOTETAN

CEFOTAXIME (Claforan)

Dose: Infection dependent:
- Usual: 1–2 g IM or IV q8–12h.
- Life-threatening infection: up to 2 g IV q4h.
- Maximum: 12 g in 24 h.

Actions: Bactericidal third-generation cephalosporin that inhibits cell wall synthesis.
- Some gram (+) coverage (but *not* MRSA or enterococci).
- Excellent gram (−) coverage (but *not Pseudomonas aeruginosa*).
- Some anaerobes, including some *Bacteroides fragilis.*
- *NOTE:* The above-mentioned antimicrobial coverage summary should be used as a guideline only; treatment decisions should take into account not only local epidemiologic patterns of antibiotic susceptibility but also, when available, culture susceptibility results.

Clearance: Metabolized via liver; renally excreted; metabolites are active in patients with end-stage renal disease.
- Moderately increase dosing interval in patients with impaired renal function.
- May need to adjust dosing interval in patients with severe liver disease.
- Supplemental dose suggested after hemodialysis but not after peritoneal dialysis.

Selected Side Effects: Local pain at IM site or phlebitis at IV site, hypersensitivity reaction, rare anaphylactic reactions.

Selected Drug Interactions: Concomitant use with amino-
glycosides increases risk of nephrotoxicity.
Cautions:
- *Contraindicated in patients with cephalosporin allergy.*
- Use with caution in patients with penicillin allergy.
Pregnancy Category: B.
Cost: $$½.

CEFOTETAN (Cefotan)
Dose: 1–3 g IM or IV q12h.
Actions:
- Bactericidal second-generation cephalosporin that inhibits
cell wall synthesis.
- Some gram (+) coverage (but *not* MRSA or enterococci).
- Excellent gram (−) coverage, including β-lactamase-produc-
ing organisms (but *not Pseudomonas aeruginosa*).
- Good anaerobic coverage, including *Bacteroides fragilis.*
- *NOTE:* The above-mentioned antimicrobial coverage sum-
mary should be used as a guideline only; treatment deci-
sions should take into account not only local epidemiologic
patterns of antibiotic susceptibility but also, when available,
culture susceptibility results.
Clearance: Primarily renally excreted.
- Moderately reduce dosage in patients with impaired renal
function.
- No change in dosage needed in patients with liver disease.
- Supplemental dose suggested after hemodialysis but not
peritoneal dialysis.
Selected Side Effects: Rare hypersensitivity and anaphy-
lactic reactions.
Selected Drug Interactions:
- Disulfiram-like reaction with alcohol.
- Concomitant use with aminoglycosides increases risk of
nephrotoxicity.
Cautions:
- *Contraindicated in patients with cephalosporin allergy.*
- Use with caution in patients with penicillin allergy.
Pregnancy Category: B.
Cost: $$.

Pearls: Is especially useful in prophylactic regimens for abdominopelvic surgery.

CEFOXITIN (Mefoxin)
Dose: 1–2 g IV q6–12h; may be given IM.
Actions: Bactericidal second-generation cephalosporin that inhibits cell wall synthesis.
- Some gram (+) coverage (but *not* enterococci).
- Good gram (−) coverage, including *Escherichia coli, Proteus, Klebsiella,* and *Haemophilus influenzae* (but *not Pseudomonas aeruginosa*).
- Excellent anaerobic coverage (including *Bacteroides fragilis*).
- *NOTE:* The above-mentioned antimicrobial coverage summary should be used as a guideline only; treatment decisions should take into account not only local epidemiologic patterns of antibiotic susceptibility but also, when available, culture susceptibility results.

Clearance: Renally excreted.
- Moderately increase dosing interval in patients with impaired renal function.
- No change in dosage required in patients with liver disease.
- Supplemental dose suggested after hemodialysis but not after peritoneal dialysis.

Selected Side Effects: Local reactions at injection site, hypersensitivity, and rare anaphylactic reactions.
Selected Drug Interactions: Concomitant use with aminoglycosides may increase risk of nephrotoxicity.
Cautions:
- *Contraindicated in patients with cephalosporin allergy.*
- Use with caution in patients with penicillin allergy.

Pregnancy Category: B.
Cost: $$.
Pearls: Can *falsely* raise measured serum creatinine levels.

CEFTAZIDIME (Fortaz, Tazicef, Tazidime)
Dose:
- 1–2 g IM or IV q8–12h.
- Usual: 1 g IV q8h.

Actions:
- Bactericidal third-generation cephalosporin that inhibits cell wall synthesis.
- Excellent gram (-) coverage, particularly for *Pseudomonas aeruginosa.*
- Poor gram (+) or anaerobic coverage.
- *NOTE:* The above-mentioned antimicrobial coverage summary should be used as a guideline only; treatment decisions should take into account not only local epidemiologic patterns of antibiotic susceptibility but also, when available, culture susceptibility results.

Clearance: Primarily renally excreted.
- Markedly increase dosing interval in patients with impaired renal function.
- No change in dosage needed in patients with liver disease.
- Supplemental dose suggested after hemodialysis or peritoneal dialysis.

Selected Side Effects: Local phlebitis, hypersensitivity, and rare anaphylactic reactions.

Selected Drug Interactions: Concomitant use with aminoglycosides may increase risk of nephrotoxicity.

Cautions:
- *Contraindicated in patients with cephalosporin allergy.*
- Use with caution in patients with penicillin allergy.

Pregnancy Category: B.

Cost: $$$.

Pearls:
- (+) CSF penetration in meningeal inflammation.
- Can be used as single-agent therapy in patients with neutropenia and a fever, pending results of cultures; otherwise, reserve the use of ceftazidime for the treatment of known or suspected *Pseudomonas aeruginosa* infections.

Ceftin: *see* CEFUROXIME

CEFTIZOXIME (Cefizox)
Dose:
- 1–2 g IV q8–12h.
- Usual: 1 g IV q8h.

Actions: Bactericidal third-generation cephalosporin that inhibits cell wall synthesis.

- Excellent gram (–) coverage (but *not Pseudomonas*).
- Some gram (+) coverage, including *Staphylococcus aureus* and strep (but *not* MRSA or enterococci).
- Some anaerobic coverage (some strains of *Bacteroides fragilis* are resistant).
- *NOTE:* The above-mentioned antimicrobial coverage summary should be used as a guideline only; treatment decisions should take into account not only local epidemiologic patterns of antibiotic susceptibility but also, when available, culture susceptibility results.

Clearance: Renally excreted.

- Markedly increase dosing interval in patients with impaired renal function.
- No change in dosage needed in patients with liver disease.
- Supplemental dose suggested after hemodialysis.

Selected Side Effects: Local phlebitis, hypersensitivity, rare anaphylactic reactions, and transient elevation of LFTs.

Selected Drug Interactions: Concomitant use with aminoglycosides may increase risk of nephrotoxicity.

Cautions:

- *Contraindicated in patients with cephalosporin allergy.*
- Use with caution in patients with penicillin allergy.

Pregnancy Category: B.

Cost: $$.

Pearls: (+) CSF penetration in meningeal inflammation.

CEFTRIAXONE (Rocephin)

Dose: Disease dependent:

- Systemic infection: 1–2 g IM or IV q12–24h.
- Usually given q24h (because of long $t_{1/2}$) except in meningitis, for which the dosage may be 2 g q12h.
- Nonsystemic gonococcal infection: single dose of 250 mg IM.

Actions: Bactericidal third-generation cephalosporin that inhibits cell wall synthesis.

- Excellent gram (–) coverage (but *not Pseudomonas*).
- Some gram (+) coverage, including *Staphylococcus aureus* and strep (but *not* MRSA, enterococci, or *Listeria*).

- Some anaerobic coverage (some strains of *Bacteroides fragilis* are resistant).
- *NOTE:* The above-mentioned antimicrobial coverage summary should be used as a guideline only; treatment decisions should take into account not only local epidemiologic patterns of antibiotic susceptibility but also, when available, culture susceptibility results.

Clearance: Secreted in bile; renally excreted (60%).
- Slightly increase dosing interval in patients with end-stage renal disease; no change needed for milder renal impairment.
- Follow patients carefully if severe liver disease.
- Give maximum of 2 g daily in patients with *both* hepatic and renal failure.
- Supplemental dose not required after hemodialysis or peritoneal dialysis.

Selected Side Effects: Local phlebitis, hypersensitivity and rare anaphylactic reactions, eosinophilia, thrombocytosis, leukopenia, elevated LFTs, precipitation of biliary tract disease (due to sludging and/or stones).

Cautions:
- *Contraindicated in patients with cephalosporin allergy.*
- Use with caution in patients with penicillin allergy.

Pregnancy Category: B.
Cost: $$½.
Pearls:
- (+) CSF penetration in meningeal inflammation.
- Consider following serum levels in patients with impaired renal function.
- Can exacerbate vitamin K deficiency in predisposed patients.
- If used for empiric coverage of meningitis in elderly or debilitated patients, many sources now recommend also using ampicillin to cover for *Listeria* (which ceftriaxone does not cover).

CEFUROXIME (PO = Ceftin; IV = Kefurox, Zinacef)

Dose: Route and patient dependent:
- Adults dosage:
  - ▶ PO tablets: 125–500 mg q12h without regard to meals.
  - ▶ IV: 750–1500 mg q8h.

- Pediatric dosage:
  - ▶ Pharyngitis or tonsillitis: 10 mg/kg bid of the suspension.
  - ▶ Acute otitis media or impetigo: 15 mg/kg bid of the suspension.
- *NOTE: Ceftin tablets and suspension are NOT bioequivalent and are not substitutable.*

PO Preparations:
- 125, 250, and 500 mg tablets of Ceftin.
- 50, 100, and 200 mL bottles of suspension containing 125 mg/5 mL (1 tsp).

Actions: Bactericidal second-generation cephalosporin that inhibits cell wall synthesis.
- Good gram (−) coverage, including β-lactamase-producing organisms (but *not Pseudomonas aeruginosa*).
- Good gram (+) coverage, including *Staphylococcus aureus* and strep (but *not* enterococci or MRSA).
- *Not* most *Bacteroides fragilis.*
- *NOTE:* The above-mentioned antimicrobial coverage summary should be used as a guideline only; treatment decisions should take into account not only local epidemiologic patterns of antibiotic susceptibility but also, when available, culture susceptibility results.

Clearance: Renally excreted.
- Markedly reduce dosage in patients with impaired renal function.
- Supplemental dose suggested after hemodialysis but not after peritoneal dialysis.

Selected Side Effects: Phlebitis, nausea and vomiting (with PO), transient elevation of LFTs, rare hypersensitivity reactions.

Selected Drug Interactions:
- Concomitant use with aminoglycosides may increase risk of nephrotoxicity.
- Probenecid may raise its serum level.

Cautions:
- *Contraindicated in patients with cephalosporin allergy.*
- Use with caution in patients with penicillin allergy.

Pregnancy Category: B.

Cost: PO $$$$ (≈ $75 for 250 mg PO bid for 10 days).

Pearls:
- Clinically ineffective in meningitis.
- *Ceftin tablets and suspension are NOT bioequivalent and are not substitutable.*

CEPHALEXIN (Keflex, Keftab)
Dose: 250–500 mg PO qid without regard to meals.
PO Preparations:
- 250 and 500 mg Pulvules.
- 100 and 200 mL bottles of suspensions containing either 125 mg/5 mL (1 tsp) or 250 mg/5 mL.

Actions: Bactericidal first-generation cephalosporin that inhibits cell wall synthesis.
- Good gram (+) coverage, including *Staphylococcus aureus* and strep (but *not* MRSA or enterococci); some gram (−) coverage, including *Escherichia coli, Proteus,* and *Klebsiella* (but *not Pseudomonas aeruginosa* or nosocomial infections).
- Poor anaerobic coverage.
- *NOTE:* The above-mentioned antimicrobial coverage summary should be used as a guideline only; treatment decisions should take into account not only local epidemiologic patterns of antibiotic susceptibility but also, when available, culture susceptibility results.

Clearance: Renally excreted, but only slightly reduce dosage in patients with impaired renal function.
- No change in dosage needed in patients with liver disease.
- Supplemental dose suggested after hemodialysis or peritoneal dialysis.

Selected Side Effects: Diarrhea, hypersensitivity, and rare anaphylactic reactions.
Cautions:
- *Contraindicated in patients with cephalosporin allergy.*
- Use with caution in patients with penicillin allergy.

Pregnancy Category: B.
Cost: $$ (≈ $25 for 250 mg qid for 10 days).

Cerumenex: *see* TRIETHANOLAMINE otic solution

CHARCOAL (ACTIVATED CHARCOAL)

Dose: Suggested regimens include: (1) 20–50 g PO or via NG tube q2–6h for 24 h. (2) 50–100 mg PO or via NG tube q4–6h for 24 h.

PO Preparations: Multiple size bottles; some preparations come premixed with sorbitol.

Actions: Inert substance that absorbs most drugs and is used to treat drug overdose.

Pearls:

- Often given repeatedly with drugs that undergo hepatobiliary excretion.
- Does *not* absorb alkalis, mineral acids, or $FeSO_4$.
- Concomitant use with cathartics may reduce its effectiveness.
- May absorb oral antidotes (ie, Mucomyst).

CHLORAMBUCIL (Leukeran)

Dose:

- Initial: 4–10 mg (0.1–0.2 mg/kg) PO qd.
- Maintenance: 2–4 mg (0.03–0.1 mg/kg) PO qd.

PO Preparations: 2 mg tablets.

Actions: Alkylating agent used to treat neoplastic diseases.

Clearance: Extensively metabolized in the liver to inactive metabolites; almost no renal excretion.

Selected Side Effects: *Myelosuppression,* rare pulmonary fibrosis, rare hepatotoxicity, rare seizures.

Pregnancy Category: D.

Cost: $$$.

Pearls:

- Myelosuppression (especially of platelets) is dose-limiting toxicity.
- WBC and platelet nadirs usually occur 14–21 days after treatment.
- Pulmonary fibrosis is a rare side effect and usually occurs months to years after prolonged treatment.
- Give before or after meals (food reduces its bioavailability).

CHLORAMPHENICOL (Chloromycetin)

Dose: 12.5–25 mg/kg PO or IV q6h (50–100 mg/kg daily).

PO Preparations: 250 mg Chloromycetin Kapseals.

Actions: Broad-spectrum antibiotic that inhibits protein synthesis.

- Used to treat serious gram (+) and gram (−) infections for which less potentially dangerous drugs are ineffective or contraindicated.
- Bacteriostatic against most organisms and bactericidal against pneumococci, *Haemophilus influenzae,* and meningococci.
- Particularly useful in meningitis and in *Salmonella typhi* and *H influenzae* infections.
- *NOTE:* The above-mentioned antimicrobial coverage summary should be used as a guideline only; treatment decisions should take into account not only local epidemiologic patterns of antibiotic susceptibility but also, when available, culture susceptibility results.

Clearance: 70–90% metabolized in the liver to inactive metabolites.

- May need to reduce dosage in cases of severe renal dysfunction.
- Decrease dosage in patients with liver disease.
- Supplemental dose suggested after hemodialysis but not after peritoneal dialysis.

Selected Side Effects: *Dose-related reversible bone marrow suppression, aplastic anemia (rare but irreversible),* hypersensitivity reactions, and anaphylaxis.

Cautions:

- *Should generally only be used to treat infections for which less potentially dangerous drugs are ineffective or contraindicated.*
- May cause "gray syndrome" in children born to pregnant women given this drug.

Pregnancy Category: *Not established, but should generally not be used in pregnant patients.*

Cost: $$ (≥ $16/day).

Pearls:

- Excellent CSF penetration.
- Risk of aplastic anemia, listed in various sources as 1/24,200 to 1/100,000, is not dose-related and occurs weeks to months after therapy.
- Follow CBC carefully during therapy.

CHLORDIAZEPOXIDE (Librium)
Dose: Disease dependent:
- Anxiety: 5–25 mg PO tid–qid (in elderly patients give 5 mg bid–qid).
- Symptomatic alcohol withdrawal: Regimens are highly variable; one regimen is 50–100 mg PO q1–2h prn to treat symptoms of withdrawal.
- Prophylaxis against alcohol withdrawal in heavy alcohol users: Regimens are highly variable; one regimen is 50–100 mg PO q6h for 24 h, then 25–50 mg PO q6h for 24–48 h, then 25 mg PO q6h for 24 h; another regimen is 25–100 mg PO q1–2h prn to treat symptoms of withdrawal.

PO Preparations: 5, 10, and 25 mg capsules.
Actions: Benzodiazepine with antianxiety, sedative, and muscle-relaxant properties, used to treat anxiety or alcohol withdrawal.
Clearance: Metabolized in the liver; active metabolites are renally excreted.
- Slightly decrease dosage in patients with impaired renal function.
- Reduce dosage in patients with liver disease (though the extent of drug accumulation may not correlate with sedative effects).
- Supplemental dose not required after hemodialysis.

Selected Side Effects: Drowsiness, ataxia, confusion.
Cautions:
- *Should not be used in early pregnancy or in potentially pregnant patients.*
- Avoid using in elderly patients.

Pregnancy Category: *Should not be used in early pregnancy or in potentially pregnant patients.*
Cost: Generic $, Librium $$$ (≈ $0.10 each 10 mg generic tablet; ≈ $0.50 each 10 mg Librium tablet).
Pearls:
- Long $t_{1/2}$ may lead to accumulation; some physicians prefer Ativan for treatment of alcohol withdrawal.

CHLOROTHIAZIDE (Diuril)
Dose: 0.5–1.0 g qd–bid PO or IV.
PO Preparations:
- 250 and 500 mg tablets.
- 237 mL bottle of suspension containing 250 mg/5 mL (1 tsp).

Actions: Thiazide diuretic that affects electrolyte reabsorption in the distal renal tubules, used to treat hypertension and edema.

Clearance: Primarily renally excreted.

- Avoid in patients with creatinine > 2.0 mg/dL.

Selected Side Effects: Azotemia, hyponatremia, hypochloremic alkalosis, hypokalemia, hypotension, hyperuricemia.

Selected Drug Interactions: May increase or decrease insulin requirements.

Cautions: Patients allergic to sulfa drugs may show cross-sensitivity.

Pregnancy Category: C

Cost: Generic $, Diuril $$ (≈ $0.10 each 500 mg generic tablet; ≈ $0.30 each 500 mg Diuril tablet).

Pearls:

- Onset of action: PO < 2 h with peak at 4 h and duration 6-12 h; IV ≈ 15 min with peak at 30 min.
- May deleteriously alter lipid and glucose metabolism (although long-term clinical significance of any lipid alterations is unclear).
- Is often used synergistically with a loop diuretic.

CHLORPHENIRAMINE (Chlor-Trimeton; *see also* Contac)

Dose: Use dependent:

- Chronic allergy (hay fever, etc.): 4 mg PO q4–6h, or 8 mg SR tablet q8h, or 12 mg SR tablet q12h.
- Some sources suggest beginning therapy at lower doses and gradually increasing to these levels.
- Acute allergic reaction: 12 mg PO in 1–3 divided doses.

PO Preparations:

- 4 mg tablets.
- 8 and 12 mg SR tablets.
- 4 oz syrup containing 2 mg/5 mL (1 tsp).

Actions: Antihistamine with anticholinergic and sedative effects, used to treat allergic reactions and allergic rhinitis.

Pregnancy Category: B.

Pearls: When taken for chronic allergies, instruct patients to use regularly and not intermittently or prn.

CHLORPROMAZINE (Thorazine)

Dose: Disease and route dependent:
- Nausea and vomiting:
  - ► PO: 10–25 mg q4–6h of regular tablets or SR capsules prn.
  - ► IM: 25 mg initially; if no hypotension occurs, may give 25–50 mg q3–4h prn.
  - ► PR: 50–100 mg suppository q6–8h prn.
- Acute psychotic disorder: 25 mg IM; if necessary, may give additional 25–50 mg IM 1 h later. Intractable hiccups: 25–50 mg PO tid–qid; if symptoms persist for 2–3 days, may give 25–50 mg IM.

PO Preparations:
- 10, 25, 50, 100, and 200 mg tablets.
- 30, 75, and 150 mg SR capsules.
- 4 oz bottle of syrup containing 10 mg/5 mL (1 tsp).
- 25 and 100 mg suppositories.

Actions: Phenothiazine used to treat (1) nausea and vomiting, (2) psychotic disorders, (3) intractable hiccups.

Clearance: Metabolized via liver.
- No change in dosage needed in patients with renal insufficiency.
- Consider reducing dosage in patients with liver disease (patients have increased CNS sensitivity to phenothiazines).
- Supplemental dose not required after hemodialysis or peritoneal dialysis.

Selected Side Effects: CNS (drowsiness, dizziness, insomnia, fatigue, extrapyramidal reactions, dystonia, akathisia, rigidity, tremor, *tardive dyskinesia, neuroleptic malignant syndrome*), peripheral anticholinergic effects (blurred vision, urine retention, constipation, etc), disulfiram-like reaction with alcohol, orthostatic hypotension, elevated LFTs and cholestatic jaundice, anorexia, muscle weakness, rare multiple hematologic abnormalities.

Selected Drug Interactions:
- Antacids inhibit its absorption.
- Barbiturates can reduce its effectiveness.
- Potentiates CNS depressant effects of other CNS depressants.
- Can shorten PT in patients taking warfarin.

Cautions:
- *Avoid using in elderly patients.*
- Use with caution in patients with history of seizures (can lower the convulsive threshold).

Pregnancy Category: Not established.

Cost: Generic $, Thorazine $$$ ($\approx$ $0.10 each 25 mg generic tablet; $\approx$ $0.55 each 25 mg Thorazine tablet).

Pearls:
- Give IM injection slowly and deeply into upper outer quadrant of buttock.
- Signs of neuroleptic malignant syndrome include extreme rise in temperature; muscle rigidity and "lead-pipe" syndrome; mental status changes; autonomic instability, including irregular pulse or BP, greatly increased HR, diaphoresis, arrhythmias, rhabdomyolysis (with increased CPK level, myoglobinuria, and acute renal failure).

CHLORPROPAMIDE (Diabinese)

Dose:
- Initial: 250 mg PO qd (100 or 125 mg PO qd in elderly patients).
- Usual maximum: 500 mg PO qd.

PO Preparations: 100 and 250 mg tablets.

Actions: Oral hypoglycemic agent of the sulfonylurea class, used to treat noninsulin-dependent diabetes.

Clearance: Renally excreted.
- Do not use if GFR < 50 mL/min.
- Supplemental dose not required after peritoneal dialysis.

Selected Side Effects: *Hypoglycemia,* diarrhea, nausea and vomiting, anorexia, pruritus and rash, Antabuse-like reaction with alcohol, hyponatremia (2° increased ADH).

Selected Drug Interactions:
- Increased hypoglycemia with concomitant use of other sulfonylureas, insulin, ASA, NSAID, sulfonamides, warfarin, MAOI, or β-blockers.
- Increased hyperglycemia when used with diuretics, steroids, thyroid hormone, phenothiazines, phenytoin, nicotinic acid, sympathomimetic drugs, calcium channel blockers, or isoniazid.

Pregnancy Category: C.

Cost: Generic $, Diabinese $$$ (~ $0.10 each 250 mg generic tablet; ≈ $0.65 each 250 mg Diabinese tablet).
Pearls:
- Hypoglycemia is increased in elderly, debilitated, or malnourished patients; in renal, hepatic, adrenal, or pituitary impairment; with alcohol; and with severe or prolonged exercise.
- Duration of action 40–72 h.

Chlor-Trimeton: *see* CHLORPHENIRAMINE

CHOLESTYRAMINE (Cholybar, Questran, Questran Light)
Dose:
- 1 packet, 1 scoop, or 1 Cholybar (each containing 4 g of resin) 1–6 times daily PO.
- 1–2 packets can be taken mixed in water or juice, up to three times daily; best taken with meals.
PO Preparations:
- Cartons of 60 packets of Questran (each 9 g packet contains 4 g cholestyramine resin).
- Cartons of 60 packets of Questran Light (each 5 g packet contains 4 g cholestyramine resin).
- 378 g cans of Questran.
- 210 g cans of Questran Light.
- Cartons containing 25 caramel- or raspberry-flavored Cholybars.
Actions: Bile acid sequestrant used to treat hypercholesterolemia.
Clearance:
- Not absorbed.
- No change in dosage needed in patients with renal insufficiency.
Selected Side Effects:
- Frequent constipation, flatulence, reduced absorption of vitamins A, D, E, and K.
- May prolong PT.
Selected Drug Interactions: Decreases intestinal absorption of digoxin, penicillin, phenobarbital, propranolol, thyroid supplements, warfarin, and fat-soluble vitamins.

Cautions: *Contraindicated in patients with biliary obstruction.*
Pregnancy Category: Not established, but patients should be watched for decreased absorption of fat-soluble vitamins.
Cost: \$\$\$\$ (1 packet of Questran ≈ \$1; 1 Cholybar ≈ \$1.40; 378 g can of Questran ≈ \$38).
Pearls:
- Rarely tolerated more than bid–tid.
- Compliance may be significantly affected by its powdery taste.
- Instruct patients to take other oral medications 1 h before or 4–6 h after each dose.
- Instruct patients to increase fluid and fiber consumption to avoid developing constipation.
- Can increase triglyceride levels.

Cholybar: *see* CHOLESTYRAMINE

CILASTATIN: *see* Primaxin

CIMETIDINE (Tagamet)
Dose:
- Acute therapy: 300 mg PO or IV qid, 400 mg PO bid, or 800 mg PO qhs.
- Maintenance therapy: 400 mg PO qhs.
PO Preparations:
- 200, 300, 400, and 800 mg tablets.
- 8 oz bottle of liquid containing 300 mg/5 mL (1 tsp).
Actions: H_2-blocker used to treat peptic ulcer disease.
Clearance: Metabolized via liver; renally excreted.
- Slightly reduce dosage in patients with impaired renal function.
- No change in dosage needed for liver failure.
- Supplemental dose not required after hemodialysis or peritoneal dialysis.
Selected Side Effects: Confusional states (usually in severely ill or elderly patients).
Selected Drug Interactions:
- Raises serum levels of phenytoin, lidocaine, propranolol, quinidine, nifedipine, procainamide, metoprolol, and aminophylline.
- Prolongs PT in patients taking warfarin.

- Magnesium and aluminum hydroxide antacids (such as Maalox and Mylanta) reduce its bioavailability and should be given at least 2 h apart from it.

Pregnancy Category: B.

Cost: $$$ (≈ $0.80 each 400 mg tablet).

Cipro: *see* CIPROFLOXACIN

CIPROFLOXACIN (Cipro)

Dose: Route dependent:
- PO: 250–750 mg bid.
- Usual PO: 500 mg bid.
- IV: 200–400 mg q12h.

PO Preparations: 250, 500, and 750 mg tablets.

Actions: Bactericidal synthetic broad-spectrum fluoroquinolone antibiotic that inhibits DNA gyrase.

- Excellent gram (−) coverage, including most *Pseudomonas aeruginosa.*
- Some gram (+) coverage, including many *Staphylococcus aureus* (including some MRSA strains) and *S epidermidis* (but less against strep and enterococci).
- Not effective against anaerobes.
- Enterococci may be resistant to Cipro.
- Increasingly, problems are developing with staph isolates resistance to Cipro.
- *NOTE:* The above-mentioned antimicrobial coverage summary should be used as a guideline only; treatment decisions should take into account not only local epidemiologic patterns of antibiotic susceptibility but also, when available, culture susceptibility results.

Clearance:
- Metabolized in liver and intestine; excreted by biliary and renal routes.
- Slightly reduce dosage or increase dosing interval in patients with impaired renal function.
- No change in dosage needed in patients with liver disease.
- Supplemental dose suggested after hemodialysis or peritoneal dialysis.

Selected Side Effects: Nausea, rare anaphylactic reactions, possible rare seizures.

Selected Drug Interactions:
- Raises serum level of theophylline.
- Zinc, iron, or calcium tablets reduce its absorption.
- Magnesium hydroxide or aluminum hydroxide antacids and sucralfate decrease its intestinal absorption.

Cautions:
- *Contraindicated in patients with a history of hypersensitivity to other quinolones.*
- Avoid in patients < 18 years old.

Pregnancy Category: C.

Cost: $$$ ($\approx$ $70 for 500 mg PO bid for 10 days).

Pearls: Can be taken without regard to meals (but *not* with magnesium- or aluminum-containing antacids).

CISAPRIDE (Propulsid)

Dose:
- 10 mg PO qid, taken at least 15 minutes before meals and at bedtime.
- Some patients may require 20 mg doses.

Preparations: 10 mg scored and 20 mg tablets.

Actions: Gastrointestinal prokinetic agent; used to treat nocturnal heartburn associated with gastroesophageal reflux disease.
- Physiologic actions include increasing lower esophageal sphincter pressure and accelerating gastric emptying.
- Mechanism of action is believed to be due to enhanced release of acetylcholine at the myenteric plexus.

Clearance: Primarily metabolized by the liver.
- Although accumulation of cisapride may be somewhat higher in patients with hepatic or renal impairment and in elderly patients, no dose adjustment is suggested.

Selected Side Effects: Modest increased rates of diarrhea and abdominal discomfort (about 3% > than in placebo-treated patients), QT prolongation, and possibly rare cases of the ventricular arrhythmia torsades de pointes.

Selected Drug Interactions:
- High dose H_2-blockers and bicarbonate therapy can reduce gastric acidity and thus decrease its absorption; however, cimetidine coadministration may also lead to a net increase in plasma concentration.

- Ketoconazole markedly elevates cisapride levels and leads to prolongation of the QT interval.
- May prolong PT in patients taking warfarin (Coumadin).
- The increased gastric emptying may affect absorption of other drugs.

Cautions:
- *Concurrent administration with ketoconazole, itraconazole, miconazole or troleandomycin is contraindicated, as this class of medications is associated with markedly elevated levels of cisapride and QT prolongation.*
- *Should not be used in patients in whom an increase in gastrointestinal motility could be harmful (GI hemorrhage, mechanical obstruction, perforation, etc).*
- Should be used with caution, if at all, in patients with prolonged QT interval, those taking medications that can prolong the QT interval, or with uncorrected electrolyte abnormalities.

Pregnancy Category: C.
Pearls: Is not used for the treatment of daytime heartburn.

Cis-P: *see* CISPLATIN

CISPLATIN (Cis-P, Platinol)
Dose: Tumor dependent.
Actions: Antineoplastic alkylating agent used to treat numerous malignancies, particularly those of the lung and ovary.
Clearance: 27–43% renally excreted; no liver metabolism.
- Do not administer if creatinine clearance < 50 mL/min.
- No change in dosage needed in patients with liver disease.
- Supplemental dose suggested after hemodialysis.

Selected Side Effects: *Myelosuppression, nephrotoxicity,* neuropathy (Lhermitte's sign), ototoxicity, marked nausea and vomiting, significant electrolyte depletion (Mg^{2+}, Ca^{2+}, K^+, PO_4^+, Na^+), anaphylactic reaction.
Selected Drug Interactions: Concomitant use with aminoglycosides increases risk of nephrotoxicity.
Pregnancy Category: Not established; however, in *PDR* states cisplatin can cause fetal harm when administered to a pregnant woman.

Cost: $$$.
Pearls:

- Nephrotoxicity and peripheral neuropathy are the major dose-limiting toxicities.
- Nephrotoxicity usually first appears during the second week after treatment.
- Neuropathy is directly related to cumulative dose.
- Usual signs of nephropathy include elevation of BUN, creatinine, and uric acid levels with decreased creatinine clearance.
- IV hydration and mannitol (or furosemide) are frequently used as premedication to decrease renal toxicity.
- Electrolyte replacement is usually necessary during therapy.
- Repeat treatment should not be given until creatinine < 1.5, BUN < 25, platelets > 100,000, and WBCs > 4000.
- Audiometric testing is recommended before treatment.
- Check BUN, creatinine, creatinine clearance, Mg^{2+}, K^+, and Ca^{2+} before treatment.
- Follow CBC, electrolytes, LFTs, and neurologic status.

Claforan: *see* **CEFOTAXIME**

CLARITHROMYCIN (Biaxin)
Dose: Disease dependent:

- Uncomplicated pneumonia: 250 mg PO bid for 7–14 days.
- Bronchitis: 250–500 mg PO bid for 7–14 days.
- Pharyngitis or tonsillitis: 250 mg PO bid for 10 days.
- Sinusitis: 500 mg PO bid for 14 days.
- Adjunctive therapy in Mycobacterium avium complex infections: 500–1000 mg PO bid.

PO Preparations: 250 and 500 mg tablets.
Actions: Bactericidal macrolide antibiotic with broad antibacterial coverage.

- Good gram (+) coverage, including *Staphylococcus aureus, S pneumoniae,* and group A strep (but *not* MRSA or enterococci).

- Some gram (−) coverage, including *Haemophilus influenzae.*
- Also covers *Mycoplasma pneumoniae, Legionella pneumophila* and *Moraxella catarrhalis.*
- *NOTE:* The above-mentioned antimicrobial coverage summary should be used as a guideline only; treatment decisions should take into account not only local epidemiologic patterns of antibiotic susceptibility but also, when available, culture susceptibility results.

Clearance: Metabolized via liver; renally excreted.
- Reduce dosage or increase dosing interval in patients with impaired renal function.
- No change in dosage needed in patients with liver disease.

Selected Side Effects: Predominantly GI, including diarrhea, nausea, abnormal taste, dyspepsia.

Selected Drug Interactions:
- Raises serum levels of theophylline and possibly carbamazepine.
- Although not reported in clinical trials with clarithromycin, erythromycin has been reported to raise serum levels of digoxin and of drugs metabolized by the cytochrome P-450 system, and to prolong PT in patients taking warfarin.

Cautions:
- *Contraindicated in patients with erythromycin allergy.*

Pregnancy Category: C.

Cost: $$$ (≈ $75 for 500 mg bid for 10 days).

Pearls:
- No cross-allergenicity in patients allergic to penicillin or cephalosporins.
- May be given without regard to meals.

Claritin: *see* LORATADINE

CLAVULANATE: *see* Augmentin, Timentin

Clearasil: *see* BENZOYL PEROXIDE

Cleocin: *see* CLINDAMYCIN

Cleocin T: *see* CLINDAMYCIN PHOSPHATE

CLINDAMYCIN (Cleocin)
Dose: 600 mg IM or IV q8h.
PO Preparations:
- 300 and 600 mg tablets.

Actions: Bacteriostatic antibiotic that reversibly inhibits protein synthesis.
- Good gram (+) coverage (but *not* enterococci or MRSA); *no* gram (−) coverage.
- Excellent anaerobic coverage (5% of *Bacteroides* are resistant).
- *NOTE:* The above-mentioned antimicrobial coverage summary should be used as a guideline only; treatment decisions should take into account not only local epidemiologic patterns of antibiotic susceptibility but also, when available, culture susceptibility results.

Clearance: Metabolized primarily in the liver to inactive and less active metabolites.
- No change in dosage needed for mild to moderate renal impairment.
- Use with caution in patients with severe renal disease.
- No change in dosage required for mild to moderate liver dysfunction; reduce dosage in moderate to severe liver disease.
- Supplemental dose not required after hemodialysis or peritoneal dialysis.

Selected Side Effects: Local phlebitis, GI upset, diarrhea, pseudomembranous colitis, elevated LFTs, hypersensitivity reactions.

Selected Drug Interactions: Enhances action of nondepolarizing muscle relaxants.

Pregnancy Category: Not established.

Cost: $$$ (PO ≈ $12/day).

Pearls:
- (−) CSF penetration.
- Has neuromuscular blocking properties that may potentiate other neuromuscular blockers.

- Carries high risk of *Clostridium difficile* diarrhea or colitis.
- Can be taken without regard to meals.

CLINDAMYCIN PHOSPHATE topical solution, lotion, and gel (Cleocin T)
Dose: Apply thin film to affected skin bid.
Preparations:
- 30 g tubes of gel containing 10 mg/mL.
- 30 mL and 60 mL bottles of solution containing 10 mg/mL.
- 60 mL plastic squeeze bottles of lotion containing 10 mg/mL.

Actions: Topical antibiotic used to treat acne vulgaris.
Selected Side Effects:
- Dry skin.
- Diarrhea, bloody diarrhea, and colitis (including pseudomembranous colitis) can occur with topical form.

Cautions: *Contraindicated in patients with history of regional enteritis, ulcerative colitis, or antibiotic-associated colitis.*
Pregnancy Category: B.
Cost: $$ (30 g tube: ≈ $22).

Clinoril: *see* SULINDAC

CLOMIPRAMINE (Anafranil)
Dose:
- Initial: 25 mg PO qd with food.
- May be gradually increased over next 2 weeks to total of 100 mg daily, given in divided doses with meals.
- May gradually titrate over next several weeks to maximum of 250 mg daily given in divided doses with meals.
- Once optimal dosage is reached, entire daily dose may be given qhs.

PO Preparations: 25, 50, and 75 mg capsules.
Actions: Tricyclic antidepressant that may inhibit serotonin reuptake, used to treat obsessive–compulsive disorders.
Clearance:
- Metabolized to the active metabolite desmethylclomipramine.

- Effects of hepatic or renal disease on its elimination have not been determined.

Selected Side Effects: CNS effects (seizure, somnolence, tremor, dizziness, nervousness, myoclonus), GI symptoms (dry mouth, constipation, nausea, anorexia, dyspepsia, weight gain), sexual dysfunction or reduced libido, orthostatic hypotension, tachycardia, visual changes, blood dyscrasias.

Cautions:

- *Contraindicated in patients with history of hypersensitivity to tricyclics and during acute recovery period following MI.*
- Should not be given within 14 days of MAOI.

Pregnancy Category: C.

Cost: $$$$ (≈ $1.20 each 50 mg capsule).

Pearls: Steady-state plasma levels may not be reached for up to 3 weeks, so allow 2–3 weeks between further dosage changes.

CLONAZEPAM (Klonopin)

Dose:

- Initial: up to 0.5 mg PO tid.
- May gradually increase until seizures are controlled.
- Maximum: 20 mg daily.

PO Preparations: 0.5, 1.0, and 2.0 mg tablets.

Actions:

- Benzodiazepine used to treat petit mal seizures.
- Also used to treat panic attacks.

Clearance:

- Metabolized via liver.
- No change in dosage needed in patients with renal insufficiency.

Selected Side Effects: CNS depression, drowsiness, ataxia, "behavioral problems."

Selected Drug Interactions: Potentiates CNS depressant effects of other CNS depressants.

Cautions: *Contraindicated in patients with liver disease or narrow-angle glaucoma.*

Pregnancy Category: Not established.

Cost: $$$$ (≈ $1 each 1 mg tablet).
Pearls:
- Abrupt withdrawal may precipitate tonic–clonic seizures.

CLONIDINE (Catapres, Catapres-TTS)

Dose: Route dependent:
- PO: Initial 0.1 mg bid (may start lower in elderly patients); may increase by 0.1 mg daily. Usual 0.1–0.3 mg bid. Maximum 1.2 mg bid.
- Catapres-TSS Patch: One TTS-1 weekly for 2 weeks, then may increase by equivalent of 0.1 mg daily each subsequent week. Maximum two TTS-3 patches per week (equivalent to 0.6 mg daily).

Preparations:
- 0.1, 0.2, and 0.3 mg tablets.
- TTS-1, TTS-2, and TTS-3 patches delivering 0.1, 0.2, and 0.3 mg daily, respectively.

Actions: Centrally acting α-antagonist used to treat hypertension.

Clearance: Metabolized via liver; renally excreted.
- Slightly reduce dosage in patients with end-stage renal disease; no change needed for milder renal impairment.
- Reduce dosage in liver dysfunction.
- Supplemental dose not required after hemodialysis.

Selected Side Effects: Dry mouth, drowsiness, dizziness, constipation, sedation.

Selected Drug Interactions:
- Tricyclics reduce its effectiveness.
- Increases CNS depressant effects of alcohol and other sedatives.

Pregnancy Category: C.

Cost: Generic $$, Catapres tablets $$$, Catapres patch $$$$ (≈ $12 each TTS-2 patch).

Pearls:
- Use PO form with caution in patients who develop localized skin sensitivity from the patch.
- Withdrawal reactions sometimes occur, usually if patients are taking > 1.2 mg daily *or* if also taking β-blockers.

- To avoid withdrawal reactions, taper over 2–4 days when indicated.
- Therapeutic drug levels are achieved with the patch after 2–3 days.

Klonopin: *see* CLONAZEPAM

CLOTRIMAZOLE (Lotrimin 1% cream, lotion, or solution, Mycelex 1% cream; *see also* Lotrisone topical cream)
Dose: Massage into skin bid.
Preparations:
- 15 and 45 g tubes of cream.
- 10 and 30 mL bottles of solution.

Actions: Topical antifungal agent.
- Cost: $$ (≈ $18 for a 30 g tube).

COBALAMIN (VITAMIN B, as either CYANOCOBALAMIN or HYDROXOCOBALAMIN)
Dose: Regimens for replacement therapy vary considerably but are most likely clinically equivalent.
- One reasonable regimen is: either cyanocobalamin or hydroxocobalamin 100–1000 μg IM daily for 7 days, then once or twice per week for 1–2 months or until hematocrit is normal. (*NOTE:* Dose is in micrograms, *not* milligrams.)
- Patients with neurologic manifestations should receive 1000 mg for at least the first week.
- Patients with pernicious anemia may require chronic treatment at 100 μg IM monthly.
- Patients with malabsorption may need chronic treatment at 1000 μg IM monthly.

Pearls: Symptoms of vitamin B deficiency include megaloblastic anemia, glossitis, and neurologic dysfunction (paresthesias, ataxia, spastic motor weakness, or reduced mentation).

CODEINE: *see also* Robitussin A-C, Tylenol with Codeine

Dose: Use dependent:
- Analgesia: 15–60 mg PO, SQ, or IM q4–6h.
- Cough suppression: 15–30 mg PO q4–6h.

PO Preparations: 15, 30, and 60 mg tablets.

Actions:
- Morphine derivative used to treat pain.
- Also has antitussive properties and can be used to treat persistent cough.

Clearance: Metabolized via liver (in part to morphine).
- Slightly reduce dosage in patients with impaired renal function.
- Decrease dosage in patients with liver disease.

Selected Side Effects: Drowsiness, sedation, respiratory depression, nausea and vomiting, constipation.

Pregnancy Category: C.

Cost: $$ ($\approx$ $0.40 per 30 mg tablet).

Cogentin: *see* BENZTROPINE

Colace: *see* DOCUSATE SODIUM

COLCHICINE

Dose: Use dependent:
- Acute gout attack, PO: 1–2 tablets initially, then 1 tablet qh or 2 tablets q2h until pain resolves or diarrhea occurs; maximum 6–8 tablets per attack.
- Acute gout attack, IV: 2 mg infused slowly (over 2–5 min); may repeat 1–2 mg in 6 h if indicated; maximum 4 mg IV.
- Prophylaxis: 1 tablet PO bid.

PO Preparations: 0.5 and 0.6 mg tablets (0.6 mg tablets are usually prescribed).

Actions: Anti-inflammatory agent that impairs leukocyte chemotaxis and synovial cell phagocytosis; used to treat gout.

Clearance: Renally excreted.
- Slightly reduce dosage in patients with end-stage renal disease.
- No change in dosage needed in patients with liver disease.
- Supplemental dose not required after hemodialysis.

Selected Side Effects:
- Nausea and vomiting, abdominal pain, frequent diarrhea.
- *Extravasation can lead to tissue necrosis.*
- Aplastic anemia and agranulocytosis can occur with prolonged use.

Selected Drug Interactions:
- Decreases absorption of vitamin B.
- Phenylbutazone can increase risk of depressed CBC.

Cost: $.

Pearls:
- *Avoid IV extravasation.*
- Some physicians discourage IV administration unless absolutely indicated.
- Most effective when used within 24 h of onset of attack.

Colestid: *see* COLESTIPOL

COLESTIPOL (Colestid)

Dose: 15–30 g PO daily, given in divided doses bid–qid before meals.

PO Preparations:
- 1 g tablets.
- Boxes of 30 or 90 packets, each packet containing 5 g.
- 300 and 500 g bottles.

Actions: Anion exchange resin, similar to cholestyramine, that binds bile acids; used to treat hypercholesterolemia.

Selected Side Effects: Constipation, GI discomfort.

Selected Drug Interactions: Can reduce absorption of propranolol, HCTZ, tetracycline, and digoxin.

Cost: $$$$ ($\approx$ $1 each 5 g packet; $\approx$ $80 each 500 g bottle); similar in cost to cholestyramine.

Compazine: *see* PROCHLORPERAZINE

Contac (CHLORPHENIRAMINE + PHENYLPROPANOLAMINE)

Dose: 1 caplet or capsule PO q12h prn.

Actions: Combination antihistamine and sympathomimetic.

Cordarone: *see* AMIODARONE

Corgard: *see* NADOLOL

CORTISONE (Cortone Acetate)
Dose:
- Initial: 25–300 mg PO or IM qd.
- Chronic therapy: 35–70 mg PO qd.

PO Preparations: 25 mg tablets.

Actions: Synthetic corticosteroid used primarily to treat adrenocortical insufficiency.

Clearance: Metabolized via liver.
- No change in dosage needed in patients with renal insufficiency.
- Dosage adjustment probably *not* needed in patients with liver disease.
- Supplemental dose not required after hemodialysis.

Pregnancy Category: Not established.

Cost: $$.

Pearls:
- Can mask signs of infection.
- With chronic use, patients may need "stress-dose" steroids during acute stress (such as infection, etc).
- Relative activity comparison of commonly used steroids:

Steroid	Relative Anti-inflammatory and Glucocorticoid Activity	Relative Mineralocorticoid Activity
Cortisone	0.8	0.8
Hydrocortisone	1.0	1.0
Prednisone	4.0	0.8
Methylprednisolone	5.0	0.5
Dexamethasone	25–30	0.0

Cortisporin Cream (POLYMYXIN B + NEOMYCIN + 0.5% HYDROCORTISONE)
Dose: Apply small quantity topically bid–qid.

Preparations: 7.5 g tube.

Actions: Combination topical antibiotic and steroid.

Selected Side Effects: Local irritation, skin sensitization and skin reactions, possible ototoxicity, nephrotoxicity, or adrenocortical suppression.
Cost: $$ (≈ $25 for a 7.5 g tube).

Cortisporin Ointment (POLYMYXIN B + BACITRACIN + NEOMYCIN + 1% HYDROCORTISONE)

Dose: Apply thin film to skin bid–qid.
PO Preparations: 15 g tube with applicator tip.
Actions: Combination topical antibiotic and steroid.
Selected Side Effects: Local irritation, skin sensitization and skin reactions, possible ototoxicity, nephrotoxicity, and adrenocortical suppression.
Pregnancy Category: C.
Cost: $$$ (0.5 oz tube: ≈ $30 retail).

Cortisporin Ophthalmic Ointment (POLYMYXIN B + BACITRACIN + NEOMYCIN + HYDROCORTISONE)

Dose: 1 or 2 drops (written "gtt") into the eye q3–4h.
PO Preparations: 1/8 oz tube.
Actions: Combination antibiotic and corticosteroid used to treat superficial ocular infections and inflammatory ocular conditions.
Pregnancy Category: C.
Cost: Generic $, Cortisporin $$ (≈ $15 each generic tube; ≈ $25 each Cortisporin tube).

Cortisporin Ophthalmic Suspension (HYDROCORTISONE + NEOMYCIN + POLYMYXIN B)

Dose: Insert 1/2 inch into the conjunctival sack tid–qid.
PO Preparations: 7.5 mL dispenser bottle.
Actions: Combination antibiotic and antiinflammatory agent used to treat inflammatory ocular conditions and infections.

Cortisporin Otic Solution (POLYMYXIN B + NEOMYCIN + HYDROCORTISONE)
Dose: 4 drops (written "gtt") into the ear tid–qid.
Preparations: 10 mL bottle with dropper.
Actions: Topical antibiotic and steroid used to treat infections of the external auditory canal.
Cost: Generic $, Cortisporin $$$ ($\approx$ $10 each generic bottle; $\approx$ $24 each Cortisporin bottle).

Cortone Acetate: *see* CORTISONE

Cotazym: *see* PANCRELIPASE

Coumadin: *see* WARFARIN

Cozaar: *see* LOSARTAN

Creon 20: *see* PANCRELIPASE

CROMOLYN SODIUM (Intal, Nasalcrom)
Dose: Route dependent:
- Aerosol: Inhale 2 puffs qid.
- Powder: Inhale 20 mg (in a capsule) qid.
- Spray: Spray into each nostril 2–6 times daily.
Preparations:
- 8.1 and 14.2 g aerosol canisters delivering at least 112 and 200 metered dose inhalers, respectively.
- 20 mg capsules.
Actions: Medication with antiasthmatic and antiallergic properties, possibly related to mast cell stabilization, used in chronic (*not acute*) treatment of certain types of asthma and rhinitic conditions.
Pregnancy Category: B.
Cost: $$$$ (14.2 g inhaler $\approx$ $55 retail); no generic form available.
Pearls:
- Can take 2–4 weeks to achieve maximum effect.
- Is one of the first-line therapies for exercise-induced asthma.

CYANOCOBALAMIN: *see* COBALAMIN

CYCLOBENZAPRINE (Flexeril)
Dose:
- 5–20 mg PO tid.
- Usual: 10 mg PO tid.

PO Preparations: 10 mg tablets.

Actions: Tricyclic amine used to treat skeletal muscle spasm of local origin.

Clearance: Metabolized via liver; renally excreted.

Selected Side Effects:
- Drowsiness, dizziness, dry mouth, and other anticholinergic effects.
- Can have tricyclic-like proarrhythmic effects.

Cautions: *Contraindicated in patients who have taken MAOI within 14 days and in patients with hyperthyroidism, recent MI, significant heart block, conduction disturbances, or arrhythmias.*

Pregnancy Category: B.

Cost: Generic $$$, Flexeril $$$$ ($\approx$ $0.55/generic tablet, $\approx$ $1.50/Flexeril tablet).

Pearls:
- Warn patients of possible sedative effects.
- Consider beginning some patients on 5 mg (half of the 10 mg tablet) PO tid.

CYCLOPHOSPHAMIDE (Cytoxan)
Dose: Extremely variable; tumor dependent. May be given PO or IV (not qhs).

PO Preparations: 25 and 50 mg tablets.

Actions: Antineoplastic alkylating agent that crosslinks tumor cell DNA; used to treat malignancies.

Clearance: Activated and metabolized via liver; 5–25% excreted unchanged in urine.
- *PDR* notes no increase in toxicity in renal failure; other sources recommend slightly reducing dosage or increasing dosing interval, or decreasing dose when creatinine clearance < 10 mL/min.

- Liver failure may affect both its activation to the active form and its metabolism to inactive products. Supplemental dose suggested after hemodialysis.

Selected Side Effects: *Myelosuppression, hemorrhagic cystitis and ureteritis,* fibrosis of urinary bladder and renal tubules, alopecia, nausea and vomiting, anorexia, ulcer of oral mucosa.

Selected Drug Interactions: Potentiates doxorubicin-induced cardiotoxicity.

Pregnancy Category: D.

Cost: $$$.

Pearls:

- Nadir occurs and WBC recovery usually begins 7–10 days after cessation of therapy.
- May necessitate additional steroids in adrenalectomized patients.
- Secondary cancers are associated with its use.
- Encourage *generous* fluid intake (2–3 quarts daily) and frequent voiding following treatment (to reduce risk of hemorrhagic cystitis).
- The cytoprotective agent mesna may be used to prevent hemorrhagic cystitis.

CYCLOSPORINE (CYCLOSPORIN A)

Dose: Variable initially; maintenance, 5–10 mg/kg PO qd.

PO Preparations:

- 25, 50, and 100 mg capsules.
- 50 mL bottles containing 100 mg/mL oral suspension.

Actions: Immunosuppressant that prolongs survival of allogenic organ transplants, most likely through T-cell suppression; used to treat transplant recipients.

Clearance: Extensively metabolized and excreted in bile; only 6% excreted in urine.

- No change in dosage needed in patients with renal insufficiency.
- May need to reduce dosage in patients with liver disease.
- Supplemental dose not required after hemodialysis or peritoneal dialysis.

Selected Side Effects: *Impaired renal function and nephrotoxicity,* hepatotoxicity, hyperkalemia, tremor, hirsutism, hypertension, hyperplasia of gums.
Selected Drug Interactions: Can significantly increase K^+ when used with K^+-sparing diuretics.
Pregnancy Category: C.
Cost: $$$.
Pearls:
- Follow LFTs and renal function.
- Periodically check cyclosporine levels.
- Adjunct steroid therapy is usually needed.

CYTARABINE: *see* CYTOSINE ARABINOSIDE

Cytosar-U: *see* CYTOSINE ARABINOSIDE

CYTOSINE ARABINOSIDE (ARA-C, CYTARABINE, Cytosar-U)

Dose: Tumor dependent; often 100 mg/m^2/day by continuous infusion for 7 days.
Actions: Antineoplastic agent that is cytotoxic to cells undergoing DNA synthesis (S-phase); used to treat malignancies, particularly acute leukemias.
Clearance: Metabolized via liver to inactive ara-U.
- No change in dosage needed in patients with renal insufficiency.
- One source recommends reducing dosage in patients with liver disease; a second recommends only following the patient carefully.
Selected Side Effects: *Bone marrow suppression,* nausea and vomiting, anorexia, fever, rash, oral and anal inflammation or ulceration, thrombophlebitis, elevated LFTs, hyperuricemia, "cytarabine syndrome" (flu-like syndrome with fever, myalgia, arthralgia, bone pain, chest pain, rash, conjunctivitis, and malaise), neurotoxicity (confusion, ataxia, seizures).
Selected Drug Interactions: Can interfere with gentamicin therapy for *Klebsiella pneumoniae.*
Pregnancy Category: D.

Cost: $$.
Pearls:
- May be given intrathecally (usual dose 3.0 mg/kg).
- A biphasic decrease in WBCs will occur: initial decline is seen within 24 h with nadir at days 7–9 followed by a second, deeper depression with nadir at days 15–24, then rapid rise to above baseline in next 10 days.
- Periodically check CBC, LFTs, renal function, and uric acid levels.
- "Cytarabine syndrome" occurs 6–12 h after administration and can be treated with steroids.

Cytotec: *see* MISOPROSTOL

Cytoxan: *see* CYCLOPHOSPHAMIDE

Dalmane: *see* FLURAZEPAM

Dantrium: *see* DANTROLENE

DANTROLENE (Dantrium)
Dose:
- Initial: 25 mg PO qd.
- Maximum: 100 mg PO bid–qid.
PO Preparations: 25, 50, and 100 mg capsules.
Actions: Skeletal muscle relaxant used to treat spasticity.
Selected Side Effects: Hepatotoxicity, drowsiness, diarrhea (which may be severe).
Cost: $$$$ ($\approx$ $2.50/day).
Pearls: Dantrolene is used now only rarely by many urologists.

DAPSONE
Dose:
- Disease dependent:
- PCP: 100 mg PO qd.
PO Preparations: 25 and 100 mg.

Actions: Antibiotic that may act by inhibiting folate synthesis; used to treat various infections.

Clearance: Acetylated in liver; undergoes enterohepatic circulation; excreted in urine.

Selected Side Effects: Dose-related hemolysis, agranulocytosis, aplastic anemia, elevated LFTs, peripheral neuropathy.

Selected Drug Interactions:

• Rifampin *markedly* increases its clearance and reduces its serum level.

• Folic acid antagonists may increase chance of hematologic reactions.

• Probenecid reduces its renal excretion, so dosage should be adjusted.

Cautions: Use with caution in G6PD deficiency and sulfone hypersensitivity.

Pregnancy Category: C.

Cost: $$$ (≈ $1/tablet).

Pearls:

• Warn patients to report any signs of infection.

• Follow CBC weekly for the first month, then monthly for 6 months, then semiannually.

• Follow LFTs.

Darvocet N-50, Darvocet N-100 (PROPOXYPHENE + ACETAMINOPHEN)

Dose: 2 tablets of Darvocet-N 50 or 1 tablet of Darvocet-N 100 q4h PO prn.

PO Preparations:

• Each Darvocet-N 50 tablet contains 50 mg propoxyphene and 325 mg acetaminophen.

• Each Darvocet-N 100 contains 100 mg propoxyphene and 650 mg acetaminophen.

Actions: Weak narcotic analgesic with antipyretic actions; used to treat mild pain.

Clearance: Metabolized primarily via liver.

• Avoid in patients with end-stage renal disease (metabolites that have lidocaine-like effects will accumulate).

• Reduce dosage in patients with liver disease.

Cautions: Use with caution in patients with liver disease (acetaminophen may be hepatotoxic in high doses).
Pregnancy Category: Not established.
Cost: Generic $$, Darvocet $$$ (≈ $0.40 each Darvocet N-50 tablet).

DAUNORUBICIN (Cerubidine)
Dose: Disease dependent:
- Often given 25–45 mg/m^2/day IV for 3 days, then the same dose given for 2 days on subsequent courses.
- Lower doses may be given in elderly patients.

Actions: Cytotoxic anthracycline that impairs DNA synthesis by inserting itself between DNA base pairs; used to treat neoplastic diseases, primarily leukemia and lymphoma.
Clearance:
- 20–30% of dose is excreted in bile; metabolized to the active metabolite daunorubicinol.
- Reduce dosage in liver or kidney disease based on bilirubin and creatinine levels, as described in *PDR*.

Selected Side Effects: *Cardiotoxicity, myelosuppression,* frequent nausea and vomiting, frequent stomatitis, alopecia, *severe local skin necrosis when extravasated,* hyperuricemia when treating leukemia.
Pregnancy Category: D.
Cost: $$$.
Pearls:
- Myelosuppression and cardiotoxicity are dose-limiting side effects.
- WBC and platelet nadirs usually occur 9–14 days after treatment with nearly complete recovery by 3 weeks.
- The major cardiotoxicity is CHF; patients with preexisting heart disease or previously treated with daunorubicin are at increased risk.
- Cardiotoxicity is rare with cumulative doses < 550 mg/m^2.
- Signs suggestive of cardiotoxicity are reduced ejection fraction or > 30% decrease in QRS voltage in limb leads.
- Obtain ejection fraction and ECG prior to initial treatment.
- Warn patients that it colors urine red up to 2 days after administration.

Daypro: *see* **OXAPROZIN**

DDAVP: *see* **DESMOPRESSIN**

ddc: *see* **ZALCITABINE**

DDI: *see* **DIDANOSINE**

Decadron: *see* **DEXAMETHASONE**

Delsym: *see* **DEXTROMETHORPHAN**

Delta-Cortef: *see* **PREDNISOLONE**

Demadex: *see* **TORSEMIDE**

Demerol: *see* **MEPERIDINE**

Deodorized Tincture of Opium (DTO)
Dose: 0.5–1.5 mL PO or via NG or feeding tube tid–qid.
PO Preparations: Tincture containing 10% opium and 19% ethanol.
Actions: Non-narcotic opioid used to treat diarrhea.
Pearls: Do not confuse with Paregoric (camphorated tincture of opium).

Depakene: *see* **VALPROIC ACID**

Depakote: *see* **VALPROIC ACID**

Depo-Medrol: *see* **METHYLPREDNISOLONE**

Depo-Provera: *see* MEDROXYPROGESTERONE

DESIPRAMINE (Norpramin)
Dose:
- Usual: 100–200 mg PO qd (25–100 mg PO qd in elderly patients).
- Maximum: 300 mg PO qd.

PO Preparations: 10, 25, 50, 75, 100, and 150 mg tablets.

Actions: Tricyclic antidepressant that may work by blocking reuptake of neurotransmitters, especially norepinephrine; used to treat depression.

Clearance: Metabolized predominantly via liver; usually metabolized more slowly in elderly patients.
- No change in dosage needed in patients with renal insufficiency.
- Supplemental dose not required after hemodialysis or peritoneal dialysis.

Selected Side Effects: Drowsiness, multiple cardiovascular effects (including effects on the conduction system, such as QT interval prolongation [similar to type Ia antiarrhythmics, such as quinidine], hypotension or postural hypotension), anticholinergic effects (dry mouth, blurred vision, tachycardia, etc), numerous psychiatric and neurologic side effects.

Selected Drug Interactions:
- Cimetidine, phenothiazines, and psychostimulants raise its serum level.
- Discontinuing cimetidine may reduce its serum level.
- Cigarette smoking as well as alcohol, barbiturates, and several other substances induce hepatic enzyme activity and depress its serum level.
- *Coadministration with MAOI may lead to hypertensive crisis, convulsions, and death.*

Cautions:
- *Contraindicated within 2 weeks of MAOI therapy and in acute post-MI recovery period.*
- Use with caution in patients with cardiovascular disease, thyroid disease, or history of urine retention, glaucoma, or seizures (lowers the seizure threshold).

Pregnancy Category: Not established.

Cost: Generic \$\$\$, Norpramin \$\$\$\$ (≈ \$0.60 each 100 mg generic tablet; ≈ \$1.80 each 100 mg Norpramin tablet).
Pearls:
- Earliest therapeutic effect may be seen in 2–5 days; full benefit usually is obtained after 2–3 weeks.
- Signs and symptoms of overdose include agitation, stupor, coma, hypotension, shock, renal shutdown, seizures, hyperactive reflexes, muscle rigidity, hyperpyrexia, vomiting, respiratory depression, and impaired conduction and arrhythmias on ECG.
- Patients with drug overdose must be monitored for arrhythmias and conduction abnormalities, with regular checks of the QRS and QT intervals, since amitriptyline has type Ia antiarrhythmic effects.

DESMOPRESSIN (DDAVP)
Dose: Bleeding disorders: 0.3 μg/kg diluted in 50 mL NS, injected slowly IV over 15–30 min. *NOTE:* Dose is in micrograms, *not* milligrams.
Actions: Synthetic analog of arginine vasopressin; used to treat certain types of platelet dysfunction.
Selected Side Effects:
- Infrequent headaches, nausea or GI distress, local burning and erythema, facial flushing, BP changes.
- Watch for possible water intoxication or hyponatremia.
Pregnancy Category: B.
Pearls:
- Monitor BP during injection.
- Mechanism of action may be related to increasing factor VIII levels in plasma.

Desogen contraceptive pills (DESOGESTREL + ETHINYL ESTRADIOL
Dose:
- 1 tablet PO qd; with 21-day regimen, take no pills on days 22–28 then begin a new cycle (3 weeks on, 1 week off).
- For 21-day and 28-day preparations, take first tablet on the first Sunday after onset of menses, or that Sunday if it is first day of menses.

Preparations: Available in 21 and 28 tablet preparations.
- Each active tablet contains 0.15 mg desogestrel and 0.03 mg ethinyl estradiol; the last seven tablets in the 28-day preparation contain inert ingredients.

Actions: Combination oral contraceptive used to prevent pregnancy.

Selected Side Effects: Serious vascular complications, menstrual changes, hypertension, gallbladder disease, liver tumors, nausea and vomiting, GI distress, breakthrough bleeding, edema, breast changes, weight changes, cervical changes, migraine headache, rash, depression, glucose intolerance, vaginal candidiasis, visual changes from alteration in corneal curvature, intolerance for contact lenses.

Selected Drug Interactions: Contraceptive effectiveness can be decreased by antibiotics (ampicillin, chloramphenicol, isoniazid, nitrofurantoin, penicillin V, rifampin, sulfonamides, tetracycline), analgesics, anxiolytics, antimigraine agents, barbiturates, and phenylbutazone.

Cautions:
- *Contraindicated in patients with thromboembolic or thrombophlebitic disorders, cardiovascular or cerebrovascular disease, vaginal bleeding of unknown cause, endometrial or other estrogen-dependent neoplasms, known or suspected breast cancer, cholestatic jaundice or jaundice with prior pill use, hepatic adenoma or carcinoma, smokers over age 35, or known or suspected pregnancy.*
- Cigarette smoking increases risk of serious cardiovascular complications; patients should be *strongly* advised not to smoke.

Pregnancy Category: X.

Cost: $$$ (≈ $20/month).

Pearls:
- Patients should undergo complete work-up prior to use with special attention to history of abnormal vaginal bleeding, BP, breast examination, and pelvic examination including cervical cytology.
- Contains a newer progestin component; is less androgenic and results in a more favorable lipid profile.

Desyrel: *see* TRAZODONE

DEXAMETHASONE (Decadron)
Dose: Disease or use dependent:
- Cerebral edema: 10 mg IM or IV initially, then 6 mg IM or IV q6h (a somewhat arbitrary dose that is frequently recommended).
- Dexamethasone suppression test for outpatient screening: Give 1 mg PO at 11:00 PM and draw plasma cortisol level at 8:00 AM the next day.
- Dexamethasone suppression test for inpatient work-up of Cushing's syndrome: Establish baseline by giving no drug on days 1 and 2. On days 3 and 4 give 0.5 mg PO q6h (low dose), and on days 5 and 6 give 2.0 mg PO q6h (high dose). Measure consecutive 24 h urinary free-cortisol levels on each of the 6 days.

PO Preparations:
- 0.25, 0.5, 0.75, 1.5, 4.0, and 6.0 mg tablets.
- 100 and 237 mL bottles of liquid containing 0.5 mg/5 mL (1 tsp).

Actions: Corticosteroid with potent anti-inflammatory actions; used primarily to treat inflammatory or allergic conditions.

Clearance: Metabolized via liver.
- No change in dosage needed in patients with renal insufficiency, and probably not in patients with liver disease.

Selected Side Effects: Increased glucose intolerance, psychiatric derangements ("steroid psychosis"), increased catabolism, worsening azotemia.

Selected Drug Interactions:
- Reduces hypoglycemic actions of insulin and oral hypoglycemic agents.
- Can increase or decrease PT in patients taking warfarin.

Pregnancy Category: Not established.
Cost: $$.
Pearls:
- Can mask signs of infection.
- Patients may need "stress doses" in times of stress.

- Used more frequently in cerebral edema caused by tumor; used less commonly, if at all, for edema secondary to cerebral hemorrhage or anoxic encephalopathy.
- Relative activity comparison of commonly used steroids:

Steroid	Relative Anti-inflammatory and Glucocorticoid Activity	Relative Mineralocorticoid Activity
Cortisone	0.8	0.8
Hydrocortisone	1.0	1.0
Prednisone	4.0	0.8
Methylprednisolone	5.0	0.5
Dexamethasone	25–30	0.0

DEXTROMETHORPHAN (Delsym; *see* also Robitussin-CF, Robitussin-DM)

Dose: Age dependent:
- Adults and children 3–12 years: 2 tsp PO q12h.
- Children 6–11 years: 1 tsp PO q12h.
- Children 2–5 years: ½ tsp PO q12h.

PO Preparations: 3 oz bottles containing 30 mg/5 mL (1 tsp) dextromethorphan.
Actions: Centrally acting non-narcotic cough suppressant.
Selected Drug Interactions: Concomitant use with MAOI can cause hyperpyretic crisis.

DiaBeta: *see* GLYBURIDE

Diabinese: *see* CHLORPROPAMIDE

Diamox: *see* ACETAZOLAMIDE

DIAZEPAM (Valium)

Dose: Disease dependent:
- Acute seizure: 5–10 mg IV initially (2.5 mg IV is sometimes given as starting dose in frail or elderly patients); may

repeat q10–15 min to maximum of 30 mg. Inject gradually (no faster than 5 mg/min).
- Muscle spasm: 5–10 mg IM or IV.
- Acute anxiety: 2–10 mg IM or IV.
- Chronic anxiety: 2–10 mg PO bid–qid.
- Symptomatic alcohol withdrawal:
  ▶ PO: 10–20 mg PO 1–2 h as needed for symptoms; average total dose requirement for symptomatic patients is 60 mg.
  ▶ Parenteral: 5–10 mg IM or IV initially; regimens from different sources vary markedly after this, with most suggesting repeat doses of 5–10 mg IM or IV at intervals varying from q5–10 min to q3–4h, depending on severity of withdrawal symptoms.
- Prophylaxis for alcohol withdrawal: 20 mg PO once, then q1–2h prn symptoms (5–10 mg IM if patient NPO).

PO Preparations:
- 2, 5, and 10 mg tablets.

Actions: Benzodiazepine with anxiolytic, antiseizure, and antispasmodic action; used to treat anxiety, seizures, and muscle spasms.

Clearance: Metabolized via liver.
- Active metabolite is renally excreted, but no change in dosage is suggested for renal disease.
- Reduce dosage or increase dosing interval in patients with liver disease.
- Supplemental dose not required after hemodialysis.

Selected Side Effects: Drowsiness, fatigue, ataxia, local thrombosis and phlebitis.

Selected Drug Interactions: Potentiates CNS depressant effects of other CNS depressants.

Cautions:
- *Contraindicated in untreated patients with narrow- or open-angle glaucoma.*
- Generally should not be used in pregnant or potentially pregnant patients.
- Use with caution in elderly patients.

Pregnancy Category: Generally should not be used in pregnant or potentially pregnant patients.

Cost: Generic $, Valium $$$ ($\approx$ $0.15 each 5 mg generic tablet; $\approx$ $).

Pearls:
- Abrupt discontinuance can cause withdrawal reactions.
- Antiseizure effects may be short-lived when used intravenously; consider starting a longer-acting anticonvulsant.
- Signs and symptoms of overdose include somnolence, confusion, diminished reflexes, and coma.

DIAZOXIDE (Hyperstat)
Dose:
- 1–3 mg/kg IV up to a maximum of 150 mg per injection. (*Individual injection doses higher than 150 mg are associated with greater side effects, particularly coronary and cerebral ischemia and infarct.*)
- Repeated similar doses can be administered at 5–15 min intervals, as clinically indicated.
- Once adequate blood pressure control is obtained, maintenance doses can be administered at intervals of 4–24 h until the patients is able to take oral antihypertensive therapy.

Actions: Relaxes smooth muscle in the peripheral arterioles, leading to vasodilation; used in the treatment of hypertensive urgency and hypertensive crisis.
- Leads to an increase in cardiac output and increased renal blood flow; coronary blood flow is not significantly changed.

Selected Side Effects: hypotension, transient hyperglycemia (occurs in most patients), sodium and water retention (after repeated injections).

Cautions:
- *Contraindicated in patients with significant aortic stenosis.*
- Use with caution in diabetic patients and those with congestive heart failure.
- Use with caution in patients with coronary artery or cerebrovascular disease (abrupt decreases in blood pressure can precipitate ischemia).

Pregnancy Category: C.
Pearls:
- Should only be administered to patients in setting in which blood pressure can be carefully monitored.

- Follow blood glucose levels, especially in diabetic patients.
- Patients who require repeated injections may retain sodium and water and may require diuretic therapy both for synergistic blood pressure reduction and to avoid congestive heart failure.

DICLOXACILLIN
Dose: 250 mg–1.0 g PO qid (usual outpatient is 250 mg PO qid).
PO Preparations:
- 250 and 500 mg capsules.
- 100 mL bottle of solution containing 62.5 mg/5 mL (1 tsp).

Actions: Bactericidal β-lactamase–resistant penicillin that inhibits cell wall synthesis.
- Good gram (+) coverage, including staph and strep (but *not* MRSA or enterococci).
- *No* gram (–) coverage.
- Poor anaerobic coverage.
- *NOTE:* The above-mentioned antimicrobial coverage summary should be used as a guideline only; treatment decisions should take into account not only local epidemiologic patterns of antibiotic susceptibility but also, when available, culture susceptibility results.

Clearance: Metabolized via liver; renally excreted.
- No change in dosage needed in patients with renal insufficiency or liver disease.
- Supplemental dose not required after hemodialysis.

Selected Side Effects: GI discomfort, rash, elevated LFTs, cholestatic jaundice.
Cautions: *Contraindicated in patients with penicillin allergy.*
Pregnancy Category: Not established.
Cost: $$ (≈ $30 for 500 mg qid for 10 days).

DIDANOSINE (DDI, DIDEOXYINOSINE, Videx)
Dose: Weight dependent:
- Patients < 60 kg: 125 mg PO of tablets or 167 mg PO of powder q12h (NOT bid).
- Patients ≥ 60 kg: 200 mg PO of tablets or 250 mg PO of powder q12h (NOT bid).

Preparations:
- 25, 50, 100, and 150 mg tablets.
- 100, 167, 250, and 375 mg buffered powder single-dose packets.

Actions: A nucleoside analogue of deoxyadenosine which, in vitro, inhibits the replication of HIV virus; used to treat advanced HIV infections in patients unresponsive to or intolerant of zidovudine (AZT).

Selected Side Effects: *Pancreatitis,* peripheral neuropathy (dose related), elevated LFTs.

Clearance: Renally excreted; other less well-studied clearance mechanisms also exist.
- Consider dose reduction in patients with renal insufficiency or liver disease.

Selected Drug Interactions: Coadministration with other drugs known to cause peripheral neuropathy or pancreatitis may increase the risk of these toxicities.

Cautions: *Should be used with extreme caution, if at all, in patients at risk for or with prior history of pancreatitis.*

Pregnancy Category: B.

Cost: $$$$$.

Pearls:
- *Pancreatitis is the major clinical toxicity associated with didanosine; this diagnosis must be considered in any patients who develop abdominal pain, nausea and vomiting, or elevated amylase level*
- At least two tablets (at each dose) need to be taken at a time to provide adequate buffering of stomach acids (since stomach acids rapidly degrade didanosine).
- Should be taken on an empty stomach.
- Doses of the powder are slightly higher than for tablet preparations because the bioavailability of the powder is less.
- DDI stands for the chemical name dideoxyinosine.

DIDEOXYCYTIDINE: *see* **ZALCITABINE**

DIDEOXYINOSINE: *see* **DIDANOSINE**

Diflucan: *see* **FLUCONAZOLE**

DIFLUNISAL (Dolobid)
Dose: Treatment dependent:
- Arthritis: 250–500 mg PO bid.
- Mild to moderate pain: 1000 mg PO initially, then 500 mg PO bid–tid.

PO Preparations: 250 and 500 mg tablets.
Actions: Nonsteroidal anti-inflammatory agent used to treat mild to moderate pain and inflammatory conditions.
Selected Side Effects: GI distress and upper GI bleeding, rash, headache, interstitial nephritis and renal papillary necrosis, hypersensitivity reactions.
Selected Drug Interactions:
- Raises serum level of acetaminophen by 50%.
- Lowers excretion of methotrexate and increases its toxicity.
- Increases toxicity of cyclosporine.
- Chronic coadministration with antacids may reduce its serum level.
- Prolongs PT in some patients taking warfarin.

Cautions:
- *Contraindicated in patients with history of hypersensitivity to aspirin or other NSAID.*
- Use with caution, if at all, in patients with history of upper GI bleeding.

Pregnancy Category: C.
Cost: $$$$ (≈ $1.20/tablet).
Pearls:
- 500 mg diflunisal has analgesic effect similar to that of 650 mg of ASA or acetaminophen.
- Has little antipyretic activity.
- Should be taken with food or antacids (to possibly decrease GI irritation and ulceration).

DIGOXIN (Lanoxin, Lanoxicaps)
Dose: Situation dependent:
- Inpatient management of atrial fibrillation or congestive heart failure: Usual regimen is 0.25–0.50 mg IV initially, followed by further doses of 0.25 mg IV q6–8h until rate control is achieved or total of 1.0–1.5 mg has been given.

Oral dose thereafter depends on heart rate (usually 0.125–0.375 mg PO qdd).

- Outpatient management of congestive heart failure: Loading dose of 1.0–1.5 mg PO, given in divided doses over 1–3 days; maintenance, usually 0.125–0.375 mg PO qd depending on renal function and clinical response (most patients with normal renal function will be maintained on 0.25 mg qd).
- Most common maintenance dose for managing atrial fibrillation or congestive heart failure is 0.25 mg PO qd (0.2 mg PO qd for Lanoxicaps).

PO Preparations:
- 0.125, 0.25, and 0.5 mg tablets.
- 0.05, 0.1, and 0.2 mg Lanoxicaps containing digoxin solution in capsules.
- 60 mL bottle of elixir containing 0.05 mg/mL.

Actions: Cardiac glycoside with direct inotropic and indirect vagomimetic effects; used to treat CHF and for rate control of supraventricular arrhythmias involving the AV node (atrial fibrillation or flutter, atrial tachycardia, or SVT).

Clearance: Renally excreted only.
- Moderately to markedly reduce dosage or moderately increase dosing interval in patients with impaired renal function; some sources recommend decreasing *loading* dose by 50% in patients with end-stage renal disease.
- No change in dosage needed in patients with liver disease.
- Supplemental dose not required after hemodialysis or peritoneal dialysis.

Selected Side Effects: Ventricular tachycardia or fibrillation, paroxysmal atrial tachycardia with block, sinoatrial and AV block, fatigue, dizziness, anorexia, nausea and vomiting, gynecomastia.

Selected Drug Interactions:
- Quinidine, verapamil, diltiazem, amiodarone, disopyramide, propafenone, flecainide, erythromycin, tetracycline, and phenytoin all raise its serum level.
- Antacids, kaolin (Kaopectate), cholestyramine, and sucralfate reduce its intestinal absorption.

Cautions: Use with caution in patients with sick sinus syndrome, AV nodal disease, WPW, or IHSS.

Pregnancy Category: C.

Cost: $ ($\approx$ $0.10 each 0.25 mg tablet; generic and brand names similarly priced).

Pearls:

- *Quinidine, verapamil, and amiodarone,* three drugs frequently used along with digoxin, can raise serum digoxin levels significantly (up to double the previous level). Many practitioners therefore empirically decrease the daily digoxin dose if these drugs are added to the patient's regimen (or, alternatively, dose reductions can be based on resulting digoxin levels). If these drugs are added, particular attention should be paid to possible increased actions of digoxin (AV block, bradycardia, etc).
- Check K^+ level before use.
- Cardioversion is contraindicated in digoxin toxicity (unless emergently necessary).
- Can cause nonischemic-mediated ECG changes during exercise testing and thus lead to false (+) test results.
- Although hemodialysis generally does not remove significant amounts of digoxin, it may be useful in overdose (particularly since K^+ levels are often substantially elevated).
- At higher doses, digoxin increases sympathetic outflow from the CNS, which may contribute to digitalis cardiotoxicity.
- Usual therapeutic level for (+) inotropy is 0.8–2.0 μg/mL.
- IV digoxin takes several hours to slow the ventricular response in atrial fibrillation. Thus, if acute rate control is required, consider using the IV preparations of verapamil, diltiazem, esmolol, propanol, atenolol, or metoprolol.
- Digoxin antibodies (Digibind) can be used to treat significant digoxin cardiotoxicity (arrhythmias or conduction abnormalities).

Dilacor XR: *see* **DILTIAZEM**

Dilantin: *see* **PHENYTOIN**

Dilatrate SR: *see* **ISOSORBIDE DINITRATE**

Dilaudid: *see* **HYDROMORPHONE**

DILTIAZEM [IV] (Cardizem; *see also* DILTIAZEM [PO])

Dose:
- Initial: 0.25 mg/kg (actual body weight) over 2 min.
- If response is inadequate, wait 15 min from first injection and then give 0.35 mg/kg (actual body weight) over 2 min.
- Maintenance: begin constant infusion of 5–15 mg/h.

Actions: Injectable calcium channel blocker used to convert paroxysmal SVT to sinus rhythm and to control ventricular rate during atrial fibrillation or flutter.

Clearance: Metabolized primarily via liver.
- Manufacturer suggests using with caution in liver or kidney disease.

Selected Side Effects: Hypotension, vasodilatation and flushing, irritation at injection site, AV block.

Selected Drug Interactions:
- Can increase bioavailability of propranolol.
- Theoretically, can have additive effects with digoxin in slowing HR and increasing AV block (although manufacturer reports that this combination of drugs has been well tolerated).

Cautions:
- *Contraindicated in sick sinus syndrome and second- or third-degree AV block except when a functioning ventricular pacemaker is in place.*
- Contraindicated in patients with severe hypotension, cardiogenic shock, VT, or patients in atrial fibrillation or atrial flutter who have an accessory bypass tract, such as in WPW syndrome or short PR syndrome.
- Be sure *any wide complex tachycardia is* not *VT before prescribing, because use in the setting of VT can precipitate hemodynamic collapse.*
- Use with caution in patients with impaired ventricular function.

Pregnancy Category: C.

Pearls:
- Ventricular rate reduction during atrial fibrillation or flutter usually occurs within 3 min and is maximal within 2–7 min.
- Duration of action for the initial bolus is usually 1–3 h.

- Patients should undergo continuous ECG monitoring and have frequent BP checks during therapy.

DILTIAZEM [PO] (Cardizem, Cardizem CR, Cardizem CD, Dilacor XR; *see also* DILTIAZEM [IV])

Dose: Preparation dependent.
- Regular pills: 30–90 mg PO tid–qid.
- Cardizem SR: 60–180 mg PO bid.
- Cardizem CD: 180–300 mg PO qd.
- Dilacor XR: 120–480 mg PO qd (this dose is for treatment of hypertension).

PO Preparations:
- 30, 60, 90, and 120 mg regular tablets of Cardizem.
- 60, 90, 120, and 180 mg long-acting Cardizem SR tablets.
- 180, 240, and 300 mg once-a-day Cardizem CD capsules.
- 120, 180, and 240 mg once-a-day Dilacor XR tablets.

Actions: Calcium channel blocker used to treat angina and hypertension.

Clearance:
- Metabolized via liver.
- No change in dosage needed in patients with renal insufficiency.

Selected Side Effects: Sinoatrial and AV block, headache, vasodilatation-induced peripheral edema, flushing, CHF, bradycardia.

Cautions: Use with caution in patients with depressed LV ejection fraction or AV block.

Selected Drug Interactions:
- Can raise serum level of digoxin.
- Concomitant use with β-blockers or digoxin increases risk of AV block.

Cautions: Use with caution in patients with depressed LV ejection fraction or AV block.

Pregnancy Category: C.

Cost: \$\$\$ (≈ \$0.50 each 60 mg tablet; ≈ \$0.90 each 120 mg Cardizem SR tablet; ≈ \$1.80 each 240 mg tablet of Cardizem CD).

DIMENHYDRINATE (Dramamine)
Dose: Route dependent:
- PO tablets: 50–100 mg q4–6h; maximum 400 mg daily.
- PO liquid (12.5 mg/5 mL): 4–8 tsp q4–6h prn, not to exceed 32 tsp in 24 h.
- PO liquid (15.62 mg/5 mL): 4–7 tsp q4–6h prn, not to exceed 26 tsp in 24 h.
- IM or IV: 50 mg prn.

PO Preparations:
- 50 mg tablets, capsules, and chewable tablets.
- 3 and 16 oz bottles containing 12.5 mg cherry flavored liquid per 4 mL.

Actions: Diphenhydramine derivative used to treat motion sickness.
Selected Side Effects: Drowsiness, anticholinergic side effects.
Pregnancy Category: B.
Cost: Generic $, Dramamine $$.
Pearls:
- First PO dose should be taken 30 min to 1 h prior to trip.
- Sold over the counter.

Dipentum: *see* OLSALAZINE SODIUM

DIPHENHYDRAMINE (Benadryl)
Dose: Disease or use dependent:
- Antihistamine: 25–50 mg PO tid–qid.
- Prophylaxis for motion sickness: 50 mg PO 30 min before exposure.
- Sleep aid: 25–50 mg PO qhs.
- Anaphylaxis or parkinsonism: 10–50 mg deep IM or IV.

PO Preparations:
- 25 and 50 mg capsules; 50 mg chewable capsules.
- 3 and 16 oz bottles of cherry-flavored liquid containing 12.5 mg/4 mL.

Actions: Antihistamine with anticholinergic and sedative properties used (1) to treat allergic conditions, motion sickness, and cough, (2) as a hypnotic, and (3) as an antiparkinsonian agent (for both idiopathic and drug-induced disease).

Clearance: Metabolized via liver.
- Slightly increase dosing interval in patients with impaired renal function.
- Reduce dosage in patients with liver disease.

Selected Side Effects: Drowsiness and sedation, epigastric distress, thickening of bronchial secretions.

Selected Drug Interactions: *Severe adverse reactions when used with MAOI.*

Cautions:
- *Contraindicated in patients taking MAOI.*
- Use with caution in narrow-angle glaucoma, symptomatic prostate hypertrophy, or bladder neck obstruction.
- Use with caution (because of atropine-like effect) in patients with history of bronchial asthma, elevated intraocular pressure, hyperthyroidism, hypertension, or cardiovascular disease.

Pregnancy Category: B.
Cost: $.
Pearls: Sold over the counter.

DIPHENOXYLATE: *see* Lomotil

Disalcid: *see* SALSALATE

DIPRIVAN (Propofol)
Dose: Use dependent:
- Induction of anesthesia:
  - ► Healthy adults < 55 years old: 40 mg every 10 s until induction onset (usually 1.5–2.5 mg/kg).
  - ► Elderly, debilitated and ASA class III or IV patients: 20 mg every 10 s until induction onset (usually 1.0–1.5 mg/kg).
- Maintenance of sedation in intubated ICU patients:
  - ► Initial: 5 µg/kg/min (*NOTE:* Dosage is in micrograms, *not* milligrams).
  - ► Infusion rate should be increased by increments of 5–10 µg/kg/min until desired level of sedation is achieved; allow at least 5 min between dose adjustments.
  - ► Usual sedative maintenance dose: 5–50 µg/kg/min; maintenance *anesthetic* doses are usually 100–200 µg/kg/min

in healthy adults < 55 years old, and 50–100 µg/kg/min in elderly or debilitated patients.

Actions: Sedative hypnotic agent; used for induction and maintenance of anesthesia or sedation.

Clearance: Metabolized via liver.

Selected Side Effects: *Respiratory depression and apnea, hypotension,* depressed cardiac output (at high doses), bradycardia, local pain at injection site.

Selected Drug Interactions: Other CNS depressants potentiate its CNS depressant effects.

Cautions:

- *Should only be used by persons trained in the administration of general anesthesia; intubation and resuscitation equipment should always be immediately available.*
- A lower induction dose and a slower maintenance rate of administration should be used in elderly or debilitated patients.

Pregnancy Category: B.

Pearls:

- Onset of action usually within 40 s.
- As preparations of Diprivan contain no antimicrobial preservatives, strict aseptic technique must be maintained during handling, and vial preparations should be used in a single-use manner only.

DIPYRIDAMOLE (Persantine)

Dose: 75–100 mg PO tid.

Preparations: 25, 50, and 75 mg tablets.

Actions: Inhibits platelet aggregation and increases coronary blood flow; used as an antiplatelet agent in various vascular conditions, and in conjunction with warfarin in patients with prosthetic valves with a prior history of embolization.

Clearance: Metabolized via liver.

- No change in dosage needed in patients with renal insufficiency.

Side Effects: Dizziness and rare hypotension.

Pearls: Does not increase risk of bleeding when given to patients taking warfarin.

Pregnancy Category: B.

Cost: Generic $$, Persantine $$$$.
Pearls: Does not increase the risk of bleeding when given to patients taking warfarin (Coumadin).

DISOPYRAMIDE (Norpace)
Dose: Delivery dependent:
- Regular pills: 100–200 mg q6–8h.
- Long-acting pills: 100–300 mg PO bid of Norpace CR.

PO Preparations:
- 100 and 150 mg regular capsules.
- 100 and 150 mg long-acting capsules.

Actions:
- Type Ia antiarrhythmic used to treat ventricular and supraventricular arrhythmias.
- Prolongation of repolarization leads to prolonged QT interval.

Clearance: Some liver metabolism; primarily renally excreted.
- Moderately increase dosing interval in patients with impaired renal function.
- May need to adjust dosage in liver dysfunction (because of prolonged $t_{1/2}$).
- Supplemental dose suggested after hemodialysis.

Selected Side Effects: Negative inotropic effects (depresses ejection fraction), hypotension, conduction abnormalities, *proarrhythmic effects, QT prolongation, and torsade de pointes,* anticholinergic effects (dry mouth, blurred vision, urinary retention, urgency or hesitancy, etc).
Selected Drug Interactions: Hepatic enzyme inducers decrease its serum level.
Cautions: Use with caution in patients taking β-blockers or calcium channel blockers.
Pregnancy Category: C.
Cost: Generic $$$, Norpace $$$$ (≈ $0.25 each 100 mg generic tablet; ≈ $0.60 each 100 mg Norpace tablet).
Pearls:
- Follow corrected QT interval (> 25% increase predisposes to development of the ventricular arrhythmia torsades de pointes).

- Give an AV blocker prior to use in patients with atrial flutter (not atrial fibrillation).
- Usual therapeutic level is 2–5 μg/mL.

DISULFIRAM (Antabuse)
Dose: 500 mg PO qd for 1–2 weeks, then 250 mg PO qd.
PO Preparations: 250 and 500 mg scored tablets.
Actions: Antioxidant that blocks oxidation of alcohol, increasing the concentration of acetaldehyde and resulting in an unpleasant reaction; used in aversion therapy for chronic alcoholism.
Selected Drug Interactions: Inhibits metabolism of alcohol, phenytoin, and warfarin.
Cautions:
- *Contraindicated in patients with severe cardiac disease, psychoses, or hypersensitivity to thiuram derivatives.*
- Contraindicated in patients currently taking metronidazole, chlorpropamide, isoniazid, phenytoin, paraldehyde, alcohol, or alcohol-containing products.
- Disulfiram should *never* be administered without a patient's full knowledge and consent.
Cost: $$$.
Pearls:
- When mixed with alcohol, causes flushing, head and neck throbbing, headache, nausea and vomiting, respiratory difficulty, sweating, chest pain, CNS effects, and so forth.
- Patients should carry identification stating that they are receiving disulfiram.
- 20% of the drug remains 1 week after therapy is discontinued.
Pregnancy Category: Not established.

Ditropan: *see* OXYBUTYNIN

Diuril: *see* CHLOROTHIAZIDE

DIVALPROEX SODIUM: *see* VALPROIC ACID

DOBUTAMINE (Dobutrex)
Dose:
- Initial: 2 µg/kg/min IV.
- Usual: 2.5–10 µg/kg/min IV.
  (NOTE: dose is in micrograms, not milligrams.)

Actions: β_2-receptor agonist that increases inotropy, HR, and BP; used to treat CHF caused by poor systolic function.

Clearance: Metabolized via liver and other tissues.

Selected Side Effects: Elevated BP, increased HR, angina, occasional hypotension.

Cautions: *Contraindicated in patients with IHSS.*

Cost: $$$.

Pearls:
- The primary action of dobutamine is positive inotropy, with relatively milder effects on heart rate and blood pressure; dobutamine usually results in a decrease in systemic vascular resistance.
- Onset of action is 1–2 min; however, the peak effect at a given infusion rate may not occur for 10 min.
- Increases AV conduction and can raise ventricular rate in patients with atrial fibrillation or atrial flutter.
- Inotropic actions may be blocked in patients who have recently received a β-blocker.
- May increase insulin requirements.

Dobutrex: *see* DOBUTAMINE

DOCUSATE SODIUM (Colace; *see also* Peri-Colace)
Dose: 50–100 mg PO qd–bid.

PO Preparations: 50 and 100 mg capsules.

Actions: Stool softener (not a laxative).

Selected Side Effects: Minimal.

Cost: Generic $, Colace $$.

Dolobid: *see* DIFLUNISAL

DOPAMINE (Intropin)
Dose:
- 2.5–20 µg/kg/min.
- Usual starting dose to increase urine output ("renal dose dopa"): 2 µg/kg/min. (*NOTE:* Dose is in micrograms, *not* milligrams.)
- Frequent starting dose for mild hypotension: 2–5 µg/kg/min; for more severe hypotension a starting dose of 5 µg/kg/min may be reasonable.

Actions: Dose dependent:
- Predominant effect at "renal doses" of 2–4 µg/kg/min is a dopaminergic receptor-mediated increase in renal blood flow.
- At doses of 5–10 µg/kg/min, a β-adrenergic receptor-mediated increase in cardiac inotropy.
- At doses > 10 µg/kg/min, an α-adrenergic receptor-mediated increase in systemic vascular resistance.

Clearance: Metabolized in liver.

Selected Side Effects: Angina, substantially increased HR, increased PVCs, reduced BP.

Cautions: Use with caution in peripheral vascular disease (may cause vasoconstriction and limb ischemia).

Pregnancy Category: C.

Cost: $.

Pearls:
- Psychotropic drugs can block dopa receptors and reduce its effectiveness.
- Doses greater than 10 µg/kg/min can decrease renal perfusion.

Doryx: *see* DOXYCYCLINE

DOXAZOSIN (Cardura)
Dose (for hypertension):
- Initial: 1 mg PO qd.
- May titrate *stepwise* to 2, 4, 8, or 16 mg PO qd.

PO Preparations: 1, 2, 4, and 8 mg scored tablets.

Actions:
- α-receptor blocker that causes peripheral dilation, used to treat hypertension.
- Also now used to treat benign prostatic hypertrophy (BPH).

Clearance: Extensively metabolized.

Selected Side Effects: Postural hypotension and dizziness, fatigue, malaise, somnolence.

Pregnancy Category: B.

Cost: $$$ (≈ $0.90 each 2 mg tablet).

Pearls:

- Many physicians give the first dose at night (in case of exaggerated hypotensive or orthostatic hypotensive effects).
- Prescribe with caution and warn patients of possible hypotensive and orthostatic effects.
- One study showed that allowing 2 weeks between dosage changes helped to minimize orthostatic effects.
- Reflex tachycardia not a common side effect with therapy.
- Consider holding diuretic therapy 1–2 days before initiating therapy (volume-depleted patients may have an exaggerated hypotensive effect).

DOXORUBICIN (Adriamycin)

Dose: Tumor dependent.

Actions: Cytotoxic anthracycline antibiotic that inhibits synthesis of nucleic acid; used to treat malignancies.

Clearance: 40–50% excreted in bile; minimal renal excretion.

- Slightly reduce dosage in patients with end-stage renal disease; no change needed for milder renal impairment.
- Clearance is reduced in liver dysfunction; adjust dosage based on serum bilirubin: for levels of 1.2–3.0 mg/dL, give 1/2 the normal dose; for levels > 3.0 mg/dL, give 1/4 the normal dose.

Selected Side Effects:

- *Cardiotoxicity,* leukopenia, frequent nausea and vomiting, reversible alopecia, mucositis (5–10 days after therapy).
- *Severe soft tissue injury with possible necrosis can occur if it is extravasated during administration.*

Selected Drug Interactions:

- Can increase hepatotoxicity of 6-mercaptopurine.
- Can exacerbate cyclophosphamide-induced hemorrhagic cystitis.
- Concomitant use with cytarabine can cause necrotizing colitis.

Pregnancy Category: Not established.
Cost: $$$.
Pearls:

- Cardiotoxicity is the major toxicity. *PDR* recommends obtaining a baseline ECG and repeating after 300 mg/m^2.
- ECG changes include T-wave flattening, ST depression, and arrhythmias, and can last up to 2 weeks after treatment; these changes generally are *not* considered an indication to discontinue therapy.
- Life-threatening arrhythmias can occur during or within a few hours after therapy.
- Significant LV failure is uncommon but can occur, especially in patients receiving a cumulative dose of >400–550 mg/m^2, mediastinal radiation therapy, or concomitant cardiotoxic agents.
- *Use extreme care to prevent extravasation during administration; central venous catheters are preferred when possible.*

DOXYCYCLINE (Doryx, Vibramycin, Vibra-Tabs)

Dose: Route dependent:

- PO: 100 mg bid on day 1, then 100 mg PO qd–bid for at least 6 more days for most infections; may be given without regard to meals, but GI side effects may decrease when taken with food.
- IV: 100 mg IV q12h.

PO Preparations:

- 50 and 100 mg capsules and 100 mg tablets.
- 1 and 16 oz bottles of flavored syrup containing 50 mg/5 mL (1 tsp).
- 2 oz bottles of flavored suspension containing 25 mg/5 mL.

Actions: Broad-spectrum bacteriostatic antibiotic that inhibits protein synthesis.

- Some gram (+) coverage.
- Some gram (−) coverage.
- Some anaerobic coverage, including most *Bacteroides fragilis.*
- Also covers *Mycoplasma, Rickettsia,* and *Chlamydia.*

- *NOTE:* The above-mentioned antimicrobial coverage summary should be used as a guideline only; treatment decisions should take into account not only local epidemiologic patterns of antibiotic susceptibility but also, when available, culture susceptibility results.

Clearance: Hepatobiliary and renally excreted.

- Slightly increase dosing interval in patients with impaired renal function.
- Reduce dosage in patients with liver disease (because of possible nephrotoxic effects).
- Supplemental dose not required after hemodialysis or peritoneal dialysis.

Selected Side Effects: Photosensitivity, *tooth discoloration in children and fetuses.*

Selected Drug Interactions:

- Prolongs PT in patients taking warfarin.
- Reduces activity of penicillin (avoid concomitant use).
- Antacids, bicarbonate, calcium, and iron supplements decrease its absorption.

Pregnancy Category: D.

Cost: $ (≈ $15 for 100 mg bid for 10 days).

Dramamine: *see* DIMENHYDRINATE

DTO: *see* Deodorized Tincture of Opium

Dulcolax: *see* BISACODYL

Duragesic: *see* FENTANYL transdermal system

Duricef: *see* CEFADROXIL

Dyazide (HYDROCHLOROTHIAZIDE + TRIAMTERENE)

Dose: 1 or 2 capsules PO qd, taken after meals.

PO Preparations: Each capsule contains 25 mg hydrochlorothiazide and 37.5 mg triamterene.

Actions: K^+-sparing diuretic combination used to treat hypertension.
Selected Drug Interactions: Can raise serum level of lithium.
Cautions:
- *Contraindicated in preexisting hyperkalemia.*
- Use with caution in patients with severe liver disease (can precipitate hepatic coma) and in patients taking ACE inhibitors (because of its K^+-sparing properties).

Pregnancy Category: C.
Cost: \$\$ ($\approx$ \$0.25/generic capsule; $\approx$ \$0.40/Dyazide capsule).

DynaCirc: *see* ISRADIPINE

Dyrenium: *see* TRIAMTERENE

Ecotrin: *see* ACETYLSALICYLIC ACID

Effexor: *see* VENLAFAXINE

Elavil: *see* AMITRIPTYLINE

ELDEPRYL: *see* SELEGILINE

Eminase: *see* ANISTREPLASE

E-Mycin: *see* ERYTHROMYCIN

ENALAPRIL (Vasotec)
Dose: Delivery dependent:
- PO: First (test) dose 2.5–5.0 mg; usual dose 5–40 mg qd.
- IV: 1.25 mg given over 5 min q6h (0.625 mg q6h in renal failure or for patients taking diuretics).

PO Preparations: 2.5, 5, 10, and 20 mg tablets.

Actions: ACE inhibitor that causes peripheral dilatation; used to treat CHF and hypertension.

Clearance: Some liver metabolism; primarily renally excreted.

- Slightly reduce dosage in patients with impaired renal function.
- No change needed in patients with liver disease.

Selected Side Effects: Hypotension and dizziness, hyperkalemia (especially in patients with impaired renal function or taking K^+-sparing drugs or K^+ supplements), nonproductive cough, impairment of renal function, angioedema, rare neutropenia.

Cautions:

- *Contraindicated during second and third trimesters of pregnancy and in patients with significant aortic stenosis or hyperkalemia.*
- Patients should almost never be given both an ACE inhibitor and a K^+ supplement, unless clearly indicated by serial serum K^+ testing.

Pregnancy Category: D.

Cost: $$$ ($\approx$ $0.90 each 10 mg tablet).

Pearls:

- Diuretics potentiate its antihypertensive effects; the risk of hypotension is increased in volume-depleted and elderly patients.
- Follow BUN, creatinine, and K when beginning therapy.
- Patients should be instructed not to use potassium supplements or salt substitutes containing potassium.
- Patients should be made aware of the possibility of developing a nonproductive cough and of developing angioedema.
- The nonproductive cough with ACE inhibitors is presumed to be due to the inhibition of the degradation of endogenous bradykinin.
- Patients who develop a cough with one ACE inhibitor usually also develop such a cough with other ACE inhibitors.
- Enalapril accumulates more than other ACE inhibitors in cases of impaired renal function (consider particularly fosinopril [Monopril] in patients with worsening renal function).

ENTERIC-COATED ASPIRIN: *see* ACETYLSALICYLIC ACID

EPINEPHRINE
Dose: Route and disease dependent:
- Status asthmaticus (in patients < 30 years old) and anaphylaxis:
  - ▶ IV: 0.3–0.5 mg (of 1:10,000 solution); may repeat q5–10 min.
  - ▶ IM: 0.3–0.5 mg (of 1:1000 solution) SQ; may repeat q20–30 min up to 3 doses.
- Cardiopulmonary resuscitation:
  - ▶ 1.0 mg (of 1:10,000 solution) IV push; may be repeated q3–5 min.
  - ▶ May be given down ET tube if no IV access is available in a dose of 2–2.5 mg.
- IV Drip: Little published data available.
  - ▶ The intensive care unit's policy at Boston University Medical Center Hospital instructs using a dose of 0.7–7.0 μg/min (*NOTE:* Dose is in micrograms, *not* milligrams).
  - ▶ In cases of *cardiac arrest* and symptomatic bradycardia with profound hypotension, the AHA/ACLS guidelines suggest that the continuous infusion rate should be comparable to the standard IV dose of epinephrine administration. The suggested regimen consists of adding 30 mg epinephrine (30 mL of a 1:1000 solution) to 250 mL of normal saline and administering at an initial rate of 100 mL/h (*NOTE:* Rate is per hour), then titrating to desired hemodynamic endpoint. This should be administered by central venous access (AHA, Advanced Cardiac Life Support, 1994).

Actions: Sympathomimetic that directly stimulates α- and β-receptors; used to treat cardiac arrest, status asthmaticus, and anaphylaxis.

Selected Side Effects: Tachyarrhythmias, tachycardia, elevated BP, necrosis of injection site.

Selected Drug Interactions: Tricyclics and MAOI can potentiate its effects.

Cautions:
- Use with caution in cardiac disease.
- Usually is not given to asthmatics > 30 years old (because of concerns about possible cardiac disease).

Pregnancy Category: C.

Pearls:
- During a "code," if no IV access is available, epinephrine can be given down the endotracheal tube at a dose of 2–2.5 mg (AHA, Advanced Cardiac Life Support, 1994).
- After peripheral administration of epinephrine in a code situation, give a 20–30 mL bolus of intravenous fluid and immediately elevate the extremity. This enhances delivery of the drug to the central circulation, which can take 1–2 min (AHA, Advanced Cardiac Life Support, 1994).
- The utility during a code of "high-dose epinephrine" is controversial. This issue was extensively reviewed at a 1992 National Conference on CPR. Although hemodialysis E may increase the rate of return of spontaneous circulation, it does not appear to improve survival rates to hospital discharge when compared with standard-dose epinephrine. The use of "high-dose epinephrine" was neither recommended nor discouraged (AHA, Advanced Cardiac Life Support, 1994). Several dosing regimens for "high-dose epinephrine" exist for use if standard-dose epinephrine is ineffective (AHA, ACLS guidelines) and include:
  - ▶ Escalating: 1 mg IV push, then 3 mg IV push, then 5 mg IV push, each administered 3 min apart.
  - ▶ Intermediate: 2–5 mg IV push q3–5 min.
  - ▶ High: 0.1 mg/kg IV push q3–5 min.
- Cardiovascular effects of epinephrine in a code situation can include (AHA, Advanced Cardiac Life Support, 1994):
  - ▶ Increased systemic vascular resistance.
  - ▶ Increased systolic and diastolic blood pressure.
  - ▶ Increased automaticity and electrical activity.
  - ▶ Increased coronary and cerebral blood flow.
  - ▶ Increased myocardial contractility.
  - ▶ Increased myocardial oxygen requirements.

Epogen: *see* ERYTHROPOIETIN

Eryc: *see* **ERYTHROMYCIN**

Erycette: *see* **ERYTHROMYCIN topical solution**

EryDerm: *see* **ERYTHROMYCIN topical solution**

Erygel: *see* **ERYTHROMYCIN topical gel**

Erymax: *see* **ERYTHROMYCIN topical solution**

EryPed: *see* **ERYTHROMYCIN ETHYLSUCCINATE**

Ery-Tab: *see* **ERYTHROMYCIN**

Erythrocin: *see* **ERYTHROMYCIN**

ERYTHROMYCIN (E-Mycin, Eryc, Ery-Tab, Erythrocin, Ilosone, PCE 333, PCE 500, etc; *see also* Benzamycin, ERYTHROMYCIN ETHYLSUCCINATE (Ery-Ped)
Dose: Route and dependent:
- Adult PO: 250 mg qid, or 333 mg tid, or 500 mg bid–qid; PCE 500 is given bid.
- Adult IV: 500 mg–1 g q6h.
- Child: *see below* under ERYTHROMYCIN ETHYLSUC-CINATE (Ery-Ped).

PO Preparations:
- Generic tablets: 250, 333, and 500 mg.
- E-Mycin: 250 and 333 mg tablets.
- Ery-Tabs: 250, 333, and 500 mg tablets.
- ERYC: 250 mg capsules containing enteric-coated pellets.
- Ilosone: 250 mg capsules; 500 mg tablets; 16 oz flavored suspension containing either 125 mg/5 mL (1 tsp) or 250 mg/5 mL.
- PCE: 333 and 500 mg particle-containing tablets.

Actions: Bacteriostatic macrolide antibiotic that reversibly inhibits protein synthesis.

- Moderate gram (+) coverage, including strep and some staph (but *not* MRSA or enterococci).
- Is drug of choice for *Legionella* and *Mycoplasma.*
- *NOTE:* The above-mentioned antimicrobial coverage summary should be used as a guideline only; treatment decisions should take into account not only local epidemiologic patterns of antibiotic susceptibility but also, when available, culture susceptibility results.

Clearance: Excreted via liver into bile.

- Slightly reduce dosage in patients with end-stage renal disease; no change needed for milder renal impairment.
- Use with caution in mild liver dysfunction; decrease dosage for moderate to severe liver disease.
- Supplemental dose not required after hemodialysis or peritoneal dialysis.

Selected Side Effects: Extremely common GI symptoms (abdominal discomfort and cramping, nausea and vomiting, diarrhea), elevated LFTs, mild allergic reaction, transient hearing loss with high doses.

- Rare cases of ventricular arrhythmias have been reported when taken with H_2-blockers.

Selected Drug Interactions:

- Can raise serum level of theophylline.
- Prolongs PT in patients taking warfarin.
- *Can cause lethal arrhythmias when taken with terfenadine (Seldane) and possibly other* H_2-*blockers.*

Pregnancy Category: Not established.

Cost: Generic and brand $$ ($\approx$ $15 for 333 mg tid for 10 days of generic or brand).

Pearls:

- When given by peripheral IV, phlebitis is common.
- GI side effects are associated with IV as well as PO dosing.
- The heavy sodium load in the IV preparation may complicate fluid management in critically ill patients.
- Generic form should be taken on an empty stomach; E-Mycin, Ery-Tab, and PCE may be taken without regard to meals.

ERYTHROMYCIN ETHYLSUCCINATE
(EryPed)

Dose: Pediatric: weight dependent; suggested usual doses for mild to moderate infections:

- Children 10–15 lb: 50 mg PO qid.
- 16–25 lb: 100 mg PO qid.
- 26–50 lb: 200 mg PO qid.
- 51–100 lb: 300 mg PO qid.
- > 100 lb: 400 mg PO qid.
- Should be given in 4 equally divided doses.

PO Preparations:

- 200 mg chewable fruit-flavored tablets (EryPed Chewable).
- 100 and 200 mL bottles of suspension (EryPed 200) containing 200 mg/5 mL (1 tsp).
- 60, 100, and 200 mL bottles of suspension (EryPed 400) containing 400 mg/5 mL (1 tsp).

Actions: Bacteriostatic macrolide antibiotic that reversibly inhibits protein synthesis.

- Moderate gram (+) coverage, including strep and some staph (but *not* MRSA or enterococci).
- Is drug of choice for *Legionella* and *Mycoplasma*.

Clearance: Excreted via liver into bile.

- Slightly reduce dosage in patients with end-stage renal disease; no change needed for milder renal impairment.
- Use with caution in mild liver dysfunction; decrease dosage in moderate to severe liver disease.
- Supplemental dose not required after hemodialysis or peritoneal dialysis.

Selected Side Effects:

- Extremely common GI symptoms (abdominal discomfort and cramping, nausea and vomiting, diarrhea), elevated LFTs, mild allergic reaction, transient hearing loss with high doses.
- Rare cases of ventricular arrhythmias have been reported when taken with H_2-blockers.

Selected Drug Interactions:

- *Can raise serum level of theophylline.*
- Can cause lethal arrhythmias when taken with terfenadine (Seldane) and possibly other H_2-blockers.
- Prolongs PT in patients taking warfarin.

Cost: $$$.
Pearls:
- May be given without regard to meals.
- *NOTE:* Because it is an ethylsuccinate preparation, recommended doses are higher than for other erythromycin preparations (which consist of erythromycin as a free base).

ERYTHROMYCIN ophthalmic ointment (Ilotycin)
Dose: Apply to infected structure qd or more frequently.
Preparations: 1/8 oz tube containing 0.5% erythromycin.
Actions: Topical antibiotic used to treat corneal and conjunctival infections.
Cost: $$ (1/8 oz tube: generic ≈ $5, Ilotycin ≈ $8).
Pregnancy Category: B.

ERYTHROMYCIN topical solution and gel (Erycette, EryDerm, Erygel, Erymax)
Dose: Apply to cleansed, dried skin bid.
Preparations: All contain 2% erythromycin.
- Erycette solution available in boxes containing 60 individual-dose swabs.
- EryDerm solution available in 60 mL bottles with applicator.
- Erygel cream available in 30 and 60 g plastic tubes.
- Erymax solution available in 60 and 120 mL bottles.
Actions: Topical antibiotic used to treat acne vulgaris.
Pregnancy Category: Not established.
Cost: Generic $$, brands $$$ (generic ≈ $10 retail per bottle, brands ≈ $20 retail per bottle or tube).

ERYTHROPOIETIN (Epogen)
Dose:
- Initial: 50–100 units/kg given 3 times a week, IV for dialysis patients, IV or SQ for patients with chronic renal failure who are not on dialysis.

- Maintenance: Highly individualized.
- Some physicians begin with a lower initial dose of 20–40 units/kg (in part for financial and reimbursement reasons).
- Decrease dosage when target hematocrit is reached or if hematocrit increases 34% in any 2-week period.

Actions: Recombinant human glycoprotein that stimulates RBC production; used to treat anemia in chronic renal failure.

Selected Side Effects: Elevated BP (especially after initial therapy), headache, arthralgias, iron deficiency, thrombocytosis.

Cautions: *Contraindicated in patients with uncontrolled hypertension or with hypersensitivity to human albumin or mammalian cell-derived products.*

Pregnancy Category: C.

Cost: $$$$.

Pearls:

- Check hematocrit twice weekly.
- Check iron stores before beginning treatment, and follow them periodically.
- Reticulocyte count should increase within 10 days and hematocrit within 2–6 weeks.
- Rate of hematocrit increase is dose dependent.
- Serum erythropoietin level is 0.01–0.03 units/mL in normal subjects and can increase 100- to 1000-fold during hypoxemia or anemia.

Esgic (BUTALBITAL, ACETAMINOPHEN + CAFFEINE)

Dose: 1 or 2 capsules or tablets PO q4h prn up to a maximum of 6 capsules or tablets in a 24 h period.

PO Preparations: Each capsule or tablet contains 50 mg butalbital, 40 mg caffeine, and 325 mg acetaminophen.

Pregnancy Category: C.

Cost: Generic $$, Esgic $$$$ (generic ≈ $0.25/tablet, Esgic ≈ $1/tablet).

Pearls: Is chemically similar to Fioricet.

COMMONLY USED DRUGS 155

Esgic-Plus (BUTALBITAL, ACETAMINOPHEN + CAFFEINE)
Dose: 1 tablet q4h prn up to 6 tablets/day.
PO Preparations: Each capsule or tablet contains 50 mg butalbital, 40 mg caffeine, and 500 mg acetaminophen.
Pregnancy Category: C.

Esidrix: *see* HYDROCHLOROTHIAZIDE

Eskalith: *see* LITHIUM CARBONATE

ESMOLOL (Brevibloc)
Dose:
- Loading: 500 µg/kg over 1 min, then give 50 µg/kg/min for 4 min. (*NOTE:* Dose is in micrograms, *not* milligrams.)
- May repeat loading dose and increase maintenance dose by 50 µg/kg/min q5min.
- Most patients respond to infusion rate of 150–200 µg/kg/min; may then gradually reduce infusion rate.

Actions: Ultra-short-acting β_1-selective β-blocker used for acute treatment of angina, arrhythmias, and other conditions.
Clearance: Metabolized by esterase in RBCs; $t_{1/2}$ is 9 min.
Selected Side Effects: *Hypotension,* increased risk of CHF, AV block, bronchospasm.
Selected Drug Interactions:
- Raises serum level of digoxin by 10–20%.
- Morphine raises its serum level 46%.

Pregnancy Category: C.
Cost: $$$$.

ESTAZOLAM (ProSom)
Dose:
- Initial: 1–2 mg PO qhs prn.
- Consider beginning with 0.5 mg in small, debilitated, or elderly patients.

PO Preparations: 1 and 2 mg scored tablets.
Actions: Benzodiazepine used to treat insomnia.

Selected Side Effects: Somnolence and sedation, hypokinesia, dizziness.

Cautions: *Should not be used in pregnant or potentially pregnant patients.*

Pregnancy Category: X.

Cost: $$ (≈ $0.80 each 1 mg tablet).

Pearls: Abrupt discontinuance can cause rebound insomnia.

ESTROGEN: *see* Premarin

ETHAMBUTOL

Dose:

- Initial treatment: 15 mg/kg PO qd.
- Retreatment: 25 mg/kg PO qd for the first 2 months, then decrease the dose to 15 mg/kg PO qd.
- Some sources recommend giving 25 mg/kg PO qd for first 2 months of treatment, or initially for severe infections.

PO Preparations: 100 and 400 mg tablets.

Actions: Bacteriostatic antitubercular agent that inhibits metabolite synthesis used to treat mycobacterial infections.

Clearance: Some excretion in feces; primarily renally excreted.

- Slightly to moderately increase dosing interval in patients with impaired renal function.
- No change in dosage needed in patients with liver disease.
- Supplemental dose suggested after hemodialysis or peritoneal dialysis.

Selected Side Effects: Decreased visual acuity (from optic neuritis).

Cautions: *Contraindicated in patients with optic neuritis.*

Pregnancy Category: Not established.

Cost: $$$$ (≈ $2/day).

Pearls:

- Initial visual check is prudent; some sources recommend regular visual examinations, especially when patients are taking 25 mg/kg qd.
- Can be taken without regard to meals.

ETHINYL ESTRADIOL: *see* Norinyl, Ortho-Novum, Tri-Levlen, Tri-Norinyl, Triphasil

Ethmozine: *see* MORICIZINE

ETHOSUXIMIDE (Zarontin)
Dose:
- Initial: 250 mg PO bid.
- May increase by 250 mg daily (not bid) every 4–7 days until effective.
- Usual maintenance: 10–20 mg/kg PO bid.
- Maximum: 1.5 g daily.

PO Preparations:
- 250 mg capsules.
- 1 pint bottle of flavored syrup containing 50 mg/mL.

Actions: Succinimide anticonvulsant used to treat petit-mal seizures.

Clearance: Primarily metabolized; some renal excretion.
- Slightly reduce dosage in patients with end-stage renal disease; no change needed for mild renal impairment.
- No change in dosage needed in patients with liver disease.
- Supplemental dose suggested after hemodialysis.

Selected Side Effects:
- GI distress, nausea and vomiting, anorexia and weight loss.
- Has been reported to cause leukopenia (rarely), SLE, aplastic anemia, and Stevens–Johnson syndrome.

Pregnancy Category: Not established for ethosuximide. Although other anticonvulsants have been shown to cause birth defects, the risks of ethosuximide during pregnancy have not been clearly established. Risks of continuing therapy must be weighed against the risk of seizures during pregnancy.

Cost: $$$$ (≈ $1 each 250 mg tablet).

ETODOLAC (Lodine)
Dose: 200 mg PO tid–qid, 300 mg PO bid–qid, or 400 mg PO bid–tid.

PO Preparations: 200, 300, and 400 mg capsules.

Actions: NSAID used to treat osteoarthritis and mild to moderate pain.

Selected Side Effects: Dyspepsia, upper GI bleeding, fluid retention, theoretical worsening of "prerenal" renal failure.

Cautions:

- *Contraindicated in patients with allergy to ASA or other NSAID.*
- Use with extreme caution, if at all, in patients with history of upper GI bleeding or ulcer disease.
- Use with caution in renal disease.

Pregnancy Category: C.

Cost: $$$$ (≈ $1.20 each 300 mg tablet).

ETOPOSIDE (VePesid, VP-16)

Dose: Variable; may be given PO or IV.

- Frequent IV regimen: 35–100 mg/m/day for 5 consecutive days or 100 mg/m on days 1, 3, and 5.

PO Preparations: 50 mg capsules.

Actions: Cell cycle-specific semisynthetic derivative of podophyllotoxin, a plant resin with cathartic and antineoplastic properties; used to treat neoplasms.

Clearance: Undergoes some metabolism, biliary excretion (16%), and urinary excretion (30–40%).

- Slightly reduce dosage in patients with impaired renal function.

Selected Side Effects: *Myelosuppression, anaphylactic reaction* (1–2%), nausea and vomiting, reversible alopecia.

Cautions: *Give slowly* (over 30–60 min) *to avoid hypotension.*

Pregnancy Category: D.

Cost: $$$.

- Bone marrow suppression is dose-limiting toxicity.
- Follow CBC.
- Granulocyte nadir occurs in 7–14 days, and platelet nadir in 9–16 days.
- Bone marrow recovery is usually complete by day 20.

Ex-Lax (unflavored), Ex-Lax Chocolate laxative, Extra Gentle Ex-Lax
Dose: 1 or 2 pills with water qhs.
PO Preparations:
- Boxes of 8, 30, and 60 unflavored pills.
- Boxes of 6, 18, 48, and 72 chewable chocolate-flavored tablets.
- Boxes of 24 Extra Gentle Ex-Lax pills.

Actions: Laxative containing active ingredient phenolphthalein; used to treat occasional constipation.

EXPECTORANTS: *see* GUAIFENESIN

FAMCICLOVIR (Famvir)
Dose: 500 mg PO q8 h for 7 d, begun as soon as possible after symptoms of herpes zoster are diagnosed.
PO Preparations: 500 mg tablets.
Actions: Antiviral agent used to shorten postherpetic neuralgia.
Clearance: Metabolized via liver; renal excretion of metabolites.
- No dose change necessary in patients with well-compensated liver disease.
- Adjust dose in patients with renal insufficiency.

Selected Drug Interactions: No significance increase in reported adverse effects when compared with those in patients receiving placebo.
Pregnancy Category: B.
Cost: $$$$ ($\approx$ $7 each 500 mg tablet).
- Can be taken without regard to meals.
- Famciclovir only minimally decreases the crusting and healing time of vesicles, does not affect the duration of acute pain (ie, before lesion healing), and does not decrease the *incidence* of postherpetic neuralgia.
- Two studies evaluated the efficacy of famciclovir in shortening postherpetic neuralgia. In one study it did shorten the duration of postherpetic neuralgia (median of 63 d with

famciclovir versus 119 d with placebo); in a second study there were no statistically significant differences in the time to loss of postherpetic neuralgia compared to placebo.
- Is more effective if started within the first 48 h of herpes zoster symptoms; efficacy has not been studied when started more than 72 h after onset of symptoms.

FAMOTIDINE (Pepcid)
Dose: Situation dependent.
- Acute therapy: 20 mg IV q12h or 40 mg PO qhs for 4–8 weeks.
- Maintenance therapy: 20 mg PO qhs.

PO Preparations:
- 20 and 40 mg tablets.
- 400 mg powder for reconstitution, giving 40 mg/5 mL (1 tsp) oral suspension.

Actions: H_2-blocker used to treat peptic ulcer disease, gastritis, esophageal reflux, and Zollinger–Ellison syndrome.

Clearance: Mainly renally excreted.
- Slightly reduce dosage in patients with impaired renal function.
- No change in dosage needed in patients with liver disease.

Selected Side Effects: Headache (rare).

Selected Drug Interactions: Magnesium- and aluminum-containing antacids, such as Maalox and Mylanta, reduce its bioavailability (give at least 2 h apart from it).

Pregnancy Category: B.

Cost: $$$$ ($\approx$ $2.70 each 40 mg tablet).

Famvir: *see* FAMCICLOVIR

Feldene: *see* PIROXICAM

FELODIPINE (Plendil)
Dose:
- Initial: 5 mg PO qd.
- Maintenance: 5–20 mg PO qd.
- Elderly patients may require lower dosage.

PO Preparations: 5 and 10 mg tablets.

Actions: Calcium channel blocker that works primarily through peripheral vasodilatation; used to treat hypertension.

Clearance: Metabolized via liver.

- No change in dosage needed in patients with renal insufficiency.
- Reduce dosage in patients with liver disease.

Selected Side Effects: Hypotension, dizziness, peripheral edema (common) palpitations, headache, flushing, gingival hyperplasia.

Selected Drug Interactions:

- Can increase serum level of digoxin.

Pregnancy Category: C.

Cost: $$$$ (≈ $1.70 each 10 mg tablet).

Pearls:

- Caution patients about possible hypotensive effects.
- Has no significant effects on cardiac conductivity.
- Studies to date have shown no significant (−) inotropic effects.

FENTANYL transdermal system (Duragesic)

Dose:

- Initial: 25 µg/h as Duragesic-25 patch applied to skin. (*NOTE:* Dose is in micrograms, *not* milligrams.)
- Change each patch after 3 days' use.
- Titrate to pain as needed.

Preparations: 25, 50, and 100 µg patches.

Actions: Topical synthetic narcotic used to treat chronic pain that requires opioid analgesia.

Selected Side Effects: Nausea and vomiting, pruritus, *hypoventilation,* CNS effects, constipation, urinary retention.

Cost: $$$$ (≈ $16 each Duragesic-50 patch).

Pregnancy Category: C.

Pearls:

- Steady-state levels are reached 5–6 days after beginning therapy and after each change in dose, so allow 1 week for equilibration before deciding on increasing the dose of fentanyl.
- Use a short-acting narcotic during first 24 h to supplement analgesic relief.

- Fentanyl is 100 times more potent than morphine.
- For total daily PO morphine dose of 45–134 mg, use transdermal fentanyl at 25 µg/h; for 500 mg dose, use fentanyl at 125–150 µg/h; for 1000 mg dose, use fentanyl at 275 µg/h.
- *Inform patients that direct exposure of the Duragesic application site to direct external heat sources (electric blankets, hot tubs, etc) while wearing the patch may increase fentanyl release from the patch.*

FENTANYL CITRATE injection (Sublimaze)
<u>Intravenous drip for severe pain control:</u>
Dose:

- Initial IV load: 50–100 µg (*NOTE:* Dosage is in micrograms, *not* milligrams) administered slowly (over 1–2 min).
- Little specific information is available on the maintenance dose for pain control (published information relates mainly to the intravenous use of fentanyl for general anesthesia). The nursing policy guidelines at Boston University Medical Center Hospital instruct using a dose of 1–4 µg/kg/h (*NOTE:* Dose is in micrograms, *not* milligrams).

Actions: Potent narcotic analgesic used for anesthesia and pain control.

Selected Side Effects: *Respiratory depression, hypotension, bradycardia,* CNS depression, muscular rigidity (especially of the chest wall).

Selected Drug Interactions:

- Other CNS depressants potentiate the CNS depressant effects of Fentanyl.
- Administration to patients who have recently taken MAO inhibitors may lead to exaggerated depressant effects of fentanyl and to hypertensive crisis.
- Clonidine potentiates its sedative and analgesic effects.

Cautions:

- Should only be administered by persons specifically trained in the use of intravenous anesthetics.
- Resuscitative equipment, oxygen, and opiate antagonists should be readily available.
- Probably should not be administered to patients taking MAO inhibitors within the prior 14 days.

Pregnancy Category: C.
Pearls:
- Fentanyl is approximately 100 times more potent than morphine; 100 μg of fentanyl is comparable to 10 mg of morphine or 75 mg of meperidine (Demerol).

Fergon: *see* FERROUS GLUCONATE

FERROUS GLUCONATE (Fergon)
Dose: 1 or 2 tablets or 1–2 tsp PO qd.
PO Preparations:
- 320 mg tablets containing 38 mg elemental ferrous iron.
- 1 pint bottles of 6% elixir.
Actions: Iron supplement.
Pregnancy Category: Generally regarded as safe during pregnancy.
Cost: $.
Pearls: May be better tolerated and produce less constipation than ferrous sulfate.

FERROUS SULFATE (IRON, FeSO$_4$)
Dose: Route dependent:
- PO: 325 mg bid–tid.
- Elixir: 1 or 2 tsp tid, preferably between meals.
PO Preparations:
- 325 mg tablets.
- 16 oz bottles of elixir containing 220 mg/5 mL (1 tsp).
Selected Side Effects: Nausea, indigestion, diarrhea, abdominal cramping, constipation.
Pregnancy Category: Generally regarded as safe during pregnancy.
Cost: $.
Pearls:
- Taking with meals reduces its GI side effects.
- Consider giving with an anticonstipation agent (Colace, Metamucil, etc).
- Turns stools black, which can be misinterpreted as melena.
- Most patients do not tolerate tid dosing, and bid dosing is recommended by some physicians for increased compliance.

- For those unable to tolerate ferrous sulfate, ferrous citrate (contained in Geritol) or ferrous gluconate may be more palatable alternatives.

Fioricet (BUTALBITAL, ACETAMINOPHEN + CAFFEINE)

Dose: 1 or 2 capsules PO q4h prn up to a maximum of 6 capsules daily.

PO Preparations: Each capsule contains 50 mg butalbital, 325 mg acetaminophen, and 40 mg caffeine.

Actions: Medication that combines analgesic properties of acetaminophen and caffeine with anxiolytic and muscle-relaxant properties of butalbital (a barbiturate); usually used to treat migraine headaches.

Selected Side Effects: Drowsiness, dizziness, lightheadedness, nausea and vomiting, mental confusion.

Selected Drug Interactions:

- Butalbital increases metabolism of warfarin and decreases serum level of tricyclics.
- Fioricet potentiates CNS depressant effects of other CNS depressants.

Cautions: Use with caution in patients with liver disease (because of potential hepatotoxicity from acetaminophen) and in patients who must perform potentially hazardous tasks.

Pregnancy Category: C.

Cost: $$$ ($\approx$ $0.60/tablet).

Pearls: May cause rebound headaches.

Fiorinal (BUTALBITAL, ASA + CAFFEINE)

Dose: 1 or 2 capsules or tablets PO q4h prn up to a maximum of 6 capsules or tablets daily.

PO Preparations: Each capsule or tablet contains 50 mg butalbital, 325 mg ASA, and 40 mg caffeine.

Actions: Medication that combines analgesic properties of ASA with anxiolytic and muscle-relaxant properties of butalbital (a barbiturate); used to treat migraine headaches.

Selected Side Effects: CNS depression, drowsiness, dizziness, impairment of mental and physical skills, lightheadedness, nausea and vomiting, flatulence.

Selected Drug Interactions:
- Butalbital increases metabolism of warfarin and reduces serum level of tricyclics.
- Fiorinal potentiates CNS depressant effects of other CNS depressants.

Cautions:
- Use with caution in peptic ulcer disease or coagulopathy and in patients who must perform potentially hazardous tasks.

Pregnancy Category: Not established.

Cost: $$$ ($\approx$ $0.55/tablet).

Flagyl: *see* METRONIDAZOLE

FLECAINIDE (Tambocor)

Dose:
- Initial: 50–100 mg PO q12h.
- Maximum: 400 mg daily (usually given in divided doses q12h).

PO Preparations: 50, 100, and 150 mg tablets.

Actions: Class Ic antiarrhythmic (blocks sodium channels, resulting in slowed impulse conduction); used to treat ventricular and supraventricular arrhythmias.

Clearance: Primarily metabolized via liver; $\approx$ 25% renally excreted.
- Slightly reduce dosage in patients with impaired renal function.
- Some sources suggest an initial dose of 50 mg PO q12h and lower maintenance doses in chronic renal failure, and lower maintenance doses or increased dosing intervals in patients with liver disease.
- Supplemental dose not required after hemodialysis.

Selected Side Effects:
- Proarrhythmic effects, (−) inotropy, CHF, neurologic side effects (dose related).
- Can raise the pacing threshold.

Selected Drug Interactions:
- Amiodarone can markedly raise its serum level.
- Concomitant use with propranolol raises serum levels of both drugs.

Cautions:
- *Contraindicated in second- or third-degree AV block and in bifascicular block unless a ventricular pacer is in place.*
- Contraindicated in patients with overt CHF.
- Use with extreme caution in patients with sick sinus syndrome.

Pregnancy Category: C.
Cost: $$$$ (≈ $1.35 each 100 mg tablet).
Pearls:
- The CAST study reported an increased mortality in post-MI patients with premature ventricular beats who were treated with flecainide.
- Should be discontinued only in hospital setting.
- Approved for the treatment of atrial arrhythmias in patients with structurally normal hearts.

Flexeril: *see* **CYCLOBENZAPRINE**

Florinef: *see* **FLUDROCORTISONE**

Floxin: *see* **OFLOXACIN**

FLUCONAZOLE (Diflucan)
Dose: Disease dependent:
- Oropharyngeal or esophageal candidiasis: 200 mg "loading dose" PO or IV, then 100 mg PO or IV qd for 2–3 weeks.
- Candidal urinary tract infections or peritonitis: doses of 50–200 mg/day have been used in studies involving a small number of patients.
- Systemic candidiasis: optimal dose not established; doses of up to 400 mg/day have been used in studies involving a small number of patients.
- Cryptococcal meningitis: 400 mg "loading dose" PO or IV, then 200 mg PO or IV qd for 10–12 weeks (maintenance suppressive therapy is necessary in immunocompromised hosts).
- Vaginal candidiasis: Single dose of 150 mg PO (this regimen used by clinicians, but, at present, not explicitly recommended by manufacturer).

COMMONLY USED DRUGS 167

PO Preparations:
- 50, 100, 150, and 200 mg tablets.
- 35 mL bottles of flavored suspension, which after reconstitution contain either 10 mg/mL or 40 mg/mL.

Actions: Antifungal antibiotic used to treat local or systemic candidiasis and cryptococcal meningitis.

Clearance: Primarily renally excreted; some excretion in feces.
- Moderately reduce dosage in patients with impaired renal function.
- No change in dosage needed in patients with liver disease.

Selected Side Effects: Nausea, headache, rash, rare elevation in LFTs and hepatitis.

Selected Drug Interactions:
- Raises serum level of phenytoin.
- Reduces metabolism and raises serum level of OHAs.
- Prolongs PT in patients taking warfarin.
- Infrequently raises serum level of cyclosporine.

Pregnancy Category: C.

Cost: $$$$ ($\approx$ $8 each 100 mg tablet).

Pearls:
- Watch patients for symptoms and signs of hepatic injury; follow LFTs.
- PO route is well absorbed; IV therapy is rarely necessary.
- Does not require low gastric pH for absorption (unlike ketoconazole); also has fewer drug interactions than other azoles.

FLUDROCORTISONE (Florinef)
Dose:
- Range: 50–200 µg PO qd. (*NOTE:* Dose is in micrograms, *not* milligrams.)
- Usual: 50 µg PO qd.

PO Preparations: 100 µg tablets.

Actions: Oral cortisol derivative with potent mineralocorticoid and moderate glucocorticoid effects used to treat adrenocortical insufficiency.

Selected Side Effects: Hypertension, edema, weight gain, CHF, hypernatremia, hypokalemia.

Cost: $$.

FLUMAZENIL (Romazicon, *formerly* Mazicon)
Dose (for suspected or known benzodiazepine overdose):

- Initial: 0.2 mg (2 mL) IV administered over 30 s.
- If desired level of consciousness is not obtained after waiting 30 s, a further dose of 0.3 mg (3 mL) IV can be administered over 30 s.
- Further doses of 0.5 mg (5 mL) IV can be administered over 30 s every 1 min up to a maximum total dose of 3 mg (patients may rarely require up to a total dose of 5 mg).

Actions: Benzodiazepine receptor antagonist; used to treat benzodiazepine overdose.

Clearance: Cleared via liver; clearance dependent on hepatic blood flow.

- Dose adjustment not necessary in renal failure.
- No supplemental dose necessary after hemodialysis.

Side Effects: Anxiety and agitation, seizures, other benzodiazepine withdrawal symptoms.

Cautions: *Contraindicated in patients who have been on benzodiazepines for life-threatening conditions (control of intracranial pressure, status epilepticus, etc) and in patients showing signs of serious cyclic antidepressant overdose.*

Pregnancy Category: C.

Pearls:

- Was formally called "Mazicon."
- Doses of approximately 0.1–0.2 mg produce partial antagonism; dose of 0.4–1.0 mg usually produce complete antagonism in patients who have received usual sedating doses of benzodiazepines; in patients with benzodiazepine overdose, 75% of such patients respond to doses of 1–3 mg.
- Patients who do not respond to doses of 3–5 mg are unlikely to respond to higher doses.
- Onset of reversal effects usually begins within 1–2 min; 80% response is achieved within 3 min; peaks effect occurs within 6–10 min.
- Watch for recurrent symptoms of resedation for several hours in patients who have taken long-acting benzodiazepines; repeat doses may be administered if needed at 20 min intervals.

FLUOCINONIDE cream, gel, ointment, and solution (Lidex)
Dose: Apply thin film to affected skin bid.
Preparations:
- 15, 30, 60, and 120 g 0.05% cream.
- 15, 30, 60, and 120 g 0.05% gel.
- 15, 30, 60, and 120 g 0.05% ointment.
- 20 and 60 mL 0.05% solution.

Actions: Topical steroid used to treat steroid-responsive dermatologic conditions.
Selected Side Effects: Local irritation, dermatitis, folliculitis, hypertrichosis, adrenal axis suppression.
Cautions:
- *Contraindicated in varicella or vaccinia infections.*
- Avoid use on the face, breasts, groin and axilla.
- Prolonged or inappropriate use of such class II steroids may lead to skin atrophy, telangiectasias, and pigmentary changes, and may suppress the adrenocortical axis.

Pregnancy Category: C.
Cost: Generic $$, Lidex $$$ (60 g retail: generic ≈ $20, Lidex ≈ $40).

FLUOROMETHOLONE ophthalmic ointment and suspension (FML, FML Forte)
Dose: Delivery dependent.
- Suspension: Instill 1 drop (written "gtt") bid–qid.
- Ointment: Apply 0.5-inch "ribbon" qd–tid.

Preparations:
- 3.5 g tube of FML ointment containing 0.1% fluorometholone.
- 1, 5, 10, and 15 mL suspensions of FML containing 0.1% fluorometholone.
- 2, 5, 10, and 15 mL suspensions of FML Forte containing 0.25% fluorometholone.

Actions: Topical corticosteroid used to treat inflammatory conditions.
Cautions: *Contraindicated in patients with possible ocular herpes simplex infection.*
Pregnancy Category: C.

5-FLUOROURACIL (5-FU)
Dose: Tumor dependent.
Actions: Antineoplastic antimetabolite that interferes with DNA and RNA synthesis; used to treat malignancies.
Clearance: Metabolized primarily via liver; 7–20% renally excreted.
- No change in dosage needed in patients with renal insufficiency.
- Use with caution in patients with liver disease.

Selected Side Effects: *Stomatitis and esophagopharyngitis, myelosuppression (especially leukopenia),* anorexia, nausea and vomiting, diarrhea, dermatitis (hand-foot syndrome or painful rash), pruritus, transient alopecia.
Selected Drug Interactions: Leucovorin can enhance its toxicity.
Cautions: *Contraindicated in patients with poor nutritional status, depressed bone marrow function, or serious infections.*
Pregnancy Category: D.
Cost: $.
Pearls:
- *PDR* recommends discontinuing therapy in patients with WBCs < 3500 or rapidly falling WBC count, intractable vomiting or diarrhea, GI ulceration and bleeding, platelets < 100,000, or clinical bleeding.
- WBC nadir generally occurs on days 9–14 and WBCs usually return to normal by day 30.
- Continuous infusion is less myelosuppressive than IV bolus therapy.

FLUOXETINE (Prozac)
Dose:
- Initial: 20 mg PO qd (one source notes a starting dose of 10 mg can be used in some patients).
- Maximum: 68–80 mg daily (80 mg dose is given 40 mg PO bid).

PO Preparations:
- 10 and 20 mg Pulvules.
- 120 mL bottle of solution containing 20 mg/5 mL (1 tsp).

Actions: Nontricyclic agent that probably inhibits serotonin reuptake; used to treat depression.

Clearance: Metabolized via liver.

- *PDR* recommends reducing dosage in patients with severe renal disease.
- $t_{1/2}$ is increased in patients with liver disease, so dosage adjustment may be needed.

Selected Side Effects: Numerous frequent CNS symptoms (including insomnia, tremor, anxiety, nervousness, abnormal dreams) decreased libido or sexual dysfunction (or both), sweating, GI complaints, altered appetite or weight loss (or both), rash or urticaria, rare SIADH.

Selected Drug Interactions:

- Severe reactions with MAOI.
- Can prolong $t_{1/2}$ of concurrently administered benzodiazepines.
- Increases plasma levels of concurrently administered tricyclic antidepressants.

Cautions: *Contraindicated in patients taking MAOI.*

Pregnancy Category: B.

Cost: $$$$ ($\approx$ $2/capsule).

Pearls:

- Allow 14 days after discontinuance of MAOI before beginning therapy.
- Allow 5 weeks after discontinuance of Prozac before beginning MAOI.

FLURAZEPAM (Dalmane)

Dose: 15–30 mg PO qhs prn.

PO Preparations: 15 and 30 mg capsules.

Actions: Long-acting benzodiazepine used to treat insomnia.

Clearance: Metabolized via liver.

- No change in dosage needed in patients with renal insufficiency.
- One source recommends reducing dosage in patients with liver disease.

Selected Side Effects: Postdose daytime hangover.

Cautions: *Should not be used in pregnant or potentially pregnant patients.*

Pregnancy Category: *Contraindicated during pregnancy.*

Cost: Generic $, Dalmane $$$ (≈ $0.15 each 15 mg generic tablet; ≈ $0.60 each 15 mg Dalmane tablet).

Pearls: May cause excessive drowsiness in elderly patients.

FLUVASTATIN (Lescol)
Dose:
- Initial: 20 mg PO qd.
- Maximum: 40 mg PO qd.

Preparations: 20 and 40 mg capsules.

Actions: HMG-CoA inhibitor that lowers total and LDL cholesterol and triglyceride levels and increases HDL cholesterol; used to treat hypercholesterolemia.

Clearance: Metabolized by the liver.

Selected Side Effects: Elevated LFTs, possible increased CPK (MM) and myopathy (especially when given with immunosuppressants, gemfibrozil, or niacin; these effects have been with other HMG-CoA reductase inhibitors), GI discomfort.

Selected Drug Interactions:
- Can prolong PT in patients taking warfarin.
- Cyclosporine, gemfibrozil, niacin, or erythromycin may increase the risk of myopathy.

Cautions:
- *Contraindicated in pregnant or potentially pregnant patients.*
- Contraindicated in patients with active liver disease or unexplained transaminase elevations.
- Use with caution in patients with history of liver disease or heavy alcohol use.

Pregnancy Category: X.

Cost: $$$ (≈ $1.15 each 20 mg tablet).

Pearls:
- Should be taken in the evening (any time from dinner to bedtime).
- Obtain LFTs and CPK level before starting therapy.
- Recommended frequency for checking liver function during treatment has been liberalized to every 6 weeks for first 3 months, then every 8 weeks for remainder of first year and approximately every 6 months thereafter.

- Discontinue if persistent LFTs > 3 times normal, substantial rise in CPK, or myositis occurs.
- Primary effects are reductions in total and LDL cholesterol; usually leads to only modest elevations of hemodialysis L cholesterol.

FML, FML Forte: *see* FLUOROMETHOLONE ophthalmic ointment and suspension

FOLIC ACID
Dose: 1 mg PO qd for 2–3 weeks.
- Some patients may need chronic replacement therapy.

PO Preparations: 0.1, 0.4, 0.8, and 1.0 mg tablets.

Pregnancy Category: Generally regarded as safe during pregnancy.

Cost: $.

Pearls:
- May prevent dysplasia of colonic epithelium in ulcerative colitis when given as therapy with sulfasalazine (Azulfidine).
- In patients who are NPO (such as alcoholics with pancreatitis), folate may be given IV by adding 1 mg of folate to the hanging bag of IV fluid.

Fortaz: *see* CEFTAZIDIME

FOSINOPRIL (Monopril)
Dose:
- Initial: 10 mg PO qd.
- Maintenance: 20–40 mg PO qd.

PO Preparations: 10 and 20 mg tablets.

Actions: ACE inhibitor used to treat hypertension.

Clearance: Metabolized via liver; excreted equally in feces and urine.
- No change in dosage needed in patients with renal insufficiency.
- Is poorly dialyzed.
- Dosage adjustment generally not required in elderly patients.

Selected Side Effects: Hypotension and dizziness, hyperkalemia (especially in patients with impaired renal function or taking K⁺-sparing drugs or K⁺ supplements), nonproductive cough, impairment of renal function, angioedema, rare neutropenia.

Cautions:
- *Contraindicated during second and third trimesters of pregnancy and in patients with significant aortic stenosis or hyperkalemia.*
- Patients should almost never be given both an ACE inhibitor and a K⁺ supplement, unless clearly indicated by serial serum K⁺ testing.

Pregnancy Category: D.

Cost: $$$ (≈ $0.75 each 20 mg tablet).

Pearls:
- Diuretics potentiate its antihypertensive effects; the risk of hypotension is increased in volume-depleted and elderly patients.
- Follow BUN, creatinine, and K⁺ when beginning therapy.
- Patients should be instructed not to use potassium supplements or salt substitutes containing potassium.
- Patients should be made aware of the possibility of developing a nonproductive cough and of developing angioedema.
- The frequently seen nonproductive cough with ACE inhibitors is presumed to be due to the inhibition of the degradation of endogenous bradykinin.
- Patients who develop a cough with one ACE inhibitor usually also develop such a cough with other ACE inhibitors.
- Absorption is not affected by food.
- Because fosinopril clearance is not affected by changes in renal function, fosinopril may be the ACE inhibitor of choice in patients with changing renal function.

5-FU: *see* 5-FLUOROURACIL

FUROSEMIDE (Lasix)
Dose:
- Initial: 10–20 mg PO or IV (higher doses are needed for patients with impaired renal function).

- Maximum: 600 mg daily.
- Usually no more than 400 mg is given at any one time.

Preparations:
- 20, 40, and 80 mg tablets.
- 60 and 120 mg bottles of flavored solution containing 10 mg/mL.

Actions: Loop diuretic that causes early increase in venodilation and later diuresis; used to treat CHF and edema.

Clearance: Some liver metabolism; primarily renally excreted.
- May need to reduce dosage in patients with liver disease.

Selected Side Effects:
- Decreased K^+ and Na^+, substantially reduced BP, hypochloremic alkalosis, ototoxicity (especially when injected too rapidly).
- Can increase ototoxicity of aminoglycosides.
- Can raise serum glucose level.

Pregnancy Category: C.

Cost: $.

Pearls:
- *Inject slowly* (< 20 mg/min) *to minimize ototoxicity.*
- Concomitant use of metolazone (Zaroxolyn) or chlorothiazide (Diuril) can potentiate its effect.
- PO peak diuretic effect occurs at 1–2 h; duration of effect 6–8 h.
- IV peak diuretic effect occurs at 30 min; duration of effect 2 h.
- Each 1 mg of furosemide administered IV is comparable in diuretic effect to 2 mg furosemide administered PO.

GABAPENTIN (Neurontin)
Dose:
- Initial: 300 mg PO on day 1, 300 mg PO bid on day 2, and then 300 mg PO tid beginning on day 3.
- Dose can then be gradually titrated upward, if clinically indicated, up to a usual maximum dose of 600 mg tid.

Preparations: 100, 300, and 400 mg capsules.

Actions: Anticonvulsant used as adjunctive therapy in the treatment of partial seizures.
- Actual mechanism of action unknown.

Clearance: Not appreciably metabolized; clearance is completely via renal excretion.
- Dose reduction required in patients with renal insufficiency.
- Probably does not need dose adjustment in patients with hepatic insufficiency.

Selected Side Effects: Somnolence, fatigue, dizziness, ataxia, diplopia, and amblyopia.

Selected Drug Interactions: Maalox reduces its absorption.

Pregnancy Category: C.

Pearls:
- Should not be abruptly discontinued (can precipitate status epilepticus).
- Can cause false (+) urine dipstick tests for protein.
- Can be taken without regard to meals.

Garamycin: *see* GENTAMICIN

Garamycin Ophthalmic: *see* GENTAMICIN SULFATE eye drops

Gas-X: *see* SIMETHICONE

G-CSF: *see* GRANULOCYTE COLONY-STIMULATING FACTOR

Gemcore: *see* GEMFIBROZIL

GEMFIBROZIL (Gemcore, Lopid)

Dose: 600 mg PO bid.

PO Preparations: 600 mg tablets.

Actions: Fibric acid derivative that inhibits hepatic triglyceride synthesis, leading to reduced VLDL and triglycerides, increased HDL, and increased or decreased LDL; used primarily to treat hypertriglyceridemia; also occasionally used to treat hypercholesterolemia.

Clearance: Metabolized via liver; renally excreted.
- Moderately reduce dosage in patients with impaired renal function.

Selected Side Effects: Dyspepsia, abdominal pain, flatulence, gallbladder disease, rare elevated LFTs, rare decrease in CBC, skin reactions.

Selected Drug Interactions:

- Can cause rhabdomyolysis if given with lovastatin (Mevacor).
- May raise the PT level in patients on anticoagulant therapy.

Cautions:

- *Contraindicated in patients with hepatic or gallbladder disease, or severe renal dysfunction.*
- Should generally not be used in patients taking HMG-CoA inhibitors, such as Lovastatin (Mevacor), Simvastatin (Zocor), and Pravastatin (Pravachol), due to increased risk of rhabdomyolysis.

Pregnancy Category: C.

Cost: Generic \$\$\$, Lopid \$\$\$\$ (≈ \$0.50/generic tablet; ≈ \$1.15/Lopid tablet).

Pearls:

- It is recommended that gemfibrozil be taken 30 min before meals.
- Main clinical uses are for elevation of HDL cholesterol and, in patients with markedly elevated triglyceride levels, reduction of such triglyceride levels.

Genoptic: *see* GENTAMICIN SULFATE eye drops

GENTAMICIN (Garamycin)

Dose:

- Loading: 2 mg/kg.
- Maintenance: 1–1.67 mg/kg q8h IM or IV.

Actions: Bactericidal aminoglycoside antibiotic that irreversibly inhibits protein synthesis.

- Excellent aerobic gram (−) coverage, including some *Pseudomonas aeruginosa* (in some institutions, nosocomial *Pseudomonas* infections may be resistant).
- May be used with a penicillin, cephalosporin, or vancomycin for synergy against staph, strep, and enterococci.
- *Not* effective against anaerobes.

- *NOTE:* The above-mentioned antimicrobial coverage summary should be used as a guideline only; treatment decisions should take into account not only local epidemiologic patterns of antibiotic susceptibility but also, when available, culture susceptibility results.

Clearance: Renally excreted.

- Markedly reduce dosage or increase dosing interval in patients with impaired renal function.
- No change in dosage needed in patients with liver disease.
- Supplemental dose suggested after hemodialysis or peritoneal dialysis.

Selected Side Effects:

- Nephrotoxicity, ototoxicity, fever.
- Can increase neuromuscular blockade.

Selected Drug Interactions: Some cephalosporins, vancomycin, loop diuretics, cisplatin, and cyclosporin increase risk of nephrotoxicity or ototoxicity.

Pregnancy Category: Not established.

Cost: $; significantly less expensive than aztreonam, amikacin, or tobramycin.

Pearls:

- No significant CSF penetration.
- Can be administered intrathecally.
- Follow serum peak and trough levels. Each hospital and source has different peak and slightly different trough ranges; reasonable generalizations are peak levels 5–10 μg/mL and trough levels 2–4 μg/mL, but *each hospital's guidelines must be followed.*.

GENTAMICIN SULFATE eye drops and ointment (Garamycin Ophthalmic, Genoptic)

Dose:

- 1 or 2 drops (written "gtt") q4h; in severe infections may give up to 2 drops hourly (as directed by an ophthalmologist).
- 0.5 inches of ointment, applied to lower eye lid of affected eye(s) bid–tid.

Preparations:

- 3.5 g tube of ointment containing 0.3% gentamicin.
- 5 mL bottle of solution containing 0.3% gentamicin.

Actions: Antibiotic eye drop.
Cost: $$ (≈ $12 for a 5 mL bottle).
Pearls: Watch for toxicity from systemic absorption.

GLIPIZIDE (Glucotrol, Glucotrol XL)
Dose:
- Initial: 5 mg PO qd (2.5 mg in elderly patients and patients with liver dysfunction).
- Maximum: 40 mg daily.
- If total daily dose is > 15 mg, divide dose of Glucotrol and administer bid; patients taking Glucotrol XL do not need to have their daily dose divided.

PO Preparations:
- 5 and 10 mg tablets of Glucotrol.
- 5 and 10 mg tablets of extended release Glucotrol XL.

Actions: Oral hypoglycemic of sulfonylurea group used to treat noninsulin-dependent diabetes.
Clearance: Metabolized via liver.
- No change in dosage needed in patients with renal insufficiency.
- Initial dose in patients with liver disease should be 2.5 mg PO qd.

Selected Side Effects: *Hypoglycemia,* skin reactions, rare hyponatremia (secondary increased ADH secretion), rare disulfiram-like (Antabuse) reactions.
Selected Drug Interactions:
- Hypoglycemia is increased with other sulfonylureas, insulin, ASA, NSAIDs, sulfonamides, warfarin, MAOI, and β-blockers.
- Hyperglycemia is increased with diuretics, steroids, thyroid hormone, phenothiazines, phenytoin, nicotinic acid, sympathomimetics, isoniazid, and calcium channel blockers.

Pregnancy Category: C.
Cost: Generic $$, Glucotrol $$$ (≈ $0.40 each 10 mg generic tablet; ≈ $0.60 each 10 mg Glucotrol tablet); tolbutamide is significantly less expensive.
Pearls:
- Ideally taken 30 min before a meal.
- Signs and symptoms of hypoglycemia can be masked in elderly patients and in patients taking β-blockers.

- Duration of action of regular Glucotrol (ie, not extended release) is 12–18 h.
- Increased hypoglycemia is more common in elderly debilitated patients or patients with renal, hepatic, adrenal, or pituitary impairment; in alcohol use; and in severe or prolonged exercise.
- Increased hyperglycemia is more common with fever, trauma, infection, surgery, or other types of stress.

GLUCAGON
Dose: 1 mg (1 unit) SQ, IM or IV.
Preparations: 1 mg (1 unit) vials.
Actions:
- Pancreatic hormone that causes the liver to release glucose into the bloodstream.
- Usually used to replenish serum levels of glucose in hypoglycemic patients when IV access for direct injection of glucose is not available.
- May also ameliorate some effects of β-blocker overdose.
Selected Side Effects: Nausea and vomiting, rash, or allergic reactions.
Pearls:
- Useful for the treatment of hypoglycemia only in patients with adequate liver stores of glycogen.
- Can cause a pheochromocytoma to release catecholamines.
- Do not combine with normal saline while injecting.

Glucophage: *see* METFORMIN

Glucotrol: *see* GLIPIZIDE

GLYBURIDE (DiaBeta, Glynase, Micronase)
Dose: Brand preparation dependent:
- DiaBeta, Micronase:
  ▶ Initial: 2.5–5.0 mg PO qd (1.25 mg in more sensitive patients).
  ▶ Maximum: 20 mg daily, usually given as 10 mg bid.

- Glynase:
  - ▶ Initial: 1.5–3 mg PO qd (0.75 mg in more sensitive patients).
  - ▶ Maximum: 12 mg PO qd (can be given either qd or bid).

PO Preparations:
- DiaBeta, Micronase: 1.25, 2.5, and 5 mg tablets.
- Glynase: 1.5, 3, and 6 mg "Prestab" tablets.

Actions: Oral hypoglycemic agent of the sulfonylurea group; used to treat noninsulin-dependent diabetes.

Clearance: Metabolized via liver.
- No change in dosage needed in patients with renal insufficiency.

Selected Side Effects: *Hypoglycemia*, skin reactions, rare hyponatremia (secondary to increased ADH secretion), rare disulfiram-like (Antabuse) reactions.

Selected Drug Interactions:
- Increased hypoglycemia with other sulfonyl ureas, insulin, ASA, NSAIDs, sulfonamides, warfarin, MAOI, and β-blockers.
- Increased hyperglycemia with diuretics, steroids, thyroid hormone, phenothiazines, phenytoin, nicotinic acid, sympathomimetic drugs, isoniazid, and calcium channel blockers.

Pregnancy Category: B.

Cost: Generic $$, DiaBeta $$$ (≈ $0.35 each 5 mg generic tablet; ≈ $0.45 each 5 mg DiaBeta tablet); tolbutamide is significantly less expensive.

Pearls:
- *The bioavailability of glyburide is not equivalent between Glynase and the two other glyburide preparations (DiaBeta, Micronase), and thus if physician is switching between Glynase and these other brands, the optimal dose of these drugs must be reiterated.*
- Give with morning meal.
- Effectiveness decreases in many patients over time.
- Increases hypoglycemia in elderly, debilitated, or malnourished patients; in patients with renal, hepatic, adrenal, or pituitary impairment; in cases of alcohol use; and in severe or prolonged exercise.
- Signs and symptoms of hypoglycemia can be masked in elderly patients and in patients taking β-blockers.

- Glynase preparations more potent milligram for milligram, with 3 mg Glynase equivalent to 5 mg glyburide.

GLYCERIN suppository
Dose: 1 suppository (2.7 g) PR.
Actions: Laxative.
Pearls:
- Onset of action is 2–60 min.
- Should be retained in colon for 15–20 min.

Glynase: *see* GLYBURIDE

GM-CSF: *see* GRANULOCYTE-MACROPHAGE COLONY-STIMULATING FACTOR

GoLYTELY (POLYETHYLENE GLYCOL– ELECTROLYTE SOLUTION)
Dose: 4 L (yes, liters!) PO over several hours.
PO Preparations: 4 L jugs containing powder for reconstitution with water.
Actions: Nonabsorbable osmotic agent used for bowel preparation before GI examinations.
Selected Side Effects: Nausea, bloating, cramps, vomiting.
Cautions: *Contraindicated in suspected GI obstruction or perforation.*
Pregnancy Category: C.
Pearls:
- Must aggressively encourage patients to consume 4 L.
- Should be taken chilled.

GRANULOCYTE COLONY-STIMULATING FACTOR (G-CSF, Neupogen)
Dose (in patients receiving myelosuppressive chemotherapy):
- Initial: 5 µg/kg/day SQ or IV. (*NOTE:* Dose is in micrograms, *not* milligrams.)

- May increase in 5 μg/kg increments.
- Usually effective at doses of 4–8 μg/kg/day.
- IV administration should be given via either short (15–30 min) or continuous infusion (but not single administration bolus).

Actions: Hematopoietic growth factor that promotes proliferation, maturation, and migration of neutrophils; used to decrease the incidence of infections in patients with chemotherapy-related neutropenia.

Selected Side Effects: Bone pain (usually only mild, moderately severe; is more common in patients receiving higher doses, ie, ≥ 20 μg/kg/day), elevations in uric acid, LDH, or alkaline phosphatase (or both).

Cost: $$$$.

Pearls: Pretreat patients with acetaminophen for bone pain.

GRANULOCYTE-MACROPHAGE COLONY-STIMULATING FACTOR, SARGRAMOSTIM (GM-CSF, Leukine)

Dose:

- Chemotherapy patients (to decrease neutropenia): 5 μg/kg SQ daily. (*NOTE:* Dose is in micrograms, *not* milligrams.)
- Bone marrow transplant patients: 250 μg/m^2/day for 21 days after transplant.

Actions: Recombinant DNA-produced glycoprotein that stimulates proliferation and differentiation of hematopoietic progenitor cells; used to treat patients following bone marrow transplantation.

Selected Side Effects: Generally well tolerated; most side effects were no more common in treatment group than in placebo group. Watch for peripheral edema, pleural or pericardial effusion, dyspnea (from sequestration of granulocytes in pulmonary circulation), transient SVT. Fever occurs in 30% of patients and can be treated with acetaminophen.

Pregnancy Category: C.

Pearls:

- Follow CBC and differential twice weekly.
- In vitro activity includes stimulating proliferation or differentiation of progenitor cells; stimulating maturation cycle of

neutrophils, monocytes or macrophages, and eosinophils; and increasing function of mature neutrophils and monocytes or macrophages.
• Clinical effects in bone marrow transplant recipients include modest shortening of hospital stay, reduced duration of neutropenia, and possible decrease in infections and need for antibiotics.Treatment did not improve 1-year survival when compared with placebo.

GUAIFENESIN expectorant (Organidin NR, Robitussin; *see also* the various Robitussin preparations)

Dose:
• 200–400 mg PO q4h prn of Organidin NR, up to a maximum of 2400 mg in 24h.
• 2 tsp of Robitussin syrup q4h PO prn.

PO Preparations
• 200 mg tablets of Organidin NR.
• 4 and 8 oz bottles of Robitussin and many other preparations containing 100 mg/5 mL (1 tsp).

Actions: Medication that increases fluid production in the respiratory tract, which may help to liquefy and reduce viscosity of secretions; used to treat persistent cough.

Selected Side Effects: Can cause GI upset and diarrhea at higher doses.

Cautions: Preparations contain iodine; therefore patients with thyroid conditions should probably avoid use of guaifenesin.

Pregnancy Category: C.

Cost: $.

Pearls:
• Actual ability to stimulate secretions and clinical efficacy are controversial.
• Several reviews of cold medicines find little evidence to support their routine use.

GUANABENZ (Wytensin)

Dose:
• Initial: 4 mg PO bid.
• Maintenance: 4–16 mg PO bid.

PO Preparations: 4 and 8 mg tablets.

Actions: Centrally acting agent that stimulates cerebral α-receptors, causing decrease in sympathetic outflow from the brain; used to treat hypertension.

Clearance: Metabolized in liver to inactive metabolites.

- No change in dosage needed in patients with renal insufficiency.
- Reduce dosage in patients with liver disease.

Selected Side Effects: Drowsiness or sedation (frequent), dizziness, weakness, dry mouth.

Pregnancy Category: C.

Cost: $$$$ ($\approx$ $0.90 each 4 mg tablet).

Pearls:

- Abrupt discontinuance can cause rebound reaction, including elevated BP, tachycardia, anxiety, and insomnia.
- Warn patients of its sedative effects.

GUANETHIDINE (Ismelin)

Dose: 10–50 mg PO qd (some clinicians use doses up to 125 mg).

PO Preparations: 10 and 25 mg tablets.

Actions: Peripheral-acting agent that depletes presynaptic norepinephrine stores and decreases norepinephrine release, diminishing sympathetic output; used to treat hypertension.

Clearance: Metabolized via liver; renally excreted; nonrenal metabolism is increased in renal failure.

- Slightly increase dosing interval in patients with end-stage renal disease (GFR <10 mL/min); no change needed for milder renal impairment.
- Dosage should probably be reduced in patients with liver disease.

Selected Side Effects: Postural hypotension (common), impotence or retrograde ejaculation, diarrhea, nasal stuffiness, weakness, edema, bradycardia, azotemia.

Selected Drug Interactions:

- Over-the-counter drugs containing α-agonists (epinephrine, phenylpropanolamine, pseudoephedrine) can decrease its antihypertensive effect.
- Augments effects of antidiabetic agents.

Cautions:
- *Contraindicated in patients with known or suspected pheochromocytoma or hypovolemia.*
- *Avoid in heart failure and in patients taking MAOI.*
- Can worsen or exacerbate asthma.
- Can exacerbate peptic ulcer disease (through excess parasympathetic activity).
- Anesthesia can enhance hypotension and precipitate cardiovascular collapse.

Cost: $$.

Habitrol: *see* NICOTINE transdermal patch

Halcion: *see* TRIAZOLAM

Haldol: *see* HALOPERIDOL

HALOPERIDOL (Haldol)
Dose: Route and disease dependent:
- PO: 0.5–5.0 mg bid–tid.
- IM: 2–5 mg; may require further IM doses.
- "Sundowning": 0.5 mg or more PO or IM q4–6h prn; usual 1–5 mg PO or IM.

PO Preparations
- 0.5, 1, 2, 5, 10, and 20 mg tablets.
- 120 and 240 mL bottles of concentrate containing 2 mg/mL.

Actions: Butyrophenone that acts as a major tranquilizer and antipsychotic used to treat "sundowning" (the phenomenon in which elderly patients become confused at night) and many other psychological conditions.

Clearance: Metabolized via liver; renally excreted.
- No change in dosage needed in patients with renal insufficiency.
- May need to adjust dosage in patients with liver disease (these patients are more sensitive to CNS effects of phenothiazines).
- Supplemental dose not required after hemodialysis or peritoneal dialysis.

Selected Side Effects: Parkinsonian symptoms and other extrapyramidal reactions, *tardive dyskinesia, neuroleptic malignant syndrome,* confusion and numerous other CNS effects, anticholinergic effects (dry mouth, blurred vision, urine retention), cardiac effects (tachycardia, hypotension, ECG changes including QT prolongation).

Selected Drug Interactions:
- Can potentiate CNS depressant effects of other CNS depressants.
- Concomitant use with lithium can increase risk of neuroleptic malignant syndrome.

Cautions:
- *Contraindicated in Parkinson's disease.*
- Use with caution in patients with history of seizures (can lower the seizure threshold), severe cardiac disorders (can cause hypotension or angina), or thyrotoxicosis.

Pregnancy Category: C.

Cost: Generic $$, Haldol $$$$ (≈ $0.20 each 2 mg generic tablet; ≈ $90 each 2 mg Haldol tablet).

Pearls:
- Signs and symptoms of overdose include severe extrapyramidal reaction, hypotension, and oversedation.
- Signs of neuroleptic malignant syndrome include extreme rise in temperature, muscle rigidity and "lead-pipe" syndrome, mental status changes, autonomic instability, including irregular pulse or BP, greatly increased HR, diaphoresis, arrhythmias, rhabdomyolysis (with increased CPK, myoglobinuria, and acute renal failure).

HCTZ: *see* HYDROCHLOROTHIAZIDE

HEPARIN
Dose: Protocol dependent:
- SQ for DVT prophylaxis: 5000 units SQ q12h.
- Adjunctive therapy with thrombolytics for acute MI: 5000 unit IV bolus, then 1000 units/h IV; adjust maintenance drip based on PTT levels.
- Thrombotic events in which thrombolytics *are not given* (DVT, most cases of pulmonary embolus, etc): both a tradi-

tional standard-dosing regimen and a newer weight-adjusted regimen are used:

▶ Traditional standard regimen: 5000 unit IV bolus, then 1000 units/h IV; adjust maintenance drip based on PTT levels.

▶ Weight-adjusted regimen (*NOTE:* Multiple weight-adjusted regimens exist; the following is one suggested regimen: 80 units/kg IV bolus, then 18 units/kg/h IV drip. After initial maintenance drip is begun, adjust subsequent drip rates based on PTT levels).

Actions: Medication that potentiates anticoagulant action of antithrombin III; used to treat unstable angina, venous and arterial thrombosis, and many other clinical conditions.

Clearance: Metabolized via liver; renally excreted.

• No change in dosage needed in patients with renal insufficiency.

• One source that addresses dosage adjustment in patients with liver disease does not recommend any change.

• Supplemental dose not required after hemodialysis or peritoneal dialysis.

Selected Side Effects: Excess bleeding, mild decrease in platelets (common), significant decrease in platelets (rarer), thrombosis, rare hyperkalemia.

Cautions:

• *Contraindicated in patients with active bleeding, severe hypertension, ulcers, hemorrhagic CVA, pericarditis, metastases from hemorrhagic tumors, or recent surgery of the CNS or prostate.*

• Check with an ophthalmologist before giving to patients with retinopathy.

• Use with caution in patients taking platelet-inhibiting drugs.

Pregnancy Category: C.

Cost: $.

Pearls:

• *The results of several large thrombolytic trials in which weight-adjusted heparin regimens were used demonstrated an increased risk of serious bleeding complications; there-*

fore, more recent trials no longer use weight-adjusted heparin protocols as adjunctive treatment with thrombolytic therapy.

- Resistance to its effects is increased in thrombosis, phlebitis, infection, cancer, and postoperative state.
- Discontinue if the platelet count falls > 100,000/mL^3 from baseline value without other clear cause.
- Discontinue if thrombosis (also called "white clot syndrome") develops.
- A bolus dose is often not given if anticoagulating for new stroke (can increase the incidence of CNS hemorrhage).
- The search for an "ideal" PTT value for various thrombotic conditions is a continuing process, and recommendations may vary somewhat from expert to expert. At present, aiming for a PTT of 46–70 for unstable angina (and probably many other thrombotic conditions) appears reasonable. A higher value of 55–85 is being used in several trials of acute treatment of myocardial infarction involving thrombolytic ther-apy with TPA, and in patients receiving TPA, this higher PTT range of 55–85 may be a more reasonable goal to aim for.
- Dosage adjustments: There are almost as many methods for adjusting IV heparin to PTT levels as there are tired interns. The following protocol is designed to achieve a PTT in the range of 46–70. The first PTT should be drawn 6 h after initial heparin bolus, and subsequent PTTs should be drawn 6 h after any dosage changes. (*NOTE: This protocol* should not *be used in patients with acute myocardial infarction who have received thrombolytic therapy, because the "ideal" PTT range may be higher, and weight-adjusted heparinization is no longer recommended for patients receiving thrombolytic therapy.*)

PTT(s)	Adjustment
<<35	80 units/kg bolus and increase drip by 4 units/kg/h
35–45	40 unit/kg bolus and increase drip by 2 units/kg/h
46–70	No change
71–90	Reduce drip by 2 units/kg/h
90	Hold heparin for 1 h then reduce drip by 3 units/kg/h

Hismanal: *see* ASTEMIZOLE

Hivid: *see* ZALCITABINE

HYDRALAZINE (Apresoline)
Dose: Route dependent:
- PO: Initially give 10 mg PO qid for 2–4 days; then 25 mg PO qid until end of the first week of therapy; then 50 mg PO qid if clinically indicated.
- Parenteral: 20–40 mg IM or IV.

PO Preparations: 10, 25, 50, and 100 mg tablets.
Actions: Direct vasodilator; used to treat hypertension.
Clearance: Metabolized via liver; renally excreted.
- Slightly increase dosing interval in patients with end-stage renal disease; no change needed for milder renal insufficiency.
- Supplemental dose not required after hemodialysis or peritoneal dialysis.

Selected Side Effects: Postural hypotension, reflex tachycardia and palpitations or angina, systemic lupus erythematosus (SLE)-like reaction, (+) Coombs' reaction, blood dyscrasias.
Selected Drug Interactions:
- Decreases serum levels of propranolol and metoprolol.
- MAO inhibitors increase the risk of hypotension.

Cautions: *Contraindicated in patients with coronary artery disease or significant aortic stenosis*.
Pregnancy Category: C.
Cost: $ (≈ $0.06 each 50 mg tablet).
Pearls: Increases renal blood flow.

Hydrea: *see* HYDROXYUREA

HYDROCHLOROTHIAZIDE (Esidrix, HCTZ, HydroDIURIL, etc.; *see also* Aldactazide, Capozide, Dyazide, Hyzaar, Maxzide, Moduretic, Prinzide, Zestoretic)
Dose: 12.5–100 mg PO qod–qd.
PO Preparations
- 25, 50, and 100 mg tablets.

Actions: Thiazide diuretic used to treat hypertension and edema.

Clearance: Renally excreted.

- Avoid in patients with serum creatinine > 2.0 mg/dL.
- No change in dosage needed in patients with liver disease.

Selected Side Effects: Hypokalemia, hypomagnesemia, dilutional hyponatremia, orthostatic hypotension, glycosuria, hyperuricemia.

Selected Drug Interactions: Cholestyramine and colestipol reduce its absorption.

Cautions: Use with caution, if at all, in patients with history of glucose intolerance, gout, or sulfa allergy.

Pregnancy Category: B.

Cost: $.

Pearls:

- Follow serum K^+.
- Can detrimentally alter lipid and glucose metabolism (though the long-term effects and clinical relevance of lipid changes are controversial).
- 25 mg dose is as effective as higher doses in treatment of hypertension; the 12.5 mg dose may also have similar efficacy.

Hydrocodone: *see* Lorcet, Vicodin, Vicodin ES

HYDROCORTISONE (Hydrocortone, Solu-Cortef; *see also* HYDROCORTISONE suppositories, HYDROCORTISONE topical cream)

Dose: Preparation and route dependent:

- Hydrocortone (hydrocortisone sodium phosphate):
  - ▶ PO 20–240 mg qd.
  - ▶ IM or IV: 7.5–120 mg q12h.
- Solu-Cortef (hydrocortisone sodium succinate): 100–500 mg IM or IV q2–10h prn.

PO Preparations

- 10 and 20 mg tablets of Hydrocortone.

Actions:
- Corticosteroid used to treat adrenocortical insufficiency (one of two drugs of choice).
- May also be used intra-articularly and topically.

Clearance: Metabolized via liver.
- No change in dosage needed in patients with renal insufficiency.
- Dosage adjustment probably not needed in patients with liver disease.

Selected Side Effects:
- Acute: Na^+ and water retention (leading to increases in hypertension, edema, and CHF), elevated glucose, psychiatric disturbances ("steroid psychosis"), impaired wound healing, increased risk of peptic ulcer disease, increased catabolism.
- Chronic: Myopathy, osteoporosis, vertebral compression fractures, aseptic necrosis, CNS changes, edema.

Selected Drug Interactions:
- Decreases hypoglycemic effects of insulin and OHAs.
- Concomitant use with K^+-depleting diuretics increases risk of hypokalemia.
- Can prolong or shorten PT in patients taking warfarin.

Pregnancy Category: Not established.

Cost: $$.

Pearls:
- Can mask signs of infection.
- Patients may need "stress-dose" steroids during stress; usual stress dose for severe illness or surgery is 100 mg IV q8h.
- Relative activity comparison of commonly used steroids:

Steroid	Relative Anti-inflammatory and Glucocorticoid Activity	Relative Mineralocorticoid Activity
Cortisone	0.8	0.8
Hydrocortisone	1.0	1.0
Prednisone	4.0	0.8
Methylprednisolone	5.0	0.5
Dexamethasone	25–30	0.0

HYDROCORTISONE suppositories (Anusol-HC, other brands)

Dose: 1 suppository PR bid–tid.
PO Preparations: 25 mg suppositories of Anusol-HC.
Actions: Topical corticosteroid containing hydrocortisone; used to treat hemorrhoids.
Selected Side Effects:
• Local irritation and reactions.
• Can theoretically suppress adrenocortical axis if enough is absorbed.
Cost: $$$.
Pregnancy Category: C.

HYDROCORTISONE topical cream (Anusol-HC, Hytone, and many other brands)

Dose: Apply to skin bid–qid.
PO Preparations: 0.25%, 0.5%, and 1.0% are usual concentrations; Hytone available in 1 and 2.5% preparations; Anusol-HC available only as 2.5% preparation in 30 g tube.
Actions: Weak topical steroid used to treat many dermatologic conditions.
Selected Side Effects:
• Local irritation and reactions.
• Can theoretically suppress adrenocortical axis if enough is absorbed.
Pregnancy Category: C.
Cost: $.
Pearls: Concentrations of 0.25%, 0.5%, and 1.0% are available without prescription (over the counter).

Hydrocortone: *see* HYDROCORTISONE

HydroDIURIL: *see* HYDROCHLOROTHIAZIDE

HYDROMORPHONE (Dilaudid, Hydrostat IR)
Dose: Condition and route dependent:
- Analgesia:
  - ▶ PO: 2–4 mg q4–6h prn.
  - ▶ SQ or IM: Suggested starting dose is 1–2 mg q4–6h prn.
  - ▶ Suppository: 3 mg q4–6h prn.
- Cough: 5 mL of the syrup q3–4 h.

Preparations:
- 1, 2, 3, 4, and 8 mg tablets.
- 3 mg suppositories.
- 1 pint bottle of cough syrup containing 1 mg/5 mL (1 tsp).

Actions:
- Narcotic analgesic used to treat moderate to severe pain.
- Also has antitussive properties.

Clearance: Little information available; probably metabolized via liver.
- One source recommends using with caution in hepatic or renal failure.

Selected Side Effects: Drowsiness, mood changes, mental clouding, *depressed respiratory function*, depression of cough reflex, constipation, pinpoint pupils, increased parasympathetic activity, elevated CSF pressure.

Cautions:
- *Contraindicated in patients with CNS injury or lesions.*
- Use with caution in elderly or debilitated patients and in patients with impaired hepatic or renal function, hypothyroidism, Addison's disease, prostate hypertrophy, or urethral stricture.

Pregnancy Category: C.
Cost: $$ (≈ $0.35 each 2 mg tablet).
Pearls:
- Respiratory depression is the major dose-limiting side effect.
- Strong potential for addition.
- Should not be first-line therapy for cough suppression.

Hydrostat IR: *see* HYDROMORPHONE

Hydroxocobalamin: *see* COBALAMIN

HYDROXYUREA (Hydrea)
Dose: Tumor dependent. Usually given qd or q3d.
PO Preparations: 500 mg tablets.

Actions: Antineoplastic agent that probably inhibits DNA synthesis; used to treat myeloproliferative disorders.
- Now also used as adjunctive treatment for sickle cell anemia.

Clearance: Predominantly renally excreted.
- Moderately to markedly reduced dosage in patients with impaired renal function.

Selected Side Effects: *Bone marrow suppression,* stomatitis, anorexia, nausea and vomiting, diarrhea and constipation, megaloblastic erythropoiesis (not related to vitamin B_{12} or folate deficiency), occasional impairment of renal tubular function or alopecia.

Cautions: *Contraindicated if WBCs* < 2500 or platelets < 100,000.

Pregnancy Category: Not established; known teratogenic potential must be weighed against potential benefits.

Cost: $$$.

Pearls:
- Follow CBC, LFTs, BUN, and creatinine.
- Bone marrow suppression is dose-limiting side effect.
- The presence of macrocytosis and hypersegmentation of PMNs can be used to assess patient compliance.

HYDROXYZINE (Atarax, Vistaril)

Dose: Disease dependent:
- Anxiety: 50–100 mg PO qid.
- Pruritus: 25 mg PO tid–qid.
- Nausea and vomiting: 25–50 mg IM.
- Sedation before and after anesthesia: 50–100 mg PO or 25–100 mg IM.

PO Preparations
- 10, 25, 50, and 100 mg tablets.
- 4 oz and 1 pint bottles of Vistaril suspension containing 25 mg/5 mL (1 tsp).
- 1 pint bottles of Atarax syrup containing 10 mg/5 mL (1 tsp).

Actions: Drug chemically unrelated to either phenothiazines or benzodiazepines, with anxiolytic, antipruritic, and antihistamine properties; used to treat anxiety, and nausea and vomiting, and as a sedative and an antipruritic.

Clearance: Little data available for humans; undergoes extensive hepatic metabolism in rats.

Selected Side Effects: Dry mouth, drowsiness, rare tremor, and convulsions.

Selected Drug Interactions: Potentiates CNS depressant effects of other CNS depressants.

Cautions: Should not be used during early pregnancy or in potentially pregnant patients.

Pregnancy Category: *Contraindicated in early pregnancy.*

Cost: Generic $$, Vistaril $$$$ (≈ $0.20 each 20 mg generic tablet; ≈ $1 each 20 mg Vistaril tablet).

Hyperstat: *see* DIAZOXIDE

Hytrin: *see* TERAZOSIN

Hyzaar (LOSARTAN + HYDROCHLOROTHIAZIDE)

Dose:

- Initial: 1 tablet PO qd.
- Initial dose of 25 mg of losartan (a half tablet) should be used in patients with liver disease and those with possible volume depletion.
- Maximum: 100 mg of losartan PO daily.
- If antihypertensive effect at drug trough (approximately 24 h after administration) is inadequate, consider giving bid.

Preparations: Each tablet contains 50 mg losartan and 12.5 mg hydrochlorothiazide.

Actions: Combination angiotensin II receptor inhibitor and thiazide diuretic; used to treat hypertension.

Selected Side Effects: Hypokalemia, rare hyperkalemia, dizziness, possible hypotension in volume-depleted patients.

Cautions:

- *Contraindicated in pregnant patients during the second and third trimesters.*
- Use with caution in patients with liver disease.

Pregnancy Category: D. Losartan has the *potential to cause fetal damage and death during the second and third trimester of pregnancy. Therefore should not be taken during pregnancy, and should be discontinued if patient becomes pregnant.*

Cost: $$$ (≈ $1.20/tablet).
Pearls:
- Combination therapy with products such as Hyzaar should be initiated only if adequate blood pressure control is not obtained with the use of a single antihypertensive agent.
- Does not produce the chronic nonproductive cough that can occur with ACE inhibitors.
- Can be taken without regard to meals.
- In patients with severe renal impairment (creatinine clearance < 30 mL/min) thiazide diuretics are less effective, and loop diuretics are preferred therapy.

IBU, IBU-Tabs: *see* IBUPROFEN

IBUPROFEN (Advil, IBU, IBU-Tabs, Medipren, Motrin, Motrin IB, Nuprin, Rufen)
Dose: 200–800 mg PO qid.
PO Preparations:
- 200, 300, 400, 600, and 800 mg tablets.
- 4 and 16 oz bottles of Advil flavored suspension containing 100 mg/5 mL (1 tsp).

Actions: NSAID with analgesic and antipyretic activity that may work by inhibiting prostaglandin synthetase; used to treat inflammatory conditions and for pain relief.
Clearance: Metabolized via liver.
- No change in dosage needed in patients with renal insufficiency.

Selected Side Effects: GI bleeding and ulceration, fluid retention and edema, elevated LFTs, interstitial nephritis and exacerbation of "prerenal" renal failure, rash, prolonged bleeding time (from reversible platelet inhibition).
Selected Drug Interactions:
- Decreases natriuretic effect of diuretics.
- Raises serum level of lithium.
Cautions:
- *Use with* extreme *caution, if at all, in patients with history of upper GI bleeding or ulcer and in elderly patients.*
- Should not be used by women who wish to become pregnant (can cause uterine muscle contraction).

- Can cause premature closure of ductus arteriosus or complications during delivery when used during last trimester of pregnancy.

Pregnancy Category: *Use during pregnancy is not recommended.*

Cost: $$ ($\approx$ $0.20 each 800 mg tablet).

Pearls:

- 200 mg preparation is available over the counter prescription.
- Consider use of misoprostol (Cytotec) to protect the stomach during long-term therapy in patients at increased risk of upper GI bleeding.
- Should not be used during third trimester of pregnancy.
- Should ideally be taken with food or antacids (to possibly decrease GI irritation and ulceration).

IL-2: *see* INTERLEUKIN-2

IFEX: *see* IFOSFAMIDE

IFOSFAMIDE (IFEX)

Dose:

- Initial: 1.2 g/m^2 IV daily for 5 consecutive days.
- Repeat every 3 weeks or after recovery from hematologic toxicity.

Actions: Antineoplastic alkylating agent, chemically related to nitrogen mustard and a synthetic analogue of cyclophosphamide, that cross-links tumor cell DNA; used to treat malignancies.

Clearance: Hydroxylated to active metabolite by liver enzymes; activation of the inactive drug to its active metabolite may theoretically be less in patients with liver disease.

- Use with caution in patients with impaired renal function.

Selected Side Effects: *Hemorrhagic cystitis, myelosuppression,* alopecia, nausea and vomiting, CNS toxicity (somnolence, confusion, depressive psychosis, hallucinations), renal toxicity (usually tubular damage).

Selected Drug Interactions: Concomitant use with other chemotherapeutic agents increases myelosuppression.

Cautions: *Contraindicated in patients with severely depressed bone marrow or significant microscopic hematuria.*
Pregnancy Category: D.
Pearls:
- To decrease the incidence of hemorrhagic cystitis, give with an agent such as mesna (which may be included in the product preparation) and hydrate vigorously.
- If microscopic hematuria (> 10 RBCs/high-power field) is present, withhold subsequent doses until resolved. Check urinalysis periodically after treatment.
- Obtain CBC prior to use and periodically after treatment; postpone treatment for WBCs < 2000 or platelets < 50,000.

Ilotycin: *see* ERYTHROMYCIN ophthalmic ointment

Imdur: *see* ISOSORBIDE MONONITRATE

Imipenem: *see* Primaxin

IMIPRAMINE (Tofranil, Tofranil PM)
Dose (for depression):
- Hospitalized patients:
  - ▶ Initial: 100 mg PO daily, given in divided doses of Tofranil or a single dose of Tofranil PM.
  - ▶ Can increase dose gradually up to 200–300 mg PO daily, given in divided doses of Tofranil or a single dose of Tofranil PM.
- Outpatients:
  - ▶ Initial: 75 mg PO of Tofranil daily, given in divided doses of Tofranil or a single dose of Tofranil PM.
  - ▶ Usual maintenance dose is 50–150 mg PO daily, given in divided doses of Tofranil or a single dose of Tofranil PM.
  - ▶ Maximum outpatient dose is 200 mg PO daily, given in divided doses of Tofranil or a single dose of Tofranil PM.
- Doses of Tofranil PM can be taken at bedtime; higher once-a-day doses of Tofranil PM should generally only be

initiated after optimal doses are titrated using bid administration.

Preparations:
- 10, 25, and 50 mg tablets of Tofranil.
- 75, 100, 125, and 150 mg tablets of Tofranil PM.

Actions: Tricyclic antidepressant.
- Mode of action is believed to involve blocking uptake of norepinephrine at synapse.

Selected Side Effects: Drowsiness, multiple cardiovascular effects (including effects on the conduction system, such as QT interval prolongation; similar to effects of type Ia antiarrhythmics such as quinidine: hypotension or postural hypotension), anticholinergic effects (dry mouth, blurred vision, tachycardia, etc), numerous psychiatric and neurologic side effects, photosensitivity.

Selected Drug Interactions:
- *Coadministration with MAOI may lead to hypertensive crisis, convulsions, and death.*
- Cimetidine raises its serum level.
- May potentiate the effects of catecholamines (including those in decongestants).

Cautions:
- *Contraindicated within 2 weeks of MAOI therapy and in acute post-MI recovery period.*
- Use with caution in patients with cardiovascular disease, thyroid disease, or history of urine retention, glaucoma, or seizures (lowers the seizure threshold).

Pregnancy Category: Not established.

Cost: $ (≈ $0.10 each 50 mg tablet).

Pearls:
- Is the original tricyclic antidepressant.
- Contains sulfites and may precipitate allergic reaction in patients with sulfite sensitivity.
- Caution patients to avoid excessive direct sunlight due to possibility of photosensitivity.

Imodium: *see* **LOPERAMIDE**

Imuran: *see* **AZATHIOPRINE**

INDAPAMIDE (Lozol)
Dose: 2.5 mg PO qd.
PO Preparations: 1.25 and 2.5 mg tablets.
Actions: Diuretic with some additional vasodilating actions; used to treat hypertension and CHF.
Selected Side Effects: Hypokalemia, hyponatremia, hyperuricemia, possible aggravation of latent or overt diabetes.
Selected Drug Interactions: Manufacturer notes that diuretics generally should not be used concomitantly with lithium (they reduce its renal clearance and add to risk of lithium toxicity).
Pregnancy Category: B.
Cost: $$$ (≈ $0.70 each 2.5 mg tablet).
Pearls:
- Manufacturer notes that doses of 5.0 mg or higher are associated with more frequent and severe hypokalemia with no apparent additional benefit in the treatment of hypertension or CHF.
- Advantages of indapamide over hydrochlorothiazide include less K^+ wasting, less elevation of uric acid levels, and fewer adverse effects on lipid profiles and glucose tolerance; however, it is considerably more expensive.

Inderal, Inderal LA: *see* PROPRANOLOL

Indocin, Indocin SR: *see* INDOMETHACIN

INDOMETHACIN (Indocin, Indocin SR)
Dose: Preparation dependent.
- Indocin: 25–50 mg PO tid (with food or antacids) or one 50 mg rectal suppository bid—tid.
- Indocin SR: One 75 mg capsule PO qd–bid.
Preparations:
- 25 and 50 mg capsules of Indocin.
- 75 mg sustained-release capsules of Indocin SR.
- 50 mg rectal suppositories.
- 237 mL bottle of oral suspension containing 25 mg/5 mL (1 tsp).

Actions: Nonsteroidal anti-inflammatory agent with analgesic and antipyretic actions; used to treat inflammation and for pain relief.

Clearance: Metabolized via liver.

- Sources disagree on whether dosage should be changed in patients with impaired renal function.
- Supplemental dose not required after hemodialysis.

Selected Side Effects: GI irritation, nausea, dyspepsia, upper GI bleeding, proteinuria, interstitial nephritis, nephrotic syndrome, worsening of "prerenal" renal failure, prolonged bleeding time, CNS effects (especially in elderly patients).

Cautions:

- *Contraindicated in patients with salicylate sensitivity, ulcer, or history of upper GI bleeding.*
- Should not be used during third trimester of pregnancy.
- Can cause premature closure of the ductus arteriosus when used during last trimester of pregnancy.

Pregnancy Category: *Use during pregnancy is not recommended.*

Cost: Generic $$, Indocin $$$$ (generic ≈ $0.25 each 50 mg tablet, Indocin ≈ $0.80 each 50 tablet).

Pearls: Should ideally be taken with food or antacids (to possibly decrease GI irritation and ulceration).

INH: *see* ISONIAZID

Inocor: *see* AMRINONE

INSULIN

Dose: Highly variable. One suggested initial dose is 10–20 units NPH or Humulin N SQ every morning with dosage adjustments based on subsequent fingerstick glucose tests.

Preparations: *See under* **Pearls.**

Clearance: Metabolized via liver; renally excreted.

- Slight reduction in dosage in patients with impaired renal function is generally suggested.

- Special care should be taken when adjusting dosage in patients with worsening renal failure (the body's needs for insulin can sometimes rise or fall).

Selected Side Effects: Local reactions, severe systemic allergic reactions, insulin reaction (symptoms include fatigue, nervousness, confusion, trembling, headache, nausea, cold sweats), hunger, weight gain.

Selected Drug Interactions:

- Concomitant use of alcohol, disopyramide, MAOI, OHA, or high-dose salicylates increases risk of hypoglycemia.
- Concomitant use with steroids, diuretics, phenytoin, sympathomimetics, or thyroid hormone increases risk of hyperglycemia.

Pregnancy: Does not cross the placenta, and benefits of treatment probably outweigh any potential risks during pregnancy.

Cost: $$.

Pearls:

- Insulin requirements are increased in high fever, obesity, hyperthyroidism, severe infection, trauma, surgery, and Cushing's syndrome.
- Insulin requirements may be decreased in hepatic dysfunction, impaired renal function, hypothyroidism, nausea and vomiting, increased activity (exercise), hypopituitarism, and adrenal insufficiency.
- Only regular insulin can be given IV.
- Systemic and local allergic reactions are very rare now that purified human insulin is used.
  - ▶ *"Sliding-Scale" Insulin Protocol:*
  - ▶ While in the hospital, many patients are put on a "sliding-scale" regimen of regular short-acting insulin, given SQ q4h or q6h, with the dose based on fingerstick glucose levels. When such a regimen is ordered, dosage should be based on the patient's usual insulin requirements. Patients should rarely receive morning doses of longer-acting insulin while on a sliding-scale insulin regimen (both can peak at the same time and cause hypoglycemia: NPH given at 7 AM and regular insulin given at 11 AM would both peak at 3 PM). A "typical" regimen follows, though

all physicians and diabetologists have their own approach:

▶ *Regular insulin SQ, sliding scale q6h, with fingerstick glucose tests:*

Glucose Level	SQ Regular Insulin
0–180	0 Units
181–240	2 Units
241–300	3 Units
301–350	4 Units
351–400	5 Units
>>400	Call MD

• Available mixtures and kinetics (human insulin preparations):

Insulin	Onset (hours)	Peak (hours)	Duration (hours)
Regular	0.5–1	2–3	3–6
NPH	2–4	4–10	10–16
Lente	3–4	4-12	12–18
Ultralente	6–10	8–12	18–20

Intal: *see* CROMOLYN SODIUM

Intropin: *see* DOPAMINE

INTERFERON (ALPHA INTERFERON, Intron A, Roferon-A)

Dose: Dose dependent; given IM or SQ.
Actions: Naturally occurring single-chain proteins that bind to specific cell membrane receptors. Their numerous effects include enhancing synthesis of antiviral enzymes, enhancing cellular antigen expression, increasing activity of natural killer cells and phagocytic macrophages, and antitumor actions. Tumors in which interferon are used include CML, melanoma, and myeloma.

Clearance: Sources vary. *PDR* states that interferons are filtered in the glomeruli and undergo proteolytic degradation during tubular reabsorption; another source notes that the majority of a dose is thought to be metabolized with none filtered or secreted by the kidneys.

Selected Side Effects: Numerous (some quite common): Extremely frequent flu-like symptoms (including fever, fatigue, myalgia, headache, chills, arthralgias), extremely frequent GI symptoms (including anorexia, nausea and vomiting, diarrhea, abdominal pain), extremely frequent dizziness, cough, alopecia, weight loss, dryness or inflammation of the oropharynx, rash, night sweats, pruritis, change in taste, confusion and mental status changes, paresthesias and numbness, elevated LFTs, leukopenia, neutropenia, thrombocytopenia.

Cautions: Use with caution in patients with severe cardiac disease, renal disease, hepatic disease, seizure disorders, or CNS dysfunction.

Pregnancy Category: C.

Cost: $$$ 1/2 .

INTERLEUKIN-2 (IL-2, Proleukin)

Dose: Disease and regimen dependent; given IV.

Actions: Lymphokine protein that binds to T cells and, among its actions, induces mitosis and cell transformation, stimulates helper T cells, and induces production of cytotoxic lymphocytes with antitumor activity; used to treat malignancies.

Clearance: Believed to be primarily renally metabolized.

Selected Side Effects: Fever and chills, nausea and vomiting, rash and pruritus, nasal congestion, fluid retention and pulmonary edema, hypotension.

Selected Drug Interactions: Glucocorticoids block all its actions.

Cautions: Use with caution in patients with history of cardiopulmonary disease.

Pearls:

- Its hypotensive effects usually occur 2–4 h after injection.
- Follow BP and fluid status and periodically examine the lungs for signs of pulmonary edema.

Intron A: *see* INTERFERON

Intropin: *see* DOPAMINE

IPECAC syrup
Dose: 15–30 mL of syrup with 200–300 mL water.
PO Preparations: Solution containing 70 mg/mL.
Actions: Emetic that induces vomiting; used to treat recent drug overdose.
Selected Side Effects: Cardiovascular disturbances if absorbed (which can occur if not vomited within 30 min of ingestion or if chronically abused).
Selected Drug Interactions: Activated charcoal neutralizes its emetic effect.
Cautions:
• *Contraindicated in patients who have ingested caustic substances or petroleum distillates, and in those patients with diminished mental status (due to risk of aspiration with emesis).*
• Use with caution in esophageal disease.
Pearls:
• Induces vomiting within 30 min in > 90% of patients.
• Average onset of action < 20 min.

IPRATROPIUM (Atrovent)
Dose:
• Usual: 2–4 inhalations from metered-dose inhaler qid.
• Maximum: 12 inhalations in 24 h.
PO Preparations: 14 g metered-dose inhaler, supplied with mouthpiece, that provides sufficient medicine for 200 inhalations.
Actions: Anticholinergic antimuscarinic bronchodilator, chemically related to atropine, that blocks smooth muscle muscarinic receptors; used to treat reactive airway disease.
Selected Side Effects: Cough.
Cautions: Use with caution in narrow-angle glaucoma, prostate hypertrophy, or bladder neck obstruction.
Pregnancy Category: B.

Cost: $$$ (≈ $40 each inhaler).
Pearls: Now felt by some practitioners to be first-line therapy for COPD.

IRON: *see* FERROUS SULFATE

Ismelin: *see* GUANETHIDINE

Ismo: *see* ISOSORBIDE MONONITRATE

ISOETHARINE (Bronkometer, Bronkosol)
Dose: Delivery dependent.
- Bronkometer: 1 or 2 inhalations, usually no more frequently than q4h.
- Bronkosol nebulizer: 0.5 mL in 2.5 mL NS q2–4h.

Preparations: Bronkometer: available in 10 and 15 mL vials with oral nebulizer.
Actions: Short-acting sympathomimetic amine with β-receptor affinity that produces bronchodilatation; used to treat reactive airway disease.
- Primarily stimulates β_2 receptors, but also has some β_1 stimulating action.

Selected Side Effects: Headache, anxiety, restlessness, tremor, insomnia, dizziness, tachycardia, palpitations, BP changes, nausea.
Cautions: Use with caution in patients with CAD, arrhythmias, hypertension, or hyperthyroidism.
Pregnancy Category: Not established.
Cost: $$$ (≈ $37 each inhaler).

ISONIAZID (INH, Nydrazid)
Dose:
- Treatment of TB (with adjunctive therapy) 5 mg/kg PO or IM qd (up to a maximum of 300 mg qd).
- Prevention of TB: 300 mg PO or IM qd.

PO Preparations: 300 mg tablets.
Actions: Antimycobacterial antibiotic that inhibits synthesis of mycolic acid; used to treat mycobacterial infections.

Clearance: Metabolized primarily via liver; 5–30% excreted unchanged in urine.
- Slightly decrease dosage for slow acetylators with impaired renal function.
- Reduce dosage in moderate to severe liver disease.
- Supplemental dose suggested after hemodialysis or peritoneal dialysis.

Selected Side Effects: *Elevated LFTs and hepatitis (age-related),* peripheral neuropathy (especially in diabetics, alcohol abusers, and malnourished patients), pyridoxine (vitamin B) deficiency, reduced WBCs, mental status changes, (+) ANA titer.

Selected Drug Interactions: Reduces excretion of phenytoin or enhances its effects.

Cautions:
- *Contraindicated in patients with active liver disease.*
- Try to avoid in pregnant or potentially pregnant patients.

Pregnancy Category: Not established and available data conflicting; consider beginning preventive therapy *after* delivery if possible.

Cost: $.

Pearls:
- Often given with pyridoxine 10 mg PO qd to prevent peripheral neuritis.
- Follow LFTs.

Isoptin, Isoptin SR: *see* VERAPAMIL

Isordil, Isordil Tembids: *see* ISOSORBIDE DINITRATE

ISOSORBIDE DINITRATE (Dilatrate SR, Isordil, Isordil Tembids; *see also* ISOSORBIDE MONONITRATE)

Dose: Preparation dependent:
- Regular-acting preparations: 10–40 mg PO qid of Isordil.
- Long-acting preparations: 40–80 mg PO bid–tid of Isordil Tembids or Dilatrate SR.

PO Preparations:
- 5, 10, 20, 30, and 40 mg tablets.
- 40 mg long-acting Isordil Tembids and Dilatrate SR sustained release capsules.

Actions: Vasodilator (mainly of veins and coronary arteries) used to treat CAD.

Clearance: Metabolized via liver; 20% renally excreted.
- No change in dosage needed in patients with renal insufficiency.

Selected Side Effects:
- Hypotension, reflex tachycardia, headache, and flushing.
- Can cause anemia in patients with G6PD deficiency.

Pregnancy Category: C.

Cost: $.

Pearls:
- A drug-free interval is recommended to avoid developing tolerance.
- One mononitrate preparation (Imdur) has been shown to interfere with an assay of serum cholesterol levels and may cause false low measurements of serum cholesterol level.

ISOSORBIDE MONONITRATE
(Imdur, Ismo, Monoket; *see also* ISOSORBIDE DINITRATE)

Dose: Preparation dependent:
- Imdur:
  - ▶ Initial: 30-60 mg PO qd.
  - ▶ Usual maximum: 120 mg PO qd (up to 240 mg may be rarely required).
- Ismo: 20 mg PO bid, with the two doses taken 7 h apart.
- Monoket: Usual dose is 20 mg PO bid, with the two doses taken 7 h apart.

PO Preparations:
- Imdur: 60 mg scored extended release tablets.
- Ismo: 20 mg scored tablets.
- Monoket: 10 and 20 mg tablets.

Actions: Vasodilator (mainly of veins and coronary arteries) used to treat CAD.

Clearance: Metabolized via liver.
- No change in dosage needed in patients with renal insufficiency.

Selected Side Effects: Hypotension, headache, and flushing.

Pregnancy Category: B or C (surprisingly, different preparations have different ratings).

Cost: $$$ ($\approx$ $0.75 each 30 mg Ismo tablet; $\approx$ $1 each 60 mg Imdur tablet).

Pearls:
- Isosorbide mononitrate is the major active metabolite of isosorbide dinitrate.
- One preparation (Imdur) has been shown to interfere with an assay of serum cholesterol levels and may cause false low measurements of serum cholesterol level.
- Taking medication with food does not decrease overall absorption.

ISOTRETINOIN (Accutane)

Dose: 0.25–1.0 mg/kg PO bid.

PO Preparations: 10, 20, and 40 mg capsules.

Actions: Retinoid that inhibits sebaceous gland function and keratinization; used to treat recalcitrant cystic acne.

Selected Side Effects: Dry skin, cheilitis, conjunctivitis, skeletal hyperostosis, arthralgias and other musculoskeletal symptoms, elevation of triglycerides, elevated erythrocyte sedimentation rates (ESR), elevated LFTs and hepatotoxicity, elevated CPK, elevated fasting glucose.

Cautions: *Contraindicated in pregnant or potentially pregnant patients.*

Pregnancy Category: X; *has been associated with major fetal abnormalities.*

Cost: $.

Pearls:
- Patients should not take multivitamin preparations containing vitamin A (to avoid possible toxicity).
- Follow LFTs, triglycerides, and serum glucose.
- Warn patients of possible reduced tolerance for contact lenses, *of the absolute necessity to avoid pregnancy,*

of frequent side effects listed above, and to avoid donating blood during therapy and for at least 1 month afterward.

- Female patients need to use contraceptives while on isotretinoin; female patients need monthly serum HCG testing before refills are given.
- Patients should have discontinued other oral acne medications (especially tetracycline) while on isotretinoin.
- Total treatment duration usually 15–20 weeks.

ISRADIPINE (DynaCirc)
Dose:
- Initial: 2.5 mg PO bid.
- Maintenance: 2.5–10 mg PO bid.

PO Preparations: 2.5 and 5 mg capsules.
Actions: Calcium channel blocker used to treat hypertension.
Clearance: Metabolized primarily via liver.
- May need to reduce dosage in liver and renal disease (because bioavailability is increased), but starting dose should remain unchanged.

Selected Side Effects: Dizziness, edema, tachycardia, palpitations, flushing.
Pregnancy Category: C.
Cost: $$$ (≈ $0.60 each 2.5 mg capsule).
Pearls: Allow 2–4 weeks to achieve maximum antihypertensive effect before adjusting dosage.

ITRACONAZOLE (Sporanox)
Dose:
- 200 mg PO qd.
- If no response, for some infections can increase to 300 and then 400 mg PO qd.
- In cases of life-threatening infections, a loading dose of 200 mg PO tid for the first 3 days can be considered.

Preparations: 100 mg capsules.
Actions: Systemic antifungal agent that inhibits the cytochrome P-450-dependent synthesis of ergosterol, a vital component of fungal cell membranes.

Clearance: Metabolized via liver.
- No dose adjustment necessary in patients with renal insufficiency.
- Careful monitoring or dose adjustment may be prudent in patients with hepatic insufficiency.
- Supplemental dose probably not required after hemodialysis.

Selected Side Effects: Nausea and vomiting, rash, elevated LFTs, possible rare cases of hepatitis.
Selected Drug Interactions: Increases serum level of terfenadine (Seldane).
Cautions: *Coadministration of itraconazole with terfenadine (Seldane) or astemizole (Hismanal) is contraindicated.*
Pregnancy Category: C.
Cost: $$$$ (≈ $6/capsule).
Pearls: Should be taken with food to increase absorption.

Kaopectate liquid (KAOLIN + PECTIN)
Dose: 60–120 mL (4–8 tbsp) PO after each bowel movement or prn.
PO Preparations: 3, 8, 12, and 16 oz and 1 gallon bottles.
Pregnancy Category: C.
Cost: $.
Pearls: Can reduce absorption of other PO drugs.

Kaopectate tablets (300 mg ATTAPULGITE)
Dose:
- 1200 mg (4 tablets) PO after each bowel movement.
- Maximum, 14 tablets in 24 h.
- Swallow tablets whole with water.

PO Preparations: Packs of 16 tablets.

Kayexalate: *see* SODIUM POLYSTYRENE SULFONATE

K-Dur: *see* POTASSIUM CHLORIDE

K-Phos: *see* PHOSPHORUS

Keflex: *see* CEPHALEXIN

Keftab: *see* CEPHALEXIN

Kefurox: *see* CEFUROXIME

Kefzol: *see* CEFAZOLIN

KETOCONAZOLE (Nizoral); *see also* the following entry, KETOCONAZOLE topical

Dose:
- Usual lower dose: 200 mg PO qd.
- Maximum dose varies from 600–1200 mg daily with different sources.

PO Preparations: 200 mg tablets.

Actions: Synthetic agent that impairs synthesis of ergosterol (a vital component of fungal cell membranes); used to treat fungal infections.

Clearance: Metabolized via liver; excreted via biliary tract.
- No change in dosage needed in patients with renal insufficiency.
- Reduce dosage, if used at all, in significant liver disease.

Selected Side Effects: *Elevated LFTs and hepatotoxicity.*

Selected Drug Interactions:
- Coadministration of ketoconazole and the antihistamine terfenadine (Seldane) can lead to prolongation of the QT interval and life-threatening ventricular arrhythmias.
- Antacids, sucralfate, H-blockers, and omeprazole decrease its absorption (requires acidity for dissolution).
- Isoniazid and rifampin reduce its serum level.
- Can prolong PT in patients taking warfarin.
- Coadministration with phenytoin can alter metabolism of both drugs.

Cautions: *Coadministration of ketoconazole and the antihistamine terfenadine (Seldane) can lead to prolongation of the QT interval and life-threatening ventricular arrhythmias; coadministration of ketoconazole and terfenadine (Seldane) or astemizole (Hismanal) is contraindicated.*

Pregnancy Category: C.
Cost: $$$$ (≈ $3/tablet).
Pearls:
- No significant CSF penetration.
- Check LFTs before and at frequent intervals during therapy.
- May be taken without regard to meals.

KETOCONAZOLE topical (Nizoral topical)
Dose: Apply to skin qd–bid.
Preparations: 15, 30, and 60 g tubes of 2% cream.
Actions: Topical antifungal; used to treat tinea and candidal skin infections.
Selected Side Effects: Skin irritation, stinging, pruritus, allergic reactions.
Pregnancy Category: C.
Cost: $$$$ (≈ $35 for a 30 g tube).

KETOROLAC (Toradol)
Dose:
- PO: 10 mg q4–6h prn for limited duration (5–14 days).
- IM: 30–60 mg initially, then 15–30 mg q6h prn.
- IV: 30–60 mg initially, then 15–30 mg q6h prn; IV doses may be administered as either IV bolus over 1–5 min or mixed with either D5W or NS and infused over 15–30 min.

PO Preparations: 10 mg tablets.
Actions: NSAID that may be given IM for short-term management of pain.
Clearance: $t_{1/2}$ is prolonged in renal failure and in elderly patients.
- Reduce dosage in renal failure, in elderly patients, and in patients weighing 250 kg.

Selected Side Effects:
- GI distress, peptic ulceration, *GI bleeding,* edema, worsening of "prerenal" renal failure.
- Chronic use can cause kidney damage.

Cautions:
- *Contraindicated in patients with allergy to ASA or NSAIDs, nasal polyps, or history of angioedema.*

- Use with extreme caution in patients with CHF, ascites, cirrhosis, or decreased renal function, and in elderly patients.

Pregnancy Category: C.

Cost: $$.

Pearls:

- Onset of action for IM preparation is 10–15 min; peak effect occurs within 2 h.
- Can have comparable analgesic effect to meperidine and morphine (30 mg IM has analgesic efficacy comparable to morphine 12 mg IM).
- Administration of IV intravenously is currently under FDA evaluation.
- IM or IV administration is recommended for not more than 5 days; PO administration is recommended for not more than 5–14 days; if used chronically, PO doses should be taken tid or less (ie, not qid or more).
- PO doses should ideally be taken with food or antacids (to possibly decrease GI irritation and ulceration).
- Limited evidence suggests that analgesic potency is greater than its anti-inflammatory potency.
- Note that GI side effects can occur even when administered IM or IV.

Klonopin: *see* CLONAZEPAM

Kwell: *see* LINDANE cream and lotion

LABETALOL (Normodyne, Trandate)

Dose: Delivery dependent.

- PO:
  - ▶ Initial: 100 mg bid.
  - ▶ May be increased q2–3d in increments of 100 mg bid.
  - ▶ Usual maintenance: 200–400 mg bid.
  - ▶ Maximum: 600–1200 mg bid.
- IV:
  - ▶ Initial: 20 mg IV over 2 min.
  - ▶ Additional doses of 40–80 mg may be given at 10 min intervals until satisfactory response or total of 300 mg is reached.

PO Preparations: 100, 200, and 300 mg tablets.

Actions: Nonselective β-blocker that also selectively blocks α-receptors used to treat hypertension.

Clearance: Metabolized primarily via liver.

- No change in dosage needed in patients with renal insufficiency.
- Reduce dosage in patients with liver disease.
- Supplemental dose not required after hemodialysis or peritoneal dialysis.

Selected Side Effects: Fatigue, dizziness, nausea, worsening of heart failure, postural hypotension, AV block, bronchospasm, rare liver toxicity.

Selected Drug Interactions: Cimetidine increases its bioavailability.

Cautions: *Contraindicated in CHF, reactive airway disease, severe bradycardia, and second- or third-degree heart block.*

Pregnancy Category: C.

Cost: $$$ (≈ $0.50 each 100 mg tablet).

Pearls:

- Maximum effect of IV dose usually occurs within 5 min after injection.
- Does not lead to significant bradycardia.
- When discontinuing, taper gradually to avoid "β-blocker withdrawal."
- Can produce falsely elevated measured levels of urinary catecholamines and false (+) urine tests for amphetamines.

LACTULOSE

Dose: Disease dependent:

- Laxative:
  - ▶ Initial 15–30 mL PO qd.
  - ▶ May increase to 60 mL PO qd.
- Encephalopathy:
  - ▶ PO: initially 30–45 mL hourly until diarrhea occurs, then 30–45 mL tid–qid to produce 2 or 3 soft stools each day.
  - ▶ PR: 300 mL lactulose with 700 mL water q4–6h.

Preparations: 10 g/15 mL syrup.

Actions:

- Disaccharide sugar metabolized in the colon to low-molecular-weight acid metabolites that raise osmotic pressure and promote bowel evacuation.

- Also acidifies stool, inhibiting bacterial production of NH.
- Used as a laxative and to treat hepatic encephalopathy.

Clearance: > 97% not absorbed.

Selected Side Effects: Severe diarrhea, hypernatremia.

Selected Drug Interactions: Concomitant use with neomycin can reduce its effectiveness (can destroy saccharolytic bacteria in the colon).

Pregnancy Category: B.

Cost: $.

Lamictal: *see* LAMOTRIGINE

LAMOTRIGINE (Lamictal)

Dose: Dependent on whether patients are taking enzyme-inducing antiepileptic drugs or valproic acid.

- Patients not on enzyme-inducing antiepileptic drugs or valproic acid: Initial 50 mg PO qd for 2 weeks, then 100 mg PO bid for 2 weeks; can then increase dose in 50 mg bid increments (ie, 100 mg daily) up to maintenance dose of 150–250 mg PO bid.
- In patients taking enzyme-inducing antiepileptic drugs or valproic acid, the doses are lower (see package insert *PDR*, etc).

Preparations: 25, 100, 150, and 200 mg tablets.

Actions: Anticonvulsant; used as adjunctive therapy in the treatment of partial seizures and possibly other types of seizures.

Clearance: Predominantly metabolized; some renal excretion.

- Dose reduction suggested in patients with significant renal insufficiency.

Selected Side Effects: Rash (usually occurs during the first 4–6 weeks of treatment; occasionally progresses to a serious rash requiring hospitalization), headache, nausea, dizziness, rhinitis, diplopia and blurred vision, vaginitis.

Selected Drug Interactions:

- Carbamazepine, phenobarbital, primidone, and phenytoin all significantly decrease its serum concentration.
- Valproic acid doubles its serum concentration.

Pregnancy Category: C.
Pearls:
- Should not be abruptly discontinued.
- Absorption not impaired by food.
- Advise patients to notify their physician immediately if they develop a skin rash.

Lanoxin: *see* DIGOXIN

Lanoxicaps: *see* DIGOXIN

LANSOPRAZOLE (Prevacid)
Dose:
- Duodenal ulcer: 15 mg PO qd for 4 weeks.
- Erosive esophagitis: 30 mg PO qd for up to 8 weeks.

Preparations: 15 and 30 mg delayed-release capsules.
Actions: Inhibits the proton pump in gastric parietal cells, thus inhibiting gastric acid secretion; used for the *short-term* treatment of duodenal ulcers and esophagitis.
Clearance: Metabolized via liver to inactive metabolites; no significant renal excretion.
- No dose adjustment necessary in patients with renal insufficiency.
- Consider dose reduction in patients with severe liver disease.

Selected Side Effects: Minimal common side effects.
Selected Drug Interactions:
- Sulcrafate decreases its absorption.
- Can interfere with drugs absorbed at acid gastric pH (ketoconazole, ampicillin, iron salts, etc).

Pregnancy Category: B.
Cost: $$$$ (≈ $3 each 15 mg tablet).
Pearls:
- Should be taken before eating.
- When used to treat *Helicobacter pylori* infections, must be started at the same time as antibiotics; if started before, the eradication rate drops precipitously to 20%.
- Patients who are on long-term therapy should have their serum gastrin levels monitored; significantly elevated levels may be an indication to switch therapy to an H_2-blocker.

Lasix: *see* **FUROSEMIDE**

Lescol: *see* **FLUVASTATIN**

Leukeran: *see* **CHLORAMBUCIL**

Levlen oral contraceptive (LEVONORGESTREL + ETHINYL ESTRADIOL)

Dose: 1 tablet PO qd.

- With 21-day regimen, take no pills on days 22–28 then begin a new cycle (3 weeks on, 1 week off).
- Take first pill of Levlen 21 on day 5 of menstrual cycle.
- Take first pill of Levlen 28 the first Sunday after onset of menses, or that Sunday if it is the first day of menses.

PO Preparations: Available in 21- and 28-pill preparations.

- Last 7 pills in the 28-pill regimen contain only inert ingredients; active pills contain 0.15 mg levonorgestrel and 0.030 mg ethinyl estradiol.

Actions: Combination oral contraceptive that suppresses ovulation and causes cervical and endometrial changes; used to prevent pregnancy.

Selected Side Effects: Serious vascular complications, menstrual changes, cervical changes, breast changes, vaginal candidiasis, hypertension, edema, weight changes, gallbladder disease, GI distress, nausea and vomiting, liver tumors, migraine headache, rash, depression, glucose intolerance, visual changes from alteration in corneal curvature, intolerance for contact lenses.

Selected Drug Interactions: Contraceptive effectiveness can be decreased by antibiotics (ampicillin, chloramphenicol, isoniazid, nitrofurantoin, penicillin V, phenytoin, rifampin, sulfonamides, tetracycline), analgesics, anxiolytics, antihistamines, migraine preparations, phenylbutazone, phenytoin, and tranquilizers.

Cautions:

- *Contraindicated in thromboembolic or thrombophlebitic disorders, cardiovascular or cerebrovascular disease, geni-*

tal bleeding of unknown cause, endometrial or other estro-gen-dependent tumors, smokers over age 35, and possible pregnancy.
- Cigarette smoking increases risk of serious cardiovascular complications; patients should be *strongly* advised not to smoke.

Pregnancy Category: X.

Cost: $$$ (≈ $20/month retail); all contraceptive pills are similarly priced.

Pearls: Patients should undergo complete work-up prior to use with special attention to history of abnormal vaginal bleeding, BP, breast examination, and pelvic examination, including cervical cytology.

LEVODOPA: *see* Sinemet

LEVONORGESTREL (Norplant; *see also* Levlen, Tri-Levlen, Triphasil)

Dose: Insert 6 tubes under skin of upper arm.

PO Preparations: 6 Silastic tubes, each containing 36 mg levonorgestrel.

Actions: Contraceptive that inhibits ovulation and thickens cervical mucus; used to prevent pregnancy.

Selected Side Effects: Menstrual changes, increased number of days of bleeding and spotting, headache, depression, nervousness, breast discharge and pain, dizziness, acne, hirsutism, hair loss, weight gain, local reactions, potential difficulty with removal.

Selected Drug Interactions: Phenytoin and carbamazepine can decrease its efficacy.

Cautions: *Contraindicated in pregnant or potentially pregnant patients.*

Pregnancy Category: X.

Cost: $$$$ (≈ $350 wholesale).

Levophed: *see* NOREPINEPHRINE

LEVOTHYROXINE: *see* L-THYROXINE

Levoxine: *see* L-THYROXINE

Librium: *see* CHLORDIAZEPOXIDE

Lidex: *see* FLUOCINONIDE cream, gel, ointment, and solution

LIDOCAINE (Xylocaine)

Dose: Situation dependent (regimens based on those prescribed by AHA, Advanced Cardiac Life Support, 1994):

- Acute therapy for cardiac arrest due to pulseless ventricular tachycardia or ventricular fibrillation:
  - ▶ 1–1.5 mg/kg IV; consider repeating dose in 3–5 min if clinically indicated, up to a maximum total administration of 3 mg/kg; if patient converts, begin maintenance therapy at 2–4 mg/min; if patient converts after only one bolus administration of lidocaine a second bolus dose of 0.5 mg/kg given 10 min after the first bolus should be considered to maintain therapeutic lidocaine levels, because lidocaine distributes rapidly throughout the body.
  - ▶ After peripheral administration in a code situation, give a 20–30 mL bolus of intravenous fluid and immediately elevate the extremity. This enhances delivery of the drug to the central circulation, which can take 1–2 min.
- Acute therapy for ventricular tachycardia (noncardiac arrest, ie, with pulse):
  - ▶ 1–1.5 mg/kg IV bolus initially; if patient converts, then begin maintenance infusion at 2–4 mg/min; a second bolus dose of 0.5 mg/kg given 10 min after the first bolus should be considered to maintain therapeutic lidocaine levels, because lidocaine rapidly distributes throughout the body.
  - ▶ If patient does not convert after first bolus, additional bolus injections of 0.5–0.75 mg/kg can be given q5–10 min, up to a total dose of 3 mg/kg. If patient converts, then begin maintenance infusion at 2–4 mg/min.

Actions: Class Ib anti-arrhythmic (sodium channel blocker) used to treat ventricular arrhythmias.

Clearance: Metabolized via liver; 20% renally excreted; metabolism is reduced in liver dysfunction, CHF, and shock (because of decreased liver blood flow).

- No change in dosage needed in patients with renal insufficiency.
- In patients with liver disease, give no more than 2 mg/min and follow serum levels.
- Reduce dosage in elderly patients, those with CHF, and others who are more susceptible to lidocaine toxicity.
- Supplemental dose not required after hemodialysis.

Selected Side Effects: Sedation, irritability, seizures, coma, mental status changes (often referred to as "lidocaine toxicity" and particularly common in elderly patients), respiratory depression, hypotension.

Selected Drug Interactions:
- Cimetidine decreases its metabolism.
- β-blockers can reduce its clearance (by decreasing liver blood flow).
- Toxicity is potentiated when used with oral lidocaine congeners (mexiletine or tocainide).

Pregnancy Category: B.
Cost: $.
Pearls:
- May give 300 mg IM if no IV access is available; onset of action when given IM is 5–15 min.
- There does not appear to be any survival benefit for initiating "prophylactic therapy" in all patients with acute MI; the decision of when to begin lidocaine in patients with acute MI and ventricular ectopy or nonsustained ventricular arrhythmias is, in general, very physician-dependent.

LINDANE cream and lotion (Gamma benzene hexachloride, Kwell)
Dose: Disease dependent:
- Scabies: Apply thin layer and massage in; wash off after 8–12 h.
- Lice: Apply and work into hair; add water after 4–5 min, then rinse and towel; consider repeating treatment the following day.

Preparations:
- 2 oz cream.
- 2 oz, 1 pint, and 1 gallon lotion.
- 2 oz, 1 pint, and 1 gallon shampoo.

Actions: Topical antiparasitic agent used to treat lice and scabies.

Selected Side Effects:
- Skin irritation, pruritus.
- Excessive absorption can lead to CNS effects ranging from dizziness to convulsion.

Cautions: *Contraindicated in patients with known seizure disorders.*

Pregnancy Category: B.

Cost: Generic $$, Kwell $$$$ (1 pint generic ≈ $25, 1 pint Kwell ≈ $65).

Pearls:
- Remember to apply underneath the nails.
- Alternate therapies recommended for infants and for pregnant women.

Lioresal: *see* BACLOFEN

LISINOPRIL (Prinivil, Zestril; *see also* Prinzide, Zestoretic)

Dose:
- Initial: 10 mg PO qd (5 mg if patient is taking diuretics).
- Usual: 10–40 mg PO qd.

PO Preparations: 5, 10, 20, and 40 mg tablets.

Actions: ACE inhibitor that causes vasodilatation; used to treat hypertension and CHF.

Clearance: No liver metabolism; 100% renally excreted.
- Moderately reduce dosage in patients with impaired renal function.

Selected Side Effects: Hypotension and dizziness, hyperkalemia (especially in patients with impaired renal function or taking K^+-sparing drugs or K^+ supplements), nonproductive cough, impairment of renal function, angioedema, rare neutropenia.

Cautions:
- *Contraindicated during second and third trimesters of pregnancy and in patients with significant aortic stenosis or hyperkalemia.*
- Patients should almost never be given both an ACE inhibitor and a K^+ supplement, unless clearly indicated by serial serum K^+ testing.

Pregnancy Category: D.

Cost: $$$ ($\approx$ $0.85 each 10 mg tablet).

Pearls:
- Diuretics potentiate its antihypertensive effects; the risk of hypotension is increased in volume-depleted and elderly patients.
- Follow BUN, creatinine, and K when beginning therapy.
- Patients should be instructed not to use potassium supplements or salt substitutes containing potassium.
- Patients should be made aware of the possibility of developing a nonproductive cough and of developing angioedema.
- The nonproductive cough with ACE inhibitors is presumed to be due to the inhibition of the degradation of endogenous bradykinin.
- Patients who develop a cough with one ACE inhibitor usually also develop such a cough with other ACE inhibitors.

LITHIUM CARBONATE (Eskalith, Lithonate)
Dose:
- Loading dose: 30 mg/kg PO given in 3 divided doses.
- Maintenance: 900 mg–1.5 g PO daily, divided into tid–qid doses with regular pills or bid doses with SR pills.

PO Preparations:
- 150, 300, and 600 mg capsules.
- 450 mg sustained-release tablets.

Actions: Psychotropic agent that alters intraneural metabolism of catecholamines and can affect Na^+ transport in neural cells; used to treat manic episodes in patients with bipolar disorder.

Clearance: Renally excreted.
- Slightly to moderately reduce dosage in patients with impaired renal function.

- No change in dosage needed in patients with liver disease.
- Supplemental dose suggested after hemodialysis or peritoneal dialysis.

Selected Side Effects: Fine hand tremor and many other CNS effects, polyuria, nephrogenic diabetes insipidus, nephrotic syndrome, leukocytosis, numerous cardiovascular effects.

Selected Drug Interactions:

- $NaHCO_3$, acetazolamide, aminophylline, and osmotic diuretics all increase its excretion.
- Can potentiate response to tricyclics.

Cautions:

- *Contraindicated in significant cardiovascular or renal disease, in Na^+-depleted patients, in patients taking diuretics, and in pregnant or potentially pregnant patients.*

Pregnancy Category: *Can significantly harm the fetus when administered during pregnancy.*

Cost: $.

Pearls:

- Risk of toxicity is increased when serum level reaches 1.5 mEq/L; some patients are unusually sensitive to lithium and can exhibit toxic signs at serum levels of 1.0 mEq/L.
- Symptoms of toxicity include diarrhea, vomiting, drowsiness, muscle weakness and incoordination, giddiness, ataxia, blurred vision, tinnitus, and large output of dilute urine.

Lithonate: *see* LITHIUM CARBONATE

Lodine: *see* ETODOLAC

LOMEFLOXACIN (Maxaquin)
Dose:

- Bronchitis: 400 mg PO qd for 10 days.
- Cystitis: 400 mg PO qd for 10 days.
- Complicated UTI: 400 mg PO qd for 14 days.

Preparations: 400 mg scored tablets.

Actions: Broad-spectrum fluorinated quinolone that inhibits DNA gyrase.

- Good gram (+) coverage, including *Staphylococcus aureus* and *S epidermidis* (and methicillin-resistant strains of both organisms) but not *Streptococcus pneumoniae.*
- Very good gram (−) coverage.
- Has in vitro activity against *Legionella.*
- Does not cover most anaerobes.
- *NOTE:* The above-mentioned antimicrobial coverage summary should be used as a guideline only; treatment decisions should take into account not only local epidemiologic patterns of antibiotic susceptibility but also, when available, culture susceptibility results.

Clearance: Primarily renally excreted.

- No change in dose necessary in patients with liver disease (provided normal renal function).
- Moderate decrease in dose necessary in patients with renal insufficiency (see *PDR*).

Selected Side Effects: *Moderate or severe phototoxic reactions (rash, blisters, etc).*

Selected Drug Interactions:

- Sulcrafate, antacids, and vitamin supplements containing iron or other minerals decrease its absorption.
- Can increase the antithrombotic effects of warfarin.

Cautions: *Does* not *cover Streptococcus pneumoniae and should* not *be used for empiric coverage of bronchitis when it is probable that S pneumoniae is a causative pathogen (can be used for empiric coverage only if a* good *sputum sample demonstrates > 25 PMNs and a predominance of gram-negative organisms).*

Pregnancy Category: C.

Cost: $$$ (≈ $75 for 100 mg qd for 10 days).

Pearls:

- *Caution patients about possible phototoxic reactions, signs and symptoms of such reactions (skin burning, redness, swelling, blisters, rash, etc) and to discontinue therapy if any such signs or symptoms occur, and to avoid direct and indirect sunlight (even when using sunscreens or sunblocks) during therapy and for several days afterward.*
- Can be taken without regard to meals.

Lomotil (DIPHENOXYLATE + ATROPINE)
Dose: 2 tablets or 2 tsp PO tid–qid until diarrhea is controlled, then 1 tablet or 1 tsp PO bid–tid.

PO Preparations:
- Tablets containing 2.5 mg diphenoxylate and 25 μg atropine.
- 2 oz bottles of liquid containing 2.5 mg diphenoxylate and 25 μg atropine per 5 mL (1 tsp).

Actions: Antidiarrheal agent with narcotic-like action that slows GI motility; used to treat diarrhea.

Selected Side Effects: Paralytic ileus and toxic megacolon, atropine-related effects (tachycardia, urinary retention, etc).

Cautions: Contraindicated in advanced liver disease and in patients taking MAOI.

Pregnancy Category: C.

Cost: Generic $, Lomotil $$$ (≈ $0.20 each generic tablet; ≈ $0.50 each Lomotil tablet).

LOPERAMIDE (Imodium, Imodium AD)
Dose:
- Initial: 2 capsules (4 mg), 2 caplets (4 mg), or 4 tsp (4 mg); then 1 capsule (2 mg), 1 caplet (2 mg), or 2 tsp (2 mg) after each unformed stool.
- Maximum: 16 mg PO daily.

PO Preparations:
- 6 and 12 tablet blister packs containing 2 mg scored Imodium A-D caplets.
- 2 mg capsules and caplets.
- 2, 3, and 4 oz bottles of cherry-flavored liquid containing 1 mg/5 mL (1 tsp).

Actions: Antidiarrheal agent that slows GI peristalsis.

Clearance: Significant first-pass metabolism; excreted primarily in feces.

Selected Side Effects: Rash, abdominal distress.

Cautions: Use with caution in liver dysfunction.

Pregnancy Category: B.

Cost: Generic $$, Imodium $$$ (≈ $0.50 generic capsule; ≈ $0.80 each Imodium capsule).

Pearls: Discontinue if abdominal distention occurs in patients with ulcerative colitis or pseudomembranous colitis (agents that inhibit intestinal motility have been reported to induce toxic megacolon).

Lopid: *see* **GEMFIBROZIL**

Lopressor: *see* **METOPROLOL**

LORATADINE (Claritin)
Dose: 10 mg PO qd (10 mg PO qod in patients with liver disease.
PO Preparations: 10 mg tablets.
Actions: Long-acting antihistamine used to treat allergic conditions.
Clearance: Metabolized to an active metabolite.
• Dosing interval should be increased to qod in patients with liver disease.
Selected Side Effects: No significant increase in somnolence compared with that in patients taking placebo.
Selected Drug Interactions:
• Ketoconazole increases serum levels.
• Cimetidine, macrolide antibiotics (erythromycin, Biaxin) and other drugs that inhibit hepatic metabolism have been associated with elevated levels of other antihistamines; there are insufficient data on their effects of loratadine.
Cautions: The concurrent use of several other antihistamines (astemizole [Hismanal] and terfenadine [Seldane]) with certain drugs has been associated with QT interval prolongation and ventricular arrhythmias. Concurrent use of loratadine and ketoconazole has been demonstrated not to prolong the QT interval. Until further data become available; however, loratadine should be used with caution in patients simultaneously taking certain other medications that inhibit hepatic metabolism (including macrolide antibiotics [such as erythromycin, clarithromycin, troleandomycin], and ketoconazole and the related drugs troleandomycin, itraconazole, fluconazole, metronidazole, and miconazole).
Pregnancy Category: B.
Cost: $$$$ (≈ $2/tablet).
Pearls: Should be taken on an empty stomach.

LORAZEPAM (Ativan)
Dose:
- PO:
  - ▸ Anxiety: Initial dose of 1 mg PO bid–tid (in elderly or debilitated patients, the initial total daily dose should be 1–2 mg); can increase to 2 mg PO bid–tid (usual maximum daily dose is 6 mg).
  - ▸ Insomnia due to anxiety or stress: 2–4 mg PO qhs.
- IM: 2–4 mg (give 2 mg in elderly patients).
- IV: 1–2 mg IV.

PO Preparations: 0.5, 1, and 2 mg tablets.

Actions: Benzodiazepine with anxiolytic and sedative effects; used for the treatment of anxiety and as a sedative.

Clearance: Metabolized in the liver; the conjugated form is renally excreted.

Selected Side Effects: Pain at IM injection site, excessive drowsiness or sedation.

Selected Drug Interactions:
- Increases the CNS depressant effects of other CNS depressants.

Cautions:
- *Contraindicated in patients with acute narrow-angle glaucoma.*
- Should not be used in patients with liver or renal failure (may be used with caution in patients with lesser degrees of liver or renal disease).
- Use with caution in elderly patients—can cause disinhibition.

Pregnancy Category: D.

Cost: Generic $$, Ativan $$$$ ($\approx$ $0.14 each 1 mg generic tablet; $\approx$ $0.75 each 1 mg Ativan tablet).

Pearls: Peak serum levels after IM injection occur after 60–90 min.

Lorcet 10/650 (HYDROCODONE + ACETAMINOPHEN)
Dose: 1 tablet q4–6 h up to a maximum of 6 tablets over 24 h.

Preparations: Each tablet contains 10 mg of hydrocodone and 625 mg of acetaminophen.

Actions: Combination schedule III narcotic and acetaminophen; used to treat moderate to moderately severe pain.

Clearance: Acetaminophen is metabolized in the liver; hydrocodone is metabolized to hydromorphone in the liver.

Cautions:

- *Contraindicated in patients with liver disease.*
- Use with caution in patients with pulmonary disease.

Pregnancy Category: C.

Pearls:

- *All the cautions that apply to acetaminophen, particularly those regarding hepatotoxicity, also apply to Vicodin.*
- As with other schedule III substances, may be prescribed by telephone in most states and may be refilled up to 5 times within 6 months.
- Has fewer GI side effects than codeine.

Lorelco: *see* **PROBUCOL**

LOSARTAN (Cozaar; see also Hyzaar)

Dose:

- Initial: 50 mg PO qd.
- Initial dose of 25 mg should be used in patients with liver disease and those with possible volume depletion.
- Maximum: 100 mg PO daily.
- If antihypertensive effect at drug trough (approximately 24 h after administration) is inadequate, consider giving bid.

Preparations: 50 mg tablets.

Actions: Angiotensin II receptor blocker; used to treat hypertension.

Clearance: Metabolized to active metabolite in the liver.

- Decrease dose in patients with liver failure.

Selected Side Effects: Possible hypotension in volume-depleted patients.

Selected Drug Interactions:

Cautions: *Contraindicated in pregnant patients during the second and third trimesters.*

Pregnancy Category: D. *Has the potential to cause fetal damage and death during the second and third trimesters of pregnancy; therefore should not be taken during pregnancy, and should be discontinued if patient becomes pregnant.*

Cost: $$$ (≈ $1.25/tablet).
Pearls:
- Does not produce the chronic nonproductive cough that can occur with ACE inhibitors.
- Has been shown in most patients to be as effective as ACE inhibitors for blood pressure control.
- Can be taken without regard to meals.

Losec: *see* OMEPRAZOLE

Lotensin: *see* BENAZEPRIL

Lotensin HCT (BENAZEPRIL + HYDROCHLOROTHIAZIDE)
Dose:
- Initial: 5 mg benazepril + 6.25 mg hydrochlorothiazide PO qd.
- Maintenance: Can titrate dose upward to a maximum of 20 mg benazepril qd (administered once/day).

Preparations:
- 5 mg benazepril + 6.25 mg hydrochlorothiazide tablet.
- 10 mg benazepril + 12.5 mg hydrochlorothiazide tablet.
- 20 benazepril + 12.5 mg hydrochlorothiazide tablet.
- 20 benazepril + 25 mg hydrochlorothiazide tablet.

Actions: Combination ACE inhibitor and diuretic; used to treat hypertension.
Selected Side Effects, Cautions, Pregnancy Category, Pearls: *See* listings under benazepril and hydrochlorothiazide.
- 5 mg benazepril + 6.25 mg hydrochlorothiazide tablet.

Cost: $$$ (≈ $0.70 each 10 mg/12.5 mg tablet).

Lotrimin: *see* CLOTRIMAZOLE

Lotrisone topical cream (CLOTRIMAZOLE + BETAMETHASONE)
Dose: Apply to skin bid.
PO Preparations: 15 and 45 g tubes.

Actions: Combination topical antifungal and steroid.
Pregnancy Category: C.
Cautions: *Should not be used in intertriginous areas.*
Cost: $$$ (≈ $20 for a 15 g tube and ≈ $45 for a 45 g tube).
Pearls:

- Use of this combination medication with high potency steroid is not recommended by many dermatologists.
- Misuse or abuse of this class I steroid can lead to skin cutaneous atrophy, telangiectasias, and pigment changes.

LOVASTATIN (Mevacor)
Dose:

- Initial: 20 mg PO qd.
- Usual: 20–80 mg PO qd.
- Allow at least 4 weeks before adjusting dosage.
- Maximum dose in patients taking immunosuppressants: 20 mg daily.

PO Preparations: 10, 20, and 40 mg tablets.
Actions: HMG-CoA inhibitor that lowers total and LDL cholesterol and triglyceride levels and increases HDL cholesterol; used to treat hypercholesterolemia.
Clearance: Hydrolyzed to active form.

- No change in dosage needed in patients with impaired renal function.

Selected Side Effects: Elevated LFTs, increased CPK (MM), and myopathy (especially when given with immunosuppressants, gemfibrozil, or niacin), GI discomfort.
Selected Drug Interactions:

- Can prolong PT in patients taking warfarin.
- Cyclosporine, gemfibrozil, niacin, or erythromycin may increase the risk of myopathy.

Cautions:

- *Contraindicated in pregnant or potentially pregnant patients.*
- Contraindicated in patients with active liver disease or unexplained transaminase elevations.
- Use with caution in patients with history of liver disease or heavy alcohol use.

Pregnancy Category: X.

Cost: $$$$ (≈ $1.75 each 20 mg tablet).
Pearls:
- Should be taken with evening meal.
- Obtain LFTs and CPK level before starting therapy.
- Recommended frequency for checking liver function during treatment has been liberalized to every 6 weeks for first 3 months, then every 8 weeks for remainder of first year and approximately every 6 months thereafter.
- Discontinue if persistent LFTs > 3 times normal, substantial rise in CPK, or myositis occurs.
- Primary effects are reductions in total and LDL cholesterol; usually leads to only modest elevations of HDL cholesterol.
- Doses over 20 mg can be taken bid to increase efficacy.

Lozol: *see* INDAPAMIDE

Maalox (MAGNESIUM HYDROXIDE + ALUMINUM HYDROXIDE)
Dose: 2–4 tablets or 2–4 tsp PO qid, given 60 min after meals and qhs.

Macrobid: *see* NITROFURANTOIN

Macrodantin: *see* NITROFURANTOIN

MAGNESIUM HYDROXIDE (MILK OF MAGNESIA, M.O.M.; *see also* Maalox, Mylanta, Rolaids)
Dose: 30 mL PO q6h prn.
Actions: Osmotic laxative; used to treat constipation or dyspepsia.
Cost: $.
Pearls:
- Magnesium levels can markedly rise in patients with end-stage renal disease.
- When taken as antacid, consider alternating with an aluminum-based antacid, such as Amphojel or ALTernaGEL (repeated use can cause diarrhea).

MAGNESIUM OXIDE (Mag-Ox 400)
Dose: 1–2 tablets PO qd.
PO Preparations: Bottles of 100 or 1000 tablets; each tablet contains 400 mg magnesium oxide.
Actions: Oral magnesium supplement.
Selected Side Effects: Diarrhea.
Cost: $.
Pearls: Signs and symptoms of hypomagnesemia include weakness, convulsions, and arrhythmias.

MAGNESIUM SULFATE
Dose: 1–2 g (8–16 mEq magnesium) IV.
PO Preparations: 2 and 4 mg vials of 50% solution containing 8 or 16 mEq magnesium, respectively.
Actions: IV magnesium supplement.
Pearls: Can usually be ordered as 1–2 "amps" IV.

Mag-Ox: *see* MAGNESIUM OXIDE

MANNITOL
Dose: 25–75 g or 1 g/kg of 20% solution IV; may repeat approximately q6h prn.
Actions: Osmotic agent that increases effective intravascular volume and diuresis.
Selected Side Effects: Necrosis if extravasated.
Cautions: Use with caution in CHF.
Pearls: Watch for signs of CHF and pulmonary edema during use.

Maxaquin: *see* LOMEFLOXACIN

Maxzide, Maxzide-25 (TRIAMTERENE + HYDROCHLOROTHIAZIDE)
Dose: 1 tablet PO qd.
PO Preparations:
• Maxzide: 75 mg triamterene and 50 mg hydrochlorothiazide.
• Maxzide-25: 37.5 mg triamterene and 25 mg hydrochlorothiazide.

Actions: Combination K⁺-sparing diuretic; used to treat hypertension.

Clearance:
- Avoid in patients with end-stage renal disease.
- Reduce dosage in patients with liver disease.

Selected Side Effects: Hyperkalemia, dilutional hyponatremia, GI discomfort.

Selected Drug Interactions:
- Increases risk of lithium toxicity.
- Heightens risk of renal failure when used with NSAIDs and of hyperkalemia when used with ACE inhibitors or K⁺ supplements.
- Potentiates antihypertensive effects of other drugs.

Pregnancy Category: C.

Cost: Generic $, Maxzide $$$ (≈ $0.20 each generic tablet; ≈ $0.85 each Maxzide tablet).

Mazicon: *see* FLUMAZENIL

MECLIZINE (Antivert)

Dose: Disease dependent:
- Vertigo: 25 mg PO tid–qid.
- Motion sickness: 25–50 mg PO taken 1 h prior to embarkation; may be repeated q24h during trip.

PO Preparations:
- 12.5, 25, and 50 mg tablets.
- 25 mg chewable tablets.

Actions: Antihistamine used to treat vertigo and motion sickness.

Selected Side Effects: Drowsiness, dry mouth, blurred vision.

Cautions: Use with caution (because of anticholinergic actions) in asthma, glaucoma, or prostate hypertrophy.

Pregnancy Category: B.

Cost: Generic $, Antivert $$$ (≈ $0.15 each 25 mg generic tablet; ≈ $0.65 each 25 mg Antivert tablet).

Medipren: *see* **IBUPROFEN**

Medrol: *see* **METHYLPREDNISOLONE**

MEDROXYPROGESTERONE (Depo-Provera); *see also* the following entry, MEDROXYPROGESTERONE (Provera)

Dose: 150 mg by deep IM injection in the gluteal or deltoid muscle every 3 months.

Actions: Inhibits the secretion of gonadotropins, which prevents follicular maturation and ovulation and results in endometrial thinning; used as a contraceptive.

Selected Side Effects: Menstrual irregularities, weight gain, rare breast tenderness or galactorrhea, possible thromboembolic disorders.

Cautions:
- *Contraindicated in patients with history of thrombophlebitis, thromboembolic disorders, liver disease, documented or suspected malignancy of breast or genital organs, vaginal bleeding of unknown cause, missed abortions, or cerebrovascular disease.*
- Contraindicated in pregnant and potentially pregnant patients.

Pregnancy Category: *Contraindicated in pregnant and potentially pregnant patients.*

Pearls:
- Give first dose during menses, or obtain a pregnancy test before administering, to ensure patient is not pregnant.
- When administered every 3 months is over 99% effective in preventing pregnancy.
- Counsel patients about possibility of irregular bleeding (especially during the first 3 months).

MEDROXYPROGESTERONE (Provera); *see also* the previous entry, MEDROXYPROGESTERONE (Depo-Provera)

Dose: Often given 5–10 mg PO qd, sometimes for 5–10 days.
- Dosing regimens vary significantly by disease.

PO Preparations: 2.5, 5, and 10 mg tablets; also available for IM injection.

Actions: Progesterone derivative that transforms estrogenic proliferative endometrium into secretory endometrium; used to treat secondary amenorrhea, abnormal uterine bleeding, and other conditions including respiratory acidosis and sleep apnea.

Clearance: Significant hepatic metabolism with 20–40% excreted in urine as metabolites, 5–15% excreted in stool.

Selected Side Effects: Menstrual irregularities, weight gain, rare breast tenderness or galactorrhea, rare skin reactions, possible thromboembolic disorders.

Cautions:
- *Contraindicated in patients with history of thrombophlebitis, thromboembolic disorders, liver disease, documented or suspected malignancy of breast or genital organs, vaginal bleeding of unknown cause, missed abortions, or cerebrovascular disease.*
- Contraindicated in pregnant and potentially pregnant patients.

Pregnancy Category: *Contraindicated in pregnant and potentially pregnant patients.*

Cost: $.

Pearls: Should be taken with food.

Mefoxin: *see* CEFOXITIN

Mellaril, Mellaril-S: *see* THIORIDAZINE

MELPHALAN (Alkeran)
Dose: Regimens are somewhat variable; often, 6 mg PO qd for induction and 2 mg PO qd for maintenance.
- For multiple myeloma, 0.25 mg/kg daily in 4-day cycles in combination with prednisone.

PO Preparations: 2 mg scored tablets.

Actions: Nitrogen mustard alkylating agent; used to treat neoplastic diseases.

Clearance: Metabolized via liver.
- One source recommends no change in dosage in patients with renal insufficiency; another suggests 50% reduction in dose for BUN > 30 or creatinine > 1.5.

Selected Side Effects: *Myelosuppression,* rare pulmonary fibrosis, rare GI distress and side effects, allergic hypersensitivity, increased incidence of secondary acute leukemia.

Pregnancy Category: D.

Cost: $$.

Pearls:

- Myelosuppression is dose-limiting toxicity.
- WBC and platelet nadirs usually occur 14–21 days after treatment.
- Should not be given with food.

MEPERIDINE (Demerol)

Dose: 50–150 mg IM, SQ, or PO q3–4h.

PO Preparations:

- 50 and 100 mg tablets.
- 50 mg/5 mL (1 tsp) syrup.

Actions: Synthetic narcotic analgesic used to treat pain.

Clearance: Metabolized predominantly via liver.

- Normeperidine, an active and neurotoxic metabolite, can accumulate in patients with end-stage renal disease and cause seizures.
- Slightly reduce dosage in patients with impaired renal function.
- Decrease dosage in patients with liver disease.

Selected Side Effects: Respiratory depression, nausea and vomiting, hypotension, sweating, constipation (minor but common).

Cautions:

- *Contraindicated in patients who have taken MAOI within 14 days.*
- Use with caution in respiratory or liver disease.
- Can aggravate preexisting convulsive disorders.

Pregnancy Category: Not established.

Cost: $$$ ($\approx$ $0.35 each 50 mg tablet).

Pearls:

- Often given IM with Vistaril to decrease nausea (usually 50 mg Demerol with 25 mg Vistaril, or 75–100 mg Demerol with 50 mg Vistaril).
- Can increase ventricular response in atrial flutter and other SVTs (because of vagolytic action).

- Can raise serum levels of amylase and lipase.
- 50–80 mg meperidine has analgesic effect approximately equal to that of 10 mg morphine.

MERCAPTOPURINE (6-MP, Purinethol)
Dose: 1.5–5.0 mg/kg PO qd.
PO Preparations: 50 mg scored tablets.
Actions: Purine analogue antimetabolite that interferes with nucleic acid synthesis; used to treat malignancies.
Clearance: Metabolized via liver to active metabolites.
- No change in dosage needed for mild renal failure; may need to reduce dosage in patients with severely decreased creatinine clearance.
- Avoid in patients with liver disease.
Selected Side Effects: *Myelosuppression,* hepatotoxicity (both cholestasis and parenchymal injury). Nausea and vomiting occur rarely.
Selected Drug Interactions:
- *Allopurinol markedly decreases its catabolism.*
- Trimethoprim + sulfamethoxazole (Bactrim, Septra) increases its bone marrow suppression.
Cautions: Reduce from 1/3 to 1/4 the normal dose when given with allopurinol.
Pregnancy Category: D.
Cost: $$.

MESNA (Mesnex)
Dose: Used in conjunction with ifosfamide therapy.
- Administered as 3 injections, each at 20% of ifosfamide dose (in mg), as follows:
- Give initial mesna dose concurrently with ifosfamide injection; repeat dose 4 and 8 h later (thus total mesna dose is 60% of the ifosfamide dose). Repeat this dosing schedule each time ifosfamide is given.
- Example: for 1.2 g/m^2 ifosfamide dose, give 240 mg/m^2 mesna simultaneously, another 240 mg/m^2 4 h later, and another 240 mg/m^2 8 h after initial injection.
Actions: Thiol agent that acts to detoxify urotoxic metabolites of ifosfamide in the kidneys; used as prophylaxis or antidote for ifosfamide-induced hemorrhagic cystitis.

Clearance: Oxidized in blood to its active metabolite mesna disulfide, which is renally excreted.
Selected Side Effects: Nausea and vomiting, diarrhea.
Cautions: *Contraindicated in patients with known allergies to thiol compounds.*
Pregnancy Category: B.
Cost: $$.
Pearls: May also be used with cyclophosphamide to reduce hemorrhagic cystitis.

Mesnex: *see* MESNA

MESTRANOL: *see* Norinyl, Ortho-Novum oral contraceptive pills

Metamucil (PSYLLIUM)
Dose: 1 rounded tsp in 8 oz liquid qd–tid.
PO Preparations:
- 7, 14, and 21 oz containers.
- Cartons of 100 single-dose packets.
- Available in sugar-free and "grit-free" preparations.

Actions: Bulk-forming fiber used to restore and maintain bowel regularity.
Pregnancy Category: Safe to use during pregnancy.
Cost: $$ (container ≈ $15 retail).
Pearls:
- Can cause allergic reaction in patients sensitive to inhaled or ingested psyllium powder (consider using Citrucel).
- Available in sugar-containing and sugar-free flavors, including orange, lemon-lime, and strawberry.

Metaprel: *see* METAPROTERENOL

METAPROTERENOL (Alupent, Metaprel)
Dose: Delivery dependent:
- PO: 20 mg tid–qid.
- Nebulizer: 0.3 mL of 5% solution in 2.5 mL NS.
- Metered-dose inhaler: 2 or 3 inhalations q3–4h up to a maximum of 12 inhalations daily.

Preparations:
- 10 and 20 mg tablets.
- 16 oz bottles of flavored syrup containing 10 mg/5 mL (1 tsp) of Alupent.
- Each Alupent inhalation aerosol contains 150 mg metaproterenol and delivers 200 inhalations.

Actions: β-stimulating bronchodilator used to treat reactive airway disease.

Selected Side Effects: Tachycardia, palpitations, hypertension, nervousness, tremor, nausea and vomiting, bad taste.

Cautions: Use with caution in patients with CAD or tachyarrhythmias.

Pregnancy Category: C.

Pearls:

Cost: $$$ ($\approx$ $25 each inhaler).

METFORMIN (Glucophage)
Dose:
- Initial 500 mg PO bid.
- Can increase dose by one 500 mg tablet each week, as clinically indicated (doses up to 2000 mg PO daily can be given as divided doses bid).
- Maximum: 2500 mg PO daily, given in divided doses tid (2 tablets with breakfast, 1 with lunch, and 2 with dinner).

PO Preparations: 500 mg tablets.

Actions: A new, nonsulfonylurea oral hypoglycemic agent; used to treat diabetes.
- Unlike most oral hypoglycemic agents, does not work by stimulating pancreatic secretion of insulin.

Selected Side Effects: GI distress (diarrhea, nausea and vomiting, bloating, flatulence) especially during initiation of therapy, rare lactic acidosis.

Cautions:
- *Contraindicated in patients with renal disease, renal insufficiency, or metabolic acidosis (due to rare occurrence of lactic acidosis).*
- Should not be taken by patients who have impaired hepatic function or who drink excessive amounts of alcohol.

Pregnancy Category: *Should not be taken by pregnant women.*

Cost: $$$ ($\approx$ $0.50/tablet).

Pearls:

- Should be taken with meals to minimize GI side effects.
- Temporarily withhold therapy in patients receiving IV iodinated contrast materials for radiologic studies.
- Has modest synergistic effects when given with a sulfonylurea (such as the oral hypoglycemic glyburide).

METHADONE

Dose: Disease dependent:

- Pain: 2.5–10 mg PO, IM, or SQ q3–4h.
- Drug detoxification:
  - ▶ Initial: 15–20 mg PO, IM, or SQ.
  - ▶ Usual: 40 mg qd or 20 mg PO, IM, or SQ bid.

PO Preparations:

- 5 and 10 mg tablets.
- 500 mg bottles of solution containing either 5 mg/5 mL (1 tsp) or 10 mg/5 mL (1 tsp).

Actions: Synthetic narcotic analgesic used to treat pain and for narcotic detoxification.

Clearance: Metabolized via liver.

- Slightly decrease dosage in patients with end-stage renal disease; no change needed for milder renal impairment.
- Reduce dosage in patients with liver disease.
- Supplemental dose not required after hemodialysis or peritoneal dialysis.

Selected Side Effects: Respiratory depression, CNS changes, hypotension, urine retention, biliary tree spasm, antidiuretic effects.

Cautions: Use with caution in patients taking other CNS depressants.

Pregnancy Category: Not established.

Cost: $.

Pearls:

- Can produce drug dependence.
- Methadone withdrawal, though qualitatively similar to morphine withdrawal, is of slower onset, has more prolonged course, and has less severe symptoms.

- Is a schedule II controlled substance.
- Is *not* an anxiolytic.
- In overdose therapy, naloxone (Narcan) is effective for only 1–3 h, whereas methadone is effective 36–48 h, so patients must be monitored for relapsing CNS depression when Narcan wears off.

METHIMAZOLE (Tapazole)
Dose:
- Recommendations for initial dose vary: *PDR* recommends 5–20 mg PO q8h; other sources suggest single daily dose of 10–30 mg PO initially for mild disease.
- Maintenance: 5–15 mg PO qd.
- Consider consulting an endocrinologist for dosing recommendations.

PO Preparations: 5 and 10 mg tablets.
Actions: Medication that blocks synthesis of thyroid hormone by inhibiting iodide organification; used to treat hyperthyroidism.
Clearance: Rapidly metabolized.
- No change in dosage needed in patients with renal insufficiency.

Selected Side Effects: Dermatologic reactions, myelosuppression (including possible granulocytopenia or agranulocytosis, thrombocytopenia or aplastic anemia), elevated LFTs, hepatitis, cholestatic jaundice, nephrotic syndrome, drug fever, SLE-like syndrome, insulin autoimmune syndrome (resulting in substantially reduced serum glucose and hypoglycemia), hypoprothrombinemia and prolongation of PT, loss of taste.
Selected Drug Interactions: Potentiates antivitamin K activity of warfarin and can prolong PT in patients taking warfarin.
Pregnancy Category: D.
Cost: $$.
Pearls:
- Monitor CBC.
- Warn patients to report signs of infection (given possible side effect of granulocytopenia or agranulocytosis).

METHOTREXATE

Dose: Tumor dependent. May be given PO, IV, or intrathecally.

Actions: Antimetabolite that inhibits dihydrofolate reductase, interfering with cell reproduction; used to treat malignancies, recalcitrant psoriasis, and rheumatoid arthritis.

Clearance: Route dependent:
- PO: hepatic and intracellularly metabolized to active metabolites.
- IV: 80–90% excreted unchanged in urine with limited biliary excretion.
- Moderately reduce dosage in patients with impaired renal function; avoid in patients with end-stage renal disease.
- Use with caution in patients with liver disease (because of hepatotoxicity).
- Supplemental dose suggested after hemodialysis but not peritoneal dialysis.

Selected Side Effects: Ulcerative stomatitis, *bone marrow depression (particularly leukopenia),* nausea and GI distress, hepatotoxicity, renal damage (when used in high doses for osteosarcoma), interstitial lung disease.

Selected Drug Interactions:
- ASA, NSAIDs, and probenecid decrease its tubular secretion and can increase its toxicity.
- ASA, phenytoin, and sulfonamides can displace protein-bound methotrexate and thus increase its toxicity.
- Trimethoprim + sulfamethoxazole (Bactrim, Septra) rarely can increase its bone marrow suppression (probably secondary to antifolate effects).

Cautions: *Contraindicated for treatment of psoriasis in pregnant or potentially pregnant patients.*

Pregnancy Category: X.

Cost: $$.

Pearls:
- Coadministration of leucovorin decreases potential for toxicity with high-dose therapy.
- Folate deficiency can increase its toxicity.
- Accumulates in and exits slowly from third space fluid collections.
- Periodically check CBC, LFTs, BUN, and creatinine.

- For severe reactions or toxicity, consider giving leucovorin to counteract the metabolic effects of methotrexate and reduce the resulting toxicity (commonly referred to as "leucovorin rescue"). *Note,* however, that leucovorin should *not* be given when methotrexate is administered intrathecally (can lead to decreased efficacy).

METHYLDOPA, METHYLDOPATE (Aldomet)
Dose:
- PO (Methyldopa):
  - ▶ Initial: 250 mg PO bid–tid for first 48 h.
  - ▶ Usual: 500 mg–2 g daily PO given bid–qid.
  - ▶ Maximum: total of 3 g PO daily.
- IV (Methyldopate):
  - ▶ Usual: 250-500 mg q6h.
  - ▶ Maximum: 1g q6h.

PO Preparations:
- 125, 250, and 500 mg tablets of methyldopa.
- 473 mL bottles of suspension of methyldopa containing 250 mg/5 mL (1 tsp).

Actions: Centrally acting agent used to treat hypertension.

Clearance: Metabolized via liver; renally excreted.
- Moderately increase dosing interval in patients with impaired renal function.
- Avoid in patients with liver disease.
- Supplemental dose suggested after hemodialysis or peritoneal dialysis.

Selected Side Effects:
- Sedation, headache, asthenia, depression, impotence, weakness, nasal congestion, frequent (+) Coombs' reaction within 6–12 months (though clinical hemolysis occurs only rarely).
- Occasional complex of fever, elevated LFTs, and eosinophilia.
- Occasional false (+) test for lupus, (+) rheumatoid factor, or (+) ANA titer.

Cautions: *Contraindicated in active hepatic disease.*

Pregnancy Category: B.

Cost: Generic $$, Aldomet $$$ (≈ $0.15 each 250 mg generic tablet; ≈ $0.35 each 250 mg methyldopa tablet).

Pearls:
- Frequently causes (+) Coombs' test but rarely causes hemolytic anemia.
- May falsely elevate urinary catecholamine levels.
- A paradoxical increase in BP that can occur with IV use reported in the product information insert, though this appears to occur only rarely, if at all, in clinical practice.
- Methyldopate is the ethyl ester of methyldopa and possesses the same pharmacologic attributes.
- When given intravenously in effective doses, blood pressure decline begins after 4–6 h and lasts 10–16 h after injection.

METHYLPREDNISOLONE (Depo-Medrol, Medrol, Solu-Medrol)

Dose: Preparation dependent.
- Medrol: 4–48 mg PO qd.
- Solu-Medrol (for asthma or COPD exacerbation): 60–125 mg IV q6h (60 mg q6h is often given for COPD exacerbation).
- Depo-Medrol:
  - ▶ Variable intra-articular dose (large joint 20–80 mg; medium joint 16–40 mg; small joint 4–10 mg).
  - ▶ May also be given 80–120 mg IM for systemic therapy.

PO Preparations:
- 2, 4, 8, 16, 24, and 32 mg tablets.
- Medrol dose pack contains 4 mg Medrol tablets beginning with 6 tablets (24 mg) the first day and tapering daily dose by 1 tablet (4 mg) each day over 6 days.

Actions: Corticosteroid with anti-inflammatory properties; used primarily to treat inflammatory and allergic conditions.

Clearance: Metabolized via liver.
- No change in dosage needed in patients with renal insufficiency.
- Dosage adjustment probably not needed in patients with liver disease.
- Supplemental dose suggested after hemodialysis.

Selected Side Effects:
- Mild NaCl and water retention (which can lead to increased hypertension, edema, and CHF), increased glucose intolerance and catabolism, decreased wound healing.
- Can aggravate peptic ulcer disease.

Pregnancy Category: Not established; observe newborns for hypoadrenalism.

Cost: Generic \$, Medrol \$\$, Medrol Dose Pack \$\$\$\$.

Pearls:

- Patients on chronic steroid use may develop adrenal suppression and may therefore need "stress steroids" in times of stress (frequently hydrocortisone 100 mg IV q8h).
- Can mask signs of infection.
- In one study, IV administration improved prognosis in patients with acute spinal cord trauma and neurologic changes who were treated within 4 h of injury. The protocol was: (1) 30 mg bolus administered over 15 min, then continuous infusion of 5.4 mg/kg/h for 23 h (*NEJM,* May 1990).
- Relative activity comparison of commonly used steroids:

Steroid	Relative Anti-inflammatory and Glucocorticoid Activity	Relative Mineralocorticoid Activity
Cortisone	0.8	0.8
Hydrocortisone	1.0	1.0
Prednisone	4.0	0.8
Methylprednisolone	5.0	0.5
Dexamethasone	25–30	0.0

METOCLOPRAMIDE (Reglan)

Dose: Disease dependent:

- GE reflux: 10–15 mg PO qid (5 mg qid in sensitive elderly patients) given 30 min before meals and qhs for 4–12 weeks.
- Diabetic gastroparesis: 10 mg PO, IM, or IV given 30 min before each meal and qhs for 2–8 weeks; oral therapy should be initiated after symptoms subside.
- Chemotherapy-induced nausea and vomiting: 1–2 mg/kg given over 15 min starting 30 min before chemotherapy; repeat dose 2, 5, 8, and 11 h after first dose.

PO Preparations:

- 5 and 10 mg tablets.
- 5 mg/5 mL (1 tsp) syrup.

Actions: Medication with central antidopaminergic and peripheral cholinergic properties that increases lower esophageal sphincter tone, enhances upper GI motility, and antagonizes dopamine-mediated nausea and vomiting; used to treat esophageal reflux and diabetic gastroparesis and to prevent chemotherapy-induced nausea and vomiting.

Clearance: Metabolized via liver; renally excreted.

- Slightly reduce dosage in patients with impaired renal function; extrapyramidal reactions are common in patients with end-stage renal disease.
- No change in dosage needed in patients with liver disease.
- Supplemental dose not required after hemodialysis or peritoneal dialysis.

Selected Side Effects: Tardive dyskinesia, acute dystonic reactions, parkinsonian-like symptoms, drowsiness, depression, confusion.

Selected Drug Interactions:

- *Concomitant use with MAOI causes hypertensive crisis.*
- Phenothiazines increase risk of extrapyramidal events.
- Anticholinergics and narcotics decrease its GI motility effects and narcotics increase its CNS depression.
- Decreases absorption of drugs absorbed in the stomach (eg, digoxin) and increases absorption of drugs absorbed in the small intestine.

Cautions:

- *Contraindicated in GI bleeding, gastric outlet or intestinal obstruction, epilepsy, pheochromocytoma, and in patients taking MAOI or drugs likely to cause extrapyramidal reactions..*
- Use with caution in hypertensive patients (can cause release of catecholamines when given IV).

Pregnancy Category: B.

Cost: Generic $$, Reglan $$$$ (≈ $0.15 each 10 mg generic tablet; ≈ $0.65 each 10 mg each Reglan tablet).

Pearls: Extrapyramidal reactions can be treated with a single dose of diphenhydramine (Benadryl) 50 mg IM.

METOLAZONE (Zaroxolyn)

Dose: Disease dependent:

- Edema: 5–20 mg PO qd.
- Hypertension: 2.5–5 mg PO qd.

PO Preparations: 2.5, 5, and 10 mg tablets.

Actions: Quinazolinone diuretic that affects electrolyte absorption in the renal tubules, similar to action of thiazides, used to treat CHF and edema, often in conjunction with furosemide.

Clearance: Predominantly excreted unchanged in urine.

- No change in dosage needed in patients with renal insufficiency; avoid in patients with end-stage renal disease.
- No change in dosage required in patients with liver disease.
- Supplemental dose not required after hemodialysis.

Selected Side Effects: Hypokalemia K^+, increased glucose and uric acid.

Cautions: *Contraindicated in anuria, hepatic coma, and gout.*

Pregnancy Category: B. The use of diuretics during pregnancy, however, is generally not recommended.

Cost: $$.

Pearls:

- Unlike thiazides, metolazone can produce diuresis in patients with GFR < 20 mL/min.
- Often works synergistically with furosemide.
- Can reactivate latent SLE.

METOPROLOL (Lopressor, Toprol XL)

Dose: Route dependent:

- PO:
  - ▶ 50–100 mg PO bid of Lopressor (can give a once daily dose when used for the treatment of hypertension).
  - ▶ 50–200 mg PO qd of long-acting Toprol XL.
- IV (in acute MI): 5 mg Lopressor q5min for total of 15 mg (as tolerated).

PO Preparations:

- Lopressor: 50 and 100 mg tablets.
- Toprol XL: 50, 100, and 200 long-acting tablets.

Actions: β_1-selective β-blocker used to treat angina and hypertension.

Clearance: Metabolized via liver.

- No change in dosage needed in patients with renal insufficiency.
- Supplemental dose suggested after hemodialysis.

Selected Side Effects: Decreased ejection fraction, hypotension, CHF, AV block, bradycardia, diarrhea, rash, pruritus, bronchospasm, depression, disorientation, impotence.

Cautions: *Contraindicated in sinus bradycardia,* second- or third-degree AV block, PR interval > 0.24 s, severely decreased ejection fraction, and bronchospastic disease.

Pregnancy Category: C.

Cost: Generic $$, Lopressor $$$ (≈ $0.50 each 100 mg metoprolol tablet; ≈ $0.75 each 100 mg Lopressor tablet; ≈ $1.50 each 200 mg Toprol XL tablet).

Pearls: Taper dose when discontinuing to avoid rebound reactions.

METRONIDAZOLE (Flagyl)

Dose: Disease dependent:

- Trichomoniasis: 2 g PO single dose, or 250 mg PO tid for 7 days.
- Intestinal amebiasis: 750 mg PO tid for 5 days.
- Giardiasis: 250 mg PO tid for 5 days.
- *Clostridium difficile* infection: 250 mg PO or IV tid for 7 days.
- Serious infection: 500 mg IV q6–8h.

PO Preparations: 250 and 500 mg tablets.

Actions: Antibiotic used to treat anaerobic bacterial infections and amebiasis, giardiasis, trichomoniasis, and *Gardnerella vaginalis* infections.

Clearance: Metabolized via liver; renally excreted.

- Slightly decrease dosage in patients with end-stage renal disease (metabolites can rarely cause an SLE-like syndrome); no change needed for milder renal impairment.
- Reduce dosage in liver dysfunction.
- Supplemental dose suggested after hemodialysis but not after peritoneal dialysis.

Selected Side Effects: GI discomfort, mild decrease in WBCs, *Antabuse-like reaction if mixed with alcohol, peripheral neuropathy and seizures (immediately discontinue for either)*, pseudomembranous colitis.

Selected Drug Interactions:

- Prolongs PT in patients taking warfarin.
- Raises serum level of lithium.

Pregnancy Category: B. *Contraindicated, however, for the treatment of trichomoniasis during the first trimester of pregnancy.*

Cost: Generic $, Flagyl $$$$ (≈ $12 for 250 mg generic tablets tid for 10 days; ≈ $52 for 250 mg Flagyl tablets tid for 10 days).

Pearls:

- Can interfere with laboratory assays of alanine and aspartate transaminase (ALT, AST), lactate dehydrogenase, and triglycerides.
- Excellent abscess penetration.
- Penicillin or clindamycin is preferred for aspiration pneumonia (metronidazole does not cover microaerophilic streptococcus, one of the anaerobic organisms associated with aspiration pneumonia).
- Warn patients to avoid alcohol ingestion during use and to discontinue medication and consult a physician if they develop any neurologic symptoms during therapy.
- Long-term use (ie, in Crohn's disease) is associated with peripheral neuropathy.

Mevacor: *see* LOVASTATIN

MEXILETINE (Mexitil)

Dose: 200–400 mg PO tid.

PO Preparations: 150, 200, and 250 mg capsules.

Actions:

- Type Ib antiarrhythmic (same category as lidocaine) used to treat ventricular arrhythmias.
- Inhibits the inward sodium current, reducing the rate of rise of the phase 0 action potential; also decreases the effective refractory period.

Clearance: Metabolized via liver; variable renally excreted.

- Slightly reduce dosage in patients with end-stage renal disease; no change needed for milder renal impairment.
- Increase dosing interval to q24h or longer in patients with liver disease.
- Supplemental dose suggested after hemodialysis but not peritoneal dialysis.

Selected Side Effects: GI distress, tremor and coordination difficulties, nervousness, dizziness/lightheadedness, proarrhythmic effects.

Selected Drug Interactions:
- Can raise serum level of theophylline.
- Hepatic enzyme inducing drugs (phenytoin, phenobarbital, rifampin, etc) decrease its serum level.

Cautions: Use with caution in patients with 2″ or 3″ heart block, sinus node dysfunction, intraventricular conduction abnormalities, hypotension, severe CHF, and liver disease.

Pregnancy Category: C.

Cost: $$$$ ($\approx$ $0.90 each 200 mg generic tablet; $\approx$ $1.10 each 100 mg Mexitil tablet).

Pearls:
- Usual therapeutic level is 0.5–2.0 µg/mL.
- Should be taken with meals.
- Degree of renal excretion is patient dependent; excretion can be reduced with alkalinization of the urine.

Mexitil: *see* MEXILETINE

MEZLOCILLIN (Mezlin)

Dose: 3 g IV q4h or 4 g IV q6h.

Actions: Bactericidal antipseudomonal penicillin that inhibits cell wall synthesis.
- Some gram (+) coverage, including enterococci and strep (but *not* staff).
- Excellent gram (−) coverage, including *Pseudomonas aeruginosa*.
- Good anaerobic coverage, including *Bacteroides fragilis.*
- *NOTE:* The above-mentioned antimicrobial coverage summary should be used as a guideline only; treatment decisions should take into account not only local epidemiologic patterns of antibiotic susceptibility but also, when available, culture susceptibility results.

Clearance: Primarily renally excreted; some hepatobiliary excretion.
- Slightly increase dosing interval in patients with impaired renal function.

- No change in dosage needed in patients with liver disease.
- Supplemental dose not required after hemodialysis or peritoneal dialysis.

Selected Side Effects: Rash, drug fever, anaphylactic reactions, interstitial nephritis, GI distress, elevated LFTs, seizures (with excessive dose), leukopenia, eosinophilia, thrombocytopenia, phlebitis.

Selected Drug Interactions: Probenecid raises its serum level.

Cautions: *Contraindicated in patients with history of hypersensitivity reactions to any of the penicillins.*

Pregnancy Category: B.

Cost: $$$.

Pearls: Contains high Na^+ load.

MICONAZOLE (Monistat Vaginal Suppositories, Monistat Vaginal Cream)

Dose: Route dependent:

- Cream: Apply qhs for 7 days (for Monistat 7).
- Suppository: Insert intravaginally qhs for 3 days (Monistat 3) or 7 days (Monistat 7).

Preparations:

- 1.59 oz tubes of Monistat 7 Vaginal Cream.
- 200 mg Monistat 3 Vaginal Suppositories.
- 100 mg Monistat 7 Vaginal Suppositories.

Actions: Fungicidal antibiotic used to treat *Candida* vaginitis.

Selected Side Effects: Vulvovaginal burning, itching, or irritation, contact dermatitis.

Cautions: Should be avoided when possible during first trimester of pregnancy (orally absorbed miconazole has been shown to have fetotoxic effects in animals).

Cost: $$

Pearls: Try to avoid in first trimester of pregnancy.

Micro-K: *see* POTASSIUM CHLORIDE

Micronase: *see* GLYBURIDE

Midamor: *see* AMILORIDE

MIDAZOLAM (Versed)
Dose:
- For preprocedure sedation and anesthesia, 0.15–0.35 mg/kg IV (approximately 1–2.5 mg for a 70 kg patient) injected over at least 20–30 s.
- May give further small doses after at least 2 min (usual interval is 3–5 min).

Actions: Short-acting benzodiazepine used in induction of anesthesia and as sedative before procedures such as endoscopy or intubation.

Selected Side Effects: *Respiratory depression, apnea,* pain at injection site, phlebitis.

Cautions: *Should be used only by experienced personnel (because of potential for respiratory arrest).*

Pregnancy Category: D.

Cost: $.

Pearls:
- Titrate *slowly* (some patients may respond to as little as 1 mg).
- *Always have oxygen and resuscitative equipment immediately available.*
- In case of accidental overdose and respiratory depression, can be reversed with flumazenil (Romazicon).
- Impairs memory of periprocedure events.
- Is 3–4 times more potent per milligram than diazepam (Valium).

MILK OF MAGNESIA: *see*
MAGNESIUM HYDROXIDE

MINERAL OIL
Dose: Delivery dependent.
- PO: 15–45 mL qd–bid.
- Enema: 60–120 mg.

PO Preparations: 16 oz bottles.

Actions: Lubricant laxative; used to treat constipation.

Cautions: Should not be used with surfactant-type stool softeners.

Cost: $.
Pearls:
- Onset of action is 48–72 h with PO therapy, immediate when given as enema.
- Decreases absorption of fat-soluble vitamins.

Minipress: *see* PRAZOSIN

Minitran: *see* NITROGLYCERIN patch

MINOXIDIL topical solution (Rogaine)
Dose:
- Apply 1 mL of solution to scalp bid.
- Maximum: 2 mL bid.

Preparations: 60 mL bottle containing 2% solution (20 mg/mL).
Actions: Topical agent that stimulates vertex hair growth and stabilizes hair loss; used to treat male-pattern baldness.
Selected Side Effects: No increase in systemic effects compared with placebo.
Pregnancy Category: C.
Cost: $$$ (≈ $60/bottle).
Pearls:
- Causes significant hair growth in only modest percentage of patients.
- Many patients need at least 4–8 months of treatment before achieving significant results.
- Remind patients who apply preparation with the fingers to wash hands after each use.

MISOPROSTOL (Cytotec)
Dose:
- Usual: 200 µg PO qid with food. (*NOTE:* Dose is in micrograms, *not* milligrams.)
- If this dose is not tolerated, can give 100 µg PO qid.

PO Preparations: 100 and 200 µg tablets.
Actions: Prostaglandin analogue used to prevent gastric ulcers in patients at high risk of complications from therapy with NSAIDs (including ASA); does *not* prevent duodenal

ulcers or the GI pain and discomfort that can be associated with NSAID use.

Clearance: De-esterified to the active compound misoprostol acid, which is primarily renally excreted.

- Dosage change not routinely needed in patients with renal insufficiency, but may be decreased if 200 μg dose is not tolerated.

Selected Side Effects: Diarrhea, abdominal pain, nausea and vomiting, possible miscarriage.

Cautions: *Contraindicated in patients with history of allergy to prostaglandins and in pregnant or potentially pregnant patients.*

Pregnancy Category: X.

Cost: $$$$ ($\approx$ $0.80 each 100 μg tablet).

Mitomycin (Mitomycin-C, Mutamycin)

Dose: 20 mg/m^2 IV.

Actions: Antibiotic that inhibits DNA synthesis; used to treat neoplastic diseases.

Clearance: Primarily metabolized in liver and other tissues; approximately 10–30% excreted unchanged in urine.

- Recommendations vary on need to adjust dosage in renal failure: one source notes it should not be used if serum creatinine > 1.7 mg/day/L; another source states no change is needed for creatinine clearance > 10 mL/min.
- No change in dosage needed in patients with liver disease.

Selected Side Effects: *Myelosuppression,* nausea and vomiting, anorexia, alopecia, stomatitis, fever, rare pulmonary toxicity, hemolytic-uremic syndrome, severe local irritation if extravasated.

Selected Drug Interactions: Concurrent use with vinca alkaloids is associated with shortness of breath and severe bronchospasm.

Pregnancy Category: Not established.

Cost: $$$$.

Pearls:

- Myelosuppression is dose-limiting toxicity.
- Average time for WBC and platelet nadirs is 4 weeks but can be as long as 8 weeks after therapy.

MODURETIC (AMILORIDE + HYDROCHLOROTHIAZIDE)

Dose: 1 or 2 tablets PO qd (can be given bid).

PO Preparations: Each tablet contains 5 mg amiloride and 50 mg hydrochlorothiazide.

Actions: Combination K^+-sparing diuretic; used to treat hypertension.

Clearance: Avoid in patients with end-stage renal disease.

Selected Side Effects: Hyperkalemia, GI discomfort, mild skin rash.

Selected Drug Interactions:

- Concomitant use with indomethacin causes elevated K^+ level.
- Increases risk of lithium toxicity.

Pregnancy Category: B.

Cost: Generic $$, Moduretic $$$ ($\approx$ $0.30 each generic tablet; $\approx$ $0.50 each Moduretic tablet).

M.O.M.: *see* MAGNESIUM HYDROXIDE

Monistat: *see* MICONAZOLE

Monoket: *see* ISOSORBIDE MONONITRATE

Monopril: *see* FOSINOPRIL

MORICIZINE (Ethmozine)

Dose:

- Usual: 200–300 mg PO tid.
- Some patients may achieve arrhythmia control with bid dose.

PO Preparations: 200, 250, and 300 mg tablets.

Actions:

- Class I anti-arrhythmic that slows the fast inward sodium current, decreasing the rate of phase 0 depolarization and slowing impulse conduction; used to treat life-threatening ventricular arrhythmias.
- Leads to a modest increase in PR and QRS duration (12–14% on average).

Clearance: Extensively metabolized via liver, metabolites excreted in feces and urine.
- Although no active metabolites are known to be renally excreted, it is recommended that patients with impaired renal function be started on a lower dose and carefully monitored.
- Reduce dosage in liver dysfunction.

Selected Side Effects: *Proarrhythmic actions,* conduction abnormalities, dizziness, nausea, headache.

Cautions:
- *Contraindicated in second- or third-degree AV block unless a pacemaker is in place.*
- May be contraindicated in bifascicular block unless a pacemaker is present.
- *Use with caution in sick sinus syndrome (can cause sinus bradycardia, sinus pause or arrest, or conduction problems).*

Pregnancy Category: B.

Cost: $$$$ ($\approx$ $1.30 each 250 mg tablet).

Pearls:
- Increased mortality rates in certain patients when used to treat post-MI PVCs in the CAST study.
- Discontinue if second- or third-degree heart block develops unless a pacemaker is in place.
- Correct K^+ and Mg abnormalities before beginning treatment.
- Is a phenothiazine derivative.

MORPHINE (MORPHINE SULFATE, MS Contin)

Dose: Highly variable.
- Initial: 2 mg IV, or 5–10 mg SQ, or 5–10 mg IM, or 5–20 mg PO.
- Maintenance: variable, with PO, SQ, and IM usually given q4h.
- Controlled-release PO (MS Contin): Divide total daily dose into either halves or thirds and give q12h or q8h, respectively.
- Acute MI: May give 2–4 mg IV at frequent intervals (avoid IM injections, which will elevate CPK levels).

- IV drip may vary between 1–4 mg/h or significantly more, especially in cancer patients.
- When converting from IV to PO, estimates of PO equivalent vary; *PDR* suggests that 3 times the IV dose may be sufficient; should titrate to pain control.
- Consider using lower initial and maintenance doses in elderly patients and in patients with respiratory or liver disease.

PO Preparations:
- 10, 15, and 30 mg tablets.
- 15, 30, 60, 100, and 200 mg tablets of MS Contin.
- 5, 10, 20, and 30 mg suppositories.
- Multiple sizes and concentrations of bottles of oral solution.

Actions: Narcotic analgesic that also promotes venous and arterial dilatation and reduces sensation of dyspnea; used to relieve pain and in acute treatment of CHF and pulmonary edema (if respiratory depression is not a significant concern).

Clearance: Metabolized via liver; $t_{1/2}$ is prolonged in liver dysfunction.
- Slightly decrease dosage in patients with impaired renal function.
- Reduce dosage in patients with liver disease.
- Supplemental dose not required after hemodialysis.

Selected Side Effects: *Respiratory depression,* nausea and vomiting, constipation, ileus, hypotension, urine retention, sedation.

Pregnancy Category: C.

Cost: Regular tablets $, MS Contin $$$$.

Pearls:
- Can cause mast cell degranulation and histamine release.
- Never crush tablets for administration via NG tube or for any other reason (may cause rapid absorption of high morphine doses).

Motrin, Motrin IB: *see* IBUPROFEN

6-MP: *see* MERCAPTOPURINE

MS Contin: *see* MORPHINE

Mucomyst: *see* ACETYLCYSTEINE

Mutamycin: *see* MITOMYCIN

Mycelex: *see* CLOTRIMAZOLE

Mycostatin: *see* NYSTATIN

**Mylanta (ALUMINUM HYDROXIDE +
MAGNESIUM HYDROXIDE + SIMETHICONE)**
Dose: 1 or 2 tablets or tsp, or 15–30 mg, between meals and qhs.

Myleran: *see* BUSULFAN

Mylicon: *see* SIMETHICONE

Mysoline: *see* PRIMIDONE

NABUMETONE (Relafen)
Dose:
- 500–2000 mg PO qd.
- Usual: 1000 mg PO given in 1 dose at night.

PO Preparations: 500 and 750 mg tablets.

Actions: Nonsteroidal anti-inflammatory agent; used to treat arthritis.

Clearance: Undergoes biotransformation in liver to active metabolite 6-MNA, which is metabolized via liver to inactive products.

- Reduce dosage in patients with severe renal disease.
- Dosage adjustment probably not needed in patients with liver disease.
- Supplemental dose not required after hemodialysis.

Selected Side Effects: GI tract ulceration and bleeding, diarrhea, dyspepsia, abdominal pain, fluid retention and worsening of CHF, exacerbation of "prerenal" renal failure or interstitial nephritis, reversible decrease in platelet aggregation, and prolongation of bleeding time.

Cautions:
- *Contraindicated in patients with salicylate sensitivity.*
- Although it may cause less upper GI bleeding or ulcers than other NSAIDs, still use with caution in patients with history of ulcer or upper GI bleeding.
- Its use during third trimester of pregnancy may cause premature closure of the ductus arteriosus.

Pregnancy Category: C.

Cost: $$$ ($1 each 500 mg tablet).

Pearls: Should be taken with food or antacids.

N-ACETYLCYSTEINE: *see* ACETYLCYSTEINE

NADOLOL (Corgard)
Dose:
- Initial: 20–40 mg PO qd.
- Usual: 40 80 mg PO qd.
- Maximum: 160–240 mg qd for angina, 240–320 mg qd for hypertension.

PO Preparations: 20, 40, 80, 120, and 160 mg tablets.

Actions: Long-acting nonselective β-blocker used to treat hypertension and angina.

Clearance: Renally excreted.
- Moderately reduce dosage in patients with impaired renal function; significant accumulation can occur in patients with end-stage renal disease.
- No change in dosage needed in patients with liver disease.
- Supplemental dose suggested after hemodialysis.

Selected Side Effects: Bradycardia, CHF, hypotension, rare but potentially serious bronchospasm, conduction abnormalities.

Cautions: *Contraindicated in bronchial asthma, sinus bradycardia, second- or third-degree heart block, or overt cardiac failure.*

Pregnancy Category: C.

Cost: Generic $$, Corgard $$$ (≈ $0.55 each 40 mg generic tablet; ≈ $0.95 each 40 mg Corgard tablet).

Pearls: Taper dose when discontinuing (to avoid rebound reactions).

NALOXONE (Narcan)
Dose:
- 0.4 mg (1 mL ampule or 1 mL prefilled syringe) IV, IM, or SQ.
- May repeat dose q2–3 min up to 10 mg.
- May be given IM or SQ if no IV access is available.

Actions: Narcotic antagonist that reverses opioid effects, including respiratory depression, sedation, and hypotension; used to treat narcotic overdose.

Clearance: Metabolized via liver; renally excreted.

Selected Side Effects: Abrupt reversal of narcotic depression can cause nausea and vomiting, sweating, tachycardia and hypertension, tremulousness, seizures and cardiac arrest, or increased PTT.

Pregnancy Category: B.

Pearls:
- Onset of action is 1–2 min when given IV, 3–5 min when given IM or SQ.
- Reevaluate diagnosis of narcotic overdose if symptoms are not reversed after total of 10 mg.
- In overdose therapy, naloxone is effective for only 1–3 h, whereas many narcotic agents have significantly longer duration of action, so patients must be continuously monitored for relapsing signs and symptoms of overdose.

NAPHAZOLINE: *see* Naphcon-A

Naphcon-A ophthalmic solution (NAPHAZOLINE + PHENIRAMINE)
Dose: 1 drop (written "gtt") in the eye up to q3–4h.

Preparations: 5 and 15 mL solutions containing 0.025% naphazoline and 0.3% pheniramine.

Actions: Ophthalmic solution used to treat ocular irritation, congestion, and allergic or inflammatory conditions.

Cautions: *Contraindicated in patients taking MAOI.*

Pregnancy Category: Not established.

Cost: Generic $, Naphcon-A $$.
Pearls: Sold without prescription (over the counter).

Naprosyn: *see* NAPROXEN

NAPROXEN (Aleve, Anaprox, Naprosyn)
Dose:
- Naprosyn: 250–500 mg PO bid.
- Anaprox: 275–550 mg PO bid (delivering 250–500 mg of naproxen bid).
- Aleve: 220 mg PO bid–tid (delivering 200 mg of Naprosyn bid–tid).

PO Preparations:
- Naprosyn: 250, 375, and 500 mg tablets.
- Anaprox: 275 and 550 mg (delivering 250 and 500 mg of naproxen, respectively).
- Aleve: 220 mg tablets (delivering 200 mg of naproxen).

Actions: Nonsteroidal anti-inflammatory agent with analgesic and antipyretic action; used to treat inflammation and pain.
Clearance: Metabolized via liver.
- No change in dosage needed in patients with renal insufficiency.
- Supplemental dose not required after hemodialysis.

Selected Side Effects: GI tract ulceration and bleeding, dyspepsia, abdominal pain, fluid retention and worsening of CHF, exacerbation of "prerenal" renal failure or interstitial nephritis, reversible decrease in platelet aggregation and prolongation of bleeding time.
Cautions:
- *Contraindicated in patients with salicylate sensitivity or history of upper GI bleeding or ulcer.*
- Should not be used during third trimester of pregnancy; can cause premature closure of the ductus arteriosus or complications during delivery.

Pregnancy Category: B. Can cause premature closure of the ductus arteriosus or complications during delivery and therefore should not be used during the third trimester of pregnancy.

Cost: Generic $$, Naprosyn $$$ (generic ≈ $0.40 each 375 mg tablet, Naprosyn ≈ $1 each 375 mg tablet).
Pearls:
- Can cause Na^+ retention.
- Should be taken with food or antacids.
- Aleve can be obtained without prescription (over the counter).

Narcan: *see* NALOXONE

Nasacort: *see* TRIAMCINOLONE nasal inhaler

Nasalcrom: *see* CROMOLYN SODIUM

Navelbine: *see* VINORELBINE

NebuPent: *see* PENTAMIDINE

Nembutal: *see* PENTOBARBITAL

NEOMYCIN SULFATE (*see also* Cortisporin, Neosporin)
Dose: Disease or use dependent.
- Hepatic encephalopathy: 1–2 g PO or via NG tube q4–6h.
- Preop: 1 g PO.
PO Preparations:
- 500 mg tablets.
- 125 mg/5 mL (1 tsp) oral solution.
Actions: Poorly absorbed aminoglycoside that decreases production of ammonia by GI bacteria; used to treat hepatic encephalopathy.
Selected Side Effects:
- Nausea and vomiting.
- Some systemic absorption can increase risk of ototoxicity or nephrotoxicity in patients with renal dysfunction.
Selected Drug Interactions: Can increase neuromuscular blockade if absorbed.
Cost: $.

Neosporin cream (POLYMYXIN B + NEOMYCIN)
Dose: Apply to skin qd–tid.
Preparations: 15 g tubes.
Actions: Topical antibiotic mixture used to prevent skin infections.
Selected Side Effects: Skin sensitization, ototoxicity, nephrotoxicity.

Neo-Synephrine: *see* PHENYLEPHRINE

Neupogen: *see* GRANULOCYTE COLONY-STIMULATING FACTOR

Neurontin: *see* GABAPENTIN

Neutra-Phos: *see* PHOSPHORUS

NIACIN: *see* NICOTINIC ACID

Niacinol: *see* NICOTINIC ACID

NICARDIPINE (Cardene, Cardene SR)
Dose:
- PO:
  - ▶ 20–40 mg PO tid of Cardene.
  - ▶ 30–60 mg PO bid of Cardene SR.
- IV (for short-term treatment of hypertension):
  - ▶ Initiate therapy at a rate of 5.0 mg/h (*NOTE:* The rate is per hour).
  - ▶ If adequate BP control is not achieved, can increase infusion rate by 2.5 mg/h every 15 min, up to a maximum infusion rate of 15.0 mg/h.
  - ▶ If more rapid BP control is necessary, can increase infusion rate every 5 min.
  - ▶ After adequate BP control achieved, the infusion rate should be decreased 3 mg/h and titrated as needed.

PO Preparations:
- Cardene: 20 and 30 mg tablets.
- Cardene SR: 30, 45, and 60 mg tablets.

Actions: Calcium channel blocker used to treat hypertension, angina, and systolic dysfunction.

Clearance: > 99% metabolized via liver, but serum level is elevated in patients with impaired renal function and is exponentially increased at higher doses.
- Use with caution in mild liver disease; reduce dosage or increase dosing interval in patients with severe liver disease.

Selected Side Effects: Hypotension, reflex tachycardia, headache, "paradoxical" increase in angina.

Cautions: *Contraindicated in patients with significant aortic stenosis.*

Pregnancy Category: C.

Cost: $$$$ (≈ $0.50 each 20 mg Cardene tablet; ≈ $1.25 each 45 mg Cardene SR tablet).

Pearls: May have less (−) inotropic effect than nifedipine.

Nicoderm: *see* NICOTINE transdermal patch

Nicolar: *see* NICOTINIC ACID

Nicotrol: *see* NICOTINE transdermal patch

NICOTINE transdermal patch (Habitrol, Nicoderm, Nicotrol, ProStep)

Dose: System dependent:
- Habitrol, Nicoderm:
  ▶ A new 21 mg/day patch applied each day for 6 weeks; then decrease to a new 14 mg/day patch applied each day for 2 weeks; then decrease to a new 7 mg/day patch applied each day for 2 weeks; then discontinue.
  ▶ Patients who weigh < 100 lb, smoke < 10 cigarettes daily, or have history of cardiovascular disease should begin with the 14 mg/day patch for 6 weeks, then decrease to the 7 mg/day patch for 2 weeks.

- ProStep:
  - ► A new 22 mg/day patch applied each day for 4–8 weeks; therapy may either then be discontinued, or, if a gradual reduction is desired, patients may be treated with a new 11 mg/day patch applied each day for 2–4 weeks; after which the patches should be discontinued.
  - ► Patients who weigh < 100 lb should begin with the 11 mg/day patches and receive treatment for 4–8 weeks; after which the patches should be discontinued.
- Nicotrol:
  - ► A new 15 mg/day patch applied each morning for 4–12 weeks ; then 10 mg/day for 2 weeks; then 5 mg/day for 2 weeks; after which the patches should be discontinued.
  - ► If symptoms of nicotine excess occur with the 15 mg/day patches, the daily dose should be decreased to 10 mg/day.
- Note that with the Nicotrol system a new patch should be applied every morning, and that patch should be taken off at bedtime (ie, is only worn during waking hours); Habitrol, Nicoderm, and ProStep patches are worn for 24 h before a new patch is applied.
- Patches should be applied to a nonhairy, clean, and dry skin site on trunk or upper outer arm.
- New patches should be applied to a *different* site; the same skin site should not be used again for at least 7 days.

Preparations:
- Habitrol, Nicoderm: Transdermal patches delivering 21, 14, or 7 mg/day of nicotine over 24 h.
- ProStep: Transdermal patches delivering 22 or 11 mg/day of nicotine over 24 h.
- Nicotrol: Transdermal patches delivering 15, 10, or 5 mg/day of nicotine over 16 h.

Actions: Transdermal system that delivers nicotine used for prophylactic treatment of nicotine withdrawal in patients attempting to stop smoking.

Clearance: Metabolized via liver; renally excreted.

Selected Side Effects: Local irritation, pruritus or erythema, diarrhea, dyspepsia, arthralgia or myalgia, somnolence, tachycardia. Nicotine toxicity is characterized by nausea and vomiting, diarrhea, abdominal pain, diaphoresis, flushing, dizziness, disturbed hearing and vision, confusion, weakness, palpitations, altered respiration, and hypotension.

Cautions:

- *Contraindicated in patients with serious arrhythmias, severe or worsening angina, and in the immediate post-MI period.*
- Should not be used by patients < 16 years old or by pregnant patients.
- Patients should be instructed to stop smoking when therapy is begun to avoid nicotine overdose.
- Use with caution in patients with peptic ulcer disease (nicotine delays healing), accelerated hypertension (nicotine increases risk of malignant hypertension), hyperthyroidism, diabetes, or pheochromocytoma (nicotine causes release of catecholamines by the adrenal medulla).

Cost: $$$$ (per initial 6 week supply: Habitrol ≈ $145, Nicoderm ≈ $170, ProStep ≈ $190, Nicotrol ≈ $160).

Pregnancy Category: D.

Pearls:

- Patients who stop smoking may require reduction in dosage of imipramine, oxazepam, theophylline, insulin, prazosin, or labetalol.
- Patients who continue to smoke while using the patch may experience increased side effects from elevated serum nicotine levels, possibly including myocardial infarction.
- Warn patients to dispose of patches carefully so that children and pets do not apply or ingest discarded patches (residual nicotine remains on the patch after 24 h).
- Patients who do not quit smoking within 4 weeks of therapy are unlikely to quit, and transdermal nicotine therapy should be discontinued.

NICOTINIC ACID (Niacin, Niacinol, Niacor, Nicolar, Slo-Niacin)

Dose:

- Initial: 250 mg following the evening meal.
- Gradually increase to 1–2 g PO tid (one source notes that one can give a 3 g dose qd).
- Usual dose of Slo-Niacin is one 750 mg tablet bid.

PO Preparations:

- 500 mg capsules of Niacinol.
- 500 mg tablets of Niacor and Nicolar.
- 250, 500, and 750 mg tablets of Slo-Niacin.

Actions: Medication that inhibits synthesis of VLDL and decreases HDL catabolism, leading to reduced LDL and triglyceride and increased HDL levels; used to treat hypercholesterolemia and hypertriglyceridemia.

Clearance: Metabolized via liver; renally excreted.

- Moderately reduce dosage in patients with impaired renal function; toxic reactions are frequent in patients with end-stage renal disease.

Selected Side Effects: Frequent flushing and pruritus (may decrease over time), GI discomfort, elevated LFTs and occasional jaundice.

Selected Drug Interactions: Adrenergic blocking drugs can substantially increase peripheral vasodilatation, causing postural hypotension.

Cautions:

- *Contraindicated in liver dysfunction, active peptic ulcer, arterial bleeding, and in patients with known idiosyncratic drug reactions.*
- Use with caution in gout or diabetes (can increase glucose levels in diabetics).

Pregnancy Category: Not established.

Cost: Generic $, brands $$$.

Pearls: Aspirin or other NSAIDs taken 30 min before initial daily dose can decrease flushing, as can taking nicotinic acid with meals.

NIFEDIPINE (Adalat, Adalat CC, Procardia, Procardia XL)

Dose: Preparation dependent.

- Regular capsules: 10–40 mg PO tid.
- Long-acting capsules: 30–90 mg PO qd of Procardia XL.
- For elderly patients beginning therapy with regular capsules, give initial 5 mg test dose, at night if possible.

PO Preparations:
- 10, 20, and 30 mg capsules of Procardia; 10 and 20 mg capsules of Adalat.
- 30, 60, and 90 mg long-acting capsules of Procardia XL and Adalat CC.

Actions: Calcium channel blocker used to treat angina and hypertension.

Clearance: Metabolized via liver.
- No change in dosage needed in patients with renal insufficiency.
- Reduce dosage in patients with liver disease.
- Supplemental dose not required after hemodialysis.

Selected Side Effects: Hypotension, dizziness or light-headedness, peripheral edema, flushing, reflex tachycardia, headache, rare (+) direct Coombs' reaction.

Selected Drug Interactions: Can raise serum level of digoxin.

Pregnancy Category: C.

Cost: $$$$ (≈ $1 each 30 mg Procardia capsules; ≈ $2.50 each 90 mg Procardia XL capsules; ≈ $1.90 each 90 mg Adalat CC capsule).
- Adalat is approximately one fourth less expensive than Procardia.

Pearls:
- May give 10 mg SL for urgent treatment of hypertension (physicians differ on whether sublingual administration actually produces quicker effect).
- Adalat preparations appears to be slightly less expensive than Procardia preparations.

NIMODIPINE (Nimotop)

Dose: For subarachnoid hemorrhage: 60 mg PO q4h for 21 days.

Preparations: 30 mg tablets.

Actions: Calcium channel blocker used to prevent ischemic stroke related to vasospasm in patients with subarachnoid hemorrhage.

Clearance: Metabolized via liver.
- Reduce dosage (to 30 mg q4h) in liver failure.

Selected Side Effects: Hypotension, headache, flushing.
Selected Drug Interactions: Can potentiate other antihypertensive agents.
Pregnancy Category: C.
Cost: $$$$ (≈ $450 retail/100 tablets).
Pearls:
- Start ASAP (within 96 h) after subarachnoid hemorrhage.
- No IV form available; give via NG tube when necessary.

Nimotop: *see* NIMODIPINE

Nipride: *see* NITROPRUSSIDE

Nitro-Dur: *see* NITROGLYCERIN patch

NITROFURANTOIN (Macrobid, Macrodantin)
Dose: Preparation dependent:
- Macrodantin: 50 mg PO qid.
- Macrobid: 100 mg PO bid for 7 days.
Preparations:
- Macrobid: 100 mg capsules.
- Macrodantin: 25, 50, and 100 mg capsules.
Actions: Bacteriostatic antibiotic that is presumed to interfere with several bacterial enzyme systems; used to treat urinary tract infections.
- Good coverage of most organisms that cause these infections, including enterococci and staph.
Clearance: Metabolized via liver; inactivated by tissue; renally excreted.
- Avoid in patients with GFR < 50 mL/min (toxic metabolites accumulate).
- Dosage should probably be adjusted in patients with liver disease.
- Supplemental dose suggested after hemodialysis.
Selected Side Effects: Nausea, acute pulmonary hypersensitivity reactions, rare chronic pulmonary reactions, hemolytic anemia.
Selected Drug Interactions: Uricosuric agents can decrease its tubular secretion, causing higher serum levels and diminished efficacy.

Cautions: *Contraindicated in anuria or oliguria, and in pregnant patients at term (38–42 weeks).*

Pregnancy Category: B. *Nitrofurantoin, however, can cause hemolytic anemia secondary to G6PD deficiency, and thus should not be administered at term.*

Cost: $$ (≈ $25 for 50 mg qid for 10 days).

Pearls: Should be taken with food (to increase absorption).

NITROGLYCERIN [IV] (NTG)
Dose:
- Usual starting dose: 20 µg/min.
- Usually increase in increments of 20 µg/min.
- Some physicians consider 400 µg/min the maximum dose, but this varies from one practitioner to another. (*NOTE:* Dose is in micrograms, *not* milligrams.)

Actions: Nitrate that relaxes vascular smooth muscle (venous > arterial) and dilates coronary arteries; used to treat angina.

Clearance: Catabolized in the liver.
- Dosage adjustment probably not needed in patients with impaired renal function.

Selected Side Effects: Headache (common), hypotension, reflex tachycardia.

Pregnancy Category: C.

Cost: $.

Pearls:
- Tolerance can quickly develop.
- Headache side effects often limits therapy.

NITROGLYCERIN paste (Nitrol 2% Ointment, Nitropaste)
Dose: Apply 1–2 inches topically q4–6h.
- Is often titrated to systolic blood pressure (ie, 2 inches for SBP > 140, 1 inch for SBP 110–140, hold for SBP < 110; or some other [fairly arbitrary] SBP parameters).

Selected Side Effects: Headache (common), lightheadedness, fainting, hypotension, nausea and vomiting, contact dermatitis.

Cost: $.

Pregnancy Category: C.

Pearls:
- Tolerance can quickly develop.
- Headache side effects often limit therapy.

NITROGLYCERIN patch (Minitran, Nitro-Dur, Transderm-Nitro)

Dose:
- Initial: 0.2–0.4 mg/h.
- Titrate upward as clinically indicated.
- Maximum: 0.8 mg/h.

Patch Sizes: 0.1, 0.2, 0.3, 0.4, 0.6, and 0.8 mg/h.

Actions: Dermal patch that slowly releases nitroglycerin, which in turn relaxes vascular smooth muscle (venous > arterial) and dilates coronary arteries; used to treat CAD.

Clearance: Metabolized via liver.
- No change in dosage needed in patients with renal insufficiency.

Selected Side Effects: Headache (common), lightheadedness, fainting, hypotension, nausea and vomiting, dermatitis.

Pregnancy Category: C.

Cost: $$$ (≈ $1.50 each 0.2 mg/h patch).

Pearls:
- Many authorities now recommend having patient remove patch at night to avoid development of tolerance.
- Tolerance can quickly develop.
- Headache side effects often limit therapy.
- Placement of patch qhs (and removal in AM) may reduce paroxysmal nocturnal dyspnea (PND) in some patients with congestive heart failure (who are not being treated with nitrates for angina).

NITROGLYCERIN spray (Nitrolingual)

Dose: Use dependent.
- Angina prophylaxis: 0.4 or 0.8 mg (1 or 2 sprayed doses) under or on the tongue 5–10 min before activity.
- Angina: 0.4 mg (1 sprayed dose) under or on the tongue q5 min up to 3 doses if necessary.

Preparations: 14.49 g metered-dose aerosol preparation that provides 200 doses.

NITROGLYCERIN sublingual tablets (Nitrostat)
Dose: Use dependent.
- Angina prophylaxis: 1 tablet SL 5–10 min before activity.
- Angina: 1 tablet SL q5min, up to 3 tablets if necessary.
- Usual prescribed pill size is 1/150 grain; consider using 1/400 grain tablet in patients very sensitive to nitroglycerin.

Preparations: 1/100, 1/150, and 1/400 grain tablets.
Selected Side Effects: Headache (common), hypotension.
Pregnancy Category: C.
Cost: $.
Pearls:
- Pills can lose their effectiveness over time; those still fresh enough to be effective often "tingle" or "bubble" when placed underneath the tongue, whereas pills that have lost their effectiveness may not.
- Because pills lose their effectiveness, patients should be instructed to obtain new pills every 3–6 months.

Nitrol: *see* NITROGLYCERIN paste

Nitrolingual: *see* NITROGLYCERIN spray

Nitropaste: *see* NITROGLYCERIN paste

NITROPRUSSIDE (Nipride)
Dose: 0.3–8.0 μg/kg/min. (*NOTE:* Dose is in micrograms, *not* milligrams.)
- Usual starting dose: 0.3–0.5 μg/kg/min.
- Can increase in increments of 0.3 μg/kg/min.
- Maximum dose: 10 μg/kg/min.

Actions: Nitrate that relaxes vascular smooth muscle (arterial > venous), causing vasodilatation; used to treat hypertension and as afterload-reducing agent.
Clearance: Decomposed by nonenzymatic processes to cyanide, much of which is converted to thiocyanate by an enzyme located in the liver and kidneys.
- One source recommends no change in dosage in patients with renal insufficiency; another source notes that risks of cyanide and thiocyanate toxicity are increased in renal or

hepatic disease. Thus, it seems prudent to use nitroprusside with caution and to monitor thiocyanate levels in patients with renal or hepatic disease.

Selected Side Effects:

- Hypotension, *thiocyanate or cyanide toxicity.*
- With prolonged use may develop *thiocyanate toxicity or, in severe liver dysfunction, rare cyanide toxicity.*

Cost: $$.

Pearls:

- Its toxic metabolite thiocyanate can cause seizure, coma, or hypothyroidism; thiocyanate levels < 10 mg/dL are usually well tolerated, whereas levels > 20 mg/dL are associated with increased toxicity.
- Cyanide inhibits the cytochrome system, leading to inhibition of aerobic metabolism and increased lactate production; metabolic acidosis may be an early sign of cyanide toxicity.

Nitrostat: *see* NITROGLYCERIN sublingual tablets

NIZATIDINE (Axid)

Dose: Use dependent.

- Active duodenal ulcer: 300 mg PO qhs or 150 mg PO bid.
- Maintenance of healed duodenal ulcer: 150 mg PO qhs.

Preparations: 150 and 300 mg Axid Pulvules.

Actions: H_2-blocker used to treat peptic ulcer disease.

Clearance: Moderately to markedly increase dosing interval in patients with impaired renal function.

Selected Side Effects: Minimal significant side effects compared with those in placebo-treated patients.

Selected Drug Interactions: Can raise serum salicylate levels in patients taking high-dose aspirin.

Pregnancy Category: C.

Cost: $$$$ ($\approx$ $3 each 300 mg tablet).

Nizoral: *see* KETOCONAZOLE

Nizoral topical: *see* KETOCONAZOLE topical

Norcuron: *see* VECURONIUM

NOREPINEPHRINE (Levophed)
Dose: Most sources recommend an initial infusion rate of 8–12 μg/min for treatment of shock; some physicians begin therapy for milder forms of hypotension with a lower infusion rate of 2–4 μg/min. In either case, dosage should be adjusted based on BP; required maintenance dose is usually 2–4 μg/min. (*NOTE:* Dose is in micrograms, *not* milligrams.)

Actions: Strong α-adrenergic stimulator that increases peripheral vascular resistance (has minimal β-adrenergic stimulation); used to treat hypotension.

Selected Side Effects: Tissue ischemia, decreased renal perfusion and urine output.

Cautions:
- *Contraindicated in occlusive vascular disease.*
- Use with extreme caution in patients taking MAOI or tricyclics (substantially increases BP).

Pregnancy Category: C.

Pearls:
- Give through a large vein or central IV when possible.
- Give phentolamine if extravasated.
- May contain sulfite.

NORETHINDRONE: *see* Norinyl, Ortho-Novum, Tri-Norinyl oral contraceptive pills

NORFLOXACIN (Noroxin)
Dose: 400 mg PO bid.

Preparations: 400 mg tablets.

Actions: Synthetic bactericidal fluoroquinolone antibiotic that inhibits DNA synthesis; used to treat urinary tract infections, including *Pseudomonas aeruginosa,* staph, strep, and enterococci.

Clearance: Metabolized via liver to active metabolites; biliary and renally excreted.
- Moderately increase dosing interval in patients with impaired renal function; avoid in patients with end-stage renal disease.

COMMONLY USED DRUGS 277

- Dosage adjustment probably not needed in patients with liver disease but good renal function.
- Supplemental dose not required after hemodialysis.

Selected Side Effects: Generally well tolerated.

Selected Drug Interactions:
- Nitrofurantoin can antagonize its actions.
- Concurrent use with antacids, sucralfate, or iron salts can decrease its absorption.
- Can potentiate effects of anticoagulants and increase theophylline toxicity and cyclosporine-induced nephrotoxicity.

Cautions:
- *Contraindicated in patients* < 18 years old.
- Should probably not be used in pregnant or potentially pregnant patients.

Pregnancy Category: C.

Cost: $$$ ($\approx$ $60 for 400 bid for 10 days).

Pearls:
- Should *not* be used to treat systemic infections (does not achieve good serum levels).
- Should be taken 1 h before or 2 h after meals.

Norinyl contraceptive pills (NORETHINDRONE + ETHINYL ESTRADIOL or NORETHINDRONE + MESTRANOL)

Dose: 1 pill PO qd, preferably qhs; with 21-day regimen, take no pills on days 22–28 then begin a new cycle (3 weeks on, 1 week off).
- Take first pill on the first Sunday after onset of menses, or that Sunday if it is first day of menses.

Preparations: Available in 21- and 28-pill preparations.
- Norinyl 1 + 35: 1 mg norethindrone and 0.035 mg ethinyl estradiol.
- Norinyl 1 + 50: 1 mg norethindrone and 0.050 mg mestranol.

Actions: Combination oral contraceptive used to prevent pregnancy.

Selected Side Effects: Serious vascular complications, menstrual changes, breakthrough bleeding, cervical and

breast changes, vaginal candidiasis, hypertension, nausea
and vomiting, liver tumors, GI distress, edema, weight
changes, migraine headache, rash, depression, glucose intolerance, visual changes from alteration in corneal curvature,
intolerance for contact lenses.

Selected Drug Interactions: Contraceptive effectiveness
can be decreased by antibiotics (ampicillin, chloramphenicol, isoniazid, nitrofurantoin, penicillin V, phenytoin, rifampin, sulfonamides, tetracycline), anxiolytics, phenylbu-
tazones, barbiturates, antimigraine medications, analgesics,
and tranquilizers.

Cautions:

• *Contraindicated in patients with thromboembolic or thrombophlebitic disorders, cardiovascular or cerebrovascular
disease, vaginal bleeding of unknown cause, endometrial
or other estrogen-dependent tumors, known or suspected
breast cancer, jaundice, hepatic tumors, smokers over age
35, or possible pregnancy.*

• Cigarette smoking increases risk of serious cardiovascular
complications; patients should be *strongly* advised not to
smoke.

Pregnancy Category: X.

Cost: $$$ (≈ $20/month).

Pearls: Patients should undergo complete work-up prior to
use, with special attention given to history of abnormal
vaginal bleeding, BP, breast examination, and pelvic exami-
nation, including cervical cytology.

Normodyne: *see* LABETALOL

Noroxin: *see* NORFLOXACIN

Norpace: *see* DISOPYRAMIDE

Norplant: *see* LEVONORGESTREL

Norpramin: *see* DESIPRAMINE

NORTRIPTYLINE (Pamelor)
Dose:
- Usual: 25 mg PO tid–qid.
- Maximum: 150 mg daily (maximum in elderly patients is 30–50 mg daily).

Preparations:
- 10, 25, 50, and 75 mg tablets.
- 16 oz bottles containing 10 mg/5 mL (1 tsp).

Actions: Tricyclic used to treat depression.

Clearance: Metabolized via liver.
- No change in dosage needed in patients with renal insufficiency.
- One source suggests slightly reducing dosage in patients with liver disease, though little data are available.
- Supplemental dose not required after hemodialysis or peritoneal dialysis.

Selected Side Effects: Prolonged conduction time, sinus tachycardia, arrhythmias, tremors, worsening of psychosis in schizophrenic patients.

Selected Drug Interactions:
- *Concomitant use with MAOI causes hyperpyretic crisis, convulsion, and death.*
- Increases risk of arrhythmia in patients receiving thyroid replacement therapy.
- Cimetidine leads to a clinically significant increase in plasma levels.

Cautions:
- *Contraindicated in patients who have taken MAOI within 2 weeks.*
- Use with caution in cardiac disease, glaucoma, or urine retention (because of its anticholinergic and conduction effects).

Pregnancy Category: Not established.

Cost: $$$ ($\approx$ $0.40 each 25 mg tablet).

Pearls:
- Consider monitoring serum level when dosage exceeds 100 mg daily.
- "Therapeutic window" is 50–150 μg/mL.
- Signs and symptoms of overdose include confusion, restlessness, agitation, vomiting, hyperpyrexia, muscle rigid-

ity, hyperactive reflexes, tachycardia, ECG evidence of impaired conduction, ventricular arrhythmias, hypotension and shock, CHF, stupor, coma, seizures, and respiratory depression.

Norvasc: *see* AMLODIPINE

NTG: *see* NITROGLYCERIN

Nuprin: *see* IBUPROFEN

Nydrazid: *see* ISONIAZID

NYSTATIN (Mycostatin cream and ointment)
Dose: Apply to skin bid.
Preparations:
- 15 and 30 g cream and ointment.
- 15 g powder.

Actions: Topical antifungal; used to treat candidiasis.

OFLOXACIN (Floxin)
Dose: Disease dependent (as recommended by manufacturer).
- Lower respiratory tract infection: 400 mg PO or IV q12h for 10 days.
- Uncomplicated urinary tract infection: 200 mg PO or IV q12h for 3 days for cystitis caused by *Escherichia coli* or *Klebsiella pneumoniae,* 7 days for cystitis caused by other organisms, or 10 days for "complicated" urinary tract infections.
- Prostatitis: 300 mg PO or IV q12h for 6 weeks.
- Acute, uncomplicated gonorrhea: Single dose of 400 mg PO or IV.
- Cervicitis and urethritis from *Chlamydia + Neisseria gonorrhoeae:* 300 mg PO or IV q12h for 7 days.
- Mild to moderate infection of skin or skin structures: 400 mg PO or IV q12h for 10 days.

Preparations: 200, 300, and 400 mg tablets.

Actions: Broad-spectrum fluoroquinolone that inhibits DNA gyrase.
- Good gram (+) coverage, including *Staphylococcus aureus* and MRSA (but *not* enterococci).
- Excellent gram (−) coverage, including *Pseudomonas aeruginosa.*
- Poor anaerobic coverage.
- Also covers *Chlamydia* (unlike Cipro) and has in vitro activity against atypical pneumonia pathogens (*Mycoplasma, Chlamydia pneumoniae* [TWAR], and *Legionella*).
- *NOTE:* The above-mentioned antimicrobial coverage summary should be used as a guideline only; treatment decisions should take into account not only local epidemiologic patterns of antibiotic susceptibility but also, when available, culture susceptibility results.

Clearance: Primarily excreted unchanged in urine.
- Adjust dosage in patients with impaired renal function: for creatinine clearance 10–50 mL/min, increase dosing interval to q24h; for creatinine clearance 210 mL/min, give 1/2 recommended dose q24h.

Selected Side Effects: Usually well tolerated. Rare side effects include nausea, diarrhea, GI distress, headache, and insomnia.

Selected Drug Interactions:
- Raises serum level of theophylline.
- Concomitant use with sucralfate, iron, multivitamins containing zinc, or antacids containing calcium, magnesium, or aluminum can substantially decrease its absorption.

Cautions: *The safety of ofloxacin in patients < 18 years old has not been established; therefore, should not be used in patients < 18 years old.*

Pregnancy Category: C.

Cost: $$$ (≈ $75 for 200 bid for 10 days).

Pearls:
- Should be taken at least 1/2 h before or at least 2 h after meals.
- IV administration does *not* provide for greater efficacy than PO administration.
- Avoid excessive exposure to sunlight (similar drugs have been associated with increased photosensitivity).

OLSALAZINE SODIUM (Dipentum)
Dose: 500 mg PO bid with food.
Preparations: 250 mg capsules.
Actions: Salicylate compound that delivers 5-ASA to the colon; used in maintenance therapy for ulcerative colitis in patients who do not tolerate sulfasalazine (Azulfidine).
Clearance: Only about 2.4% is absorbed; the rest remains in the GI tract.
Selected Side Effects: Diarrhea, abdominal cramps or pain, nausea.
Pregnancy Category: C.
Cost: $$$$ ($\approx$ $2/day).
Pearls: Unlike sulfasalazine, does not have a sulfa-containing sulfapyridine component and so is better tolerated in patients allergic or sensitive to sulfa.

OMEPRAZOLE (Prilosec, formerly Losec)
Dose: 20 mg PO qd for 4–8 weeks.
Preparations: 20 mg capsules.
Actions: Medication that inhibits H^+/K^+-ATPase of gastric parietal cells, inhibiting the proton pump; used to treat peptic ulcer disease and severe esophageal reflux.
Selected Side Effects: Minimal reported common side effects.
Selected Drug Interactions: Prolongs elimination of diazepam, warfarin, phenytoin, and other drugs that are oxidized in the liver.
Pregnancy Category: C.
Cost: $$$$ ($\approx$ $3/tablet).
Pearls:
- Can interfere with drugs absorbed at acid gastric pH (ketoconazole, ampicillin, iron salts, etc).
- Should be taken before meals.
- When used to treat *Helicobacter pylori* infections, must be started at the same time as antibiotics; if started before, the eradication rate drops precipitously to 20%.
- Patients who are on long-term therapy should have their serum gastrin levels monitored; significantly elevated levels may be an indication to switch therapy to an H_2 blocker.

ONDANSETRON (Zofran)
Dose: Three possible administration regimens:
- 32 mg dose IV infused over 15 min, beginning 30 min before chemotherapy.
- 0.15 mg/kg IV over 15 min, given 30 min before chemotherapy and repeated 4 and 8 h later (total of three 0.15 mg/kg doses).
- 8 mg dose PO given 30 min before chemotherapy and repeated 4 and 8 h later (total of three 8 mg PO doses); 8 mg PO q8h may be administered for 1–2 days after completion of chemotherapy.

Preparations: 4 and 8 mg tablets.
Actions: Selective serotonin receptor antagonist used to prevent chemotherapy-induced nausea and vomiting.
Clearance: Extensively metabolized in liver by cytochrome P-450.
- Clearance is reduced and $t_{1/2}$ prolonged in patients > 75 years old.

Selected Side Effects: Headache, dizziness, diarrhea, constipation, elevated LFTs, extrapyramidal effects.
Selected Drug Interactions: Can affect other serotonin-mediated medications (buspirone, fluoxetine, cyproheptadine, clomipramine).
Pregnancy Category: B.
Cost: \$\$\$\$\$ ($\approx$ \$20 each 8 mg tablet; $\approx$ \$200 for a 40 mg vial).
Pearls: Is not effective for "delayed nausea" (ie, 24 h after chemotherapy).

Organidin NR: *see* GUAIFENESIN

Orinase: *see* TOLBUTAMIDE

Ortho-Cyclen contraceptive pills (NORGESTIMATE + ETHINYL ESTRADIOL)
Dose: 1 tablet PO qd; with 21-day regimen, take no pills on days 22–28 then begin a new cycle (3 weeks on, 1 week off).
- For 21-day and 28-day preparations, take first tablet on the first Sunday after onset of menses, or that Sunday if it is first day of menses.

Preparations: Available in 21- and 28-tablet preparations.
- Tablets in the 21 day preparation contain 0.250 mg of norgestimate and 0.035 mg of ethinyl estradiol.
- The first 21-day tablets in the 28-day preparation are similar to those in the 21-day preparation; the last seven tablets contain inert ingredients.

Actions: Combination oral contraceptive used to prevent pregnancy.

Selected Side Effects: Serious vascular complications, menstrual changes, hypertension, gallbladder disease, liver tumors, nausea and vomiting, GI distress, breakthrough bleeding, edema, breast changes, weight changes, cervical changes, migraine headache, rash, depression, glucose intolerance, vaginal candidiasis, visual changes from alteration in corneal curvature, intolerance for contact lenses.

Selected Drug Interactions: Contraceptive effectiveness can be decreased by antibiotics (ampicillin, chloramphenicol, isoniazid, nitrofurantoin, penicillin V, rifampin, sulfonamides, tetracycline), analgesics, anxiolytics, antimigraine agents, barbiturates, and phenylbutazone.

Cautions:
- *Contraindicated in patients with thromboembolic or thrombophlebitic disorders, cardiovascular or cerebrovascular disease, vaginal bleeding of unknown cause, endometrial or other estrogen-dependent neoplasms, known or suspected breast cancer, cholestatic jaundice or jaundice with prior pill use, hepatic adenoma or carcinoma, smokers over age 35, or known or suspected pregnancy.*
- Cigarette smoking increases risk of serious cardiovascular complications; patients should be *strongly* advised not to smoke.

Pregnancy Category: X.

Cost: $$$ ($\approx$ $20/month).

Pearls:
- Patients should undergo complete work-up prior to use with special attention to history of abnormal vaginal bleeding, BP, breast examination, and pelvic examination including cervical cytology.
- Contains a newer progestin component; is less androgenic and results in a more favorable lipid profile.

Ortho-Novum contraceptive pills
(NORETHINDRONE + ETHINYL ESTRADIOL
or NORETHINDRONE + MESTRANOL)

Dose: 1 tablet PO qd; with 21-day regimen, take no pills on days 22–28 then begin a new cycle (3 weeks on, 1 week off).

- For 21-pill preparations of Ortho-Novum 7/7/7 or 10/11 and for all 28-pill preparations, take first tablet on the first Sunday after onset of menses, or that Sunday if it is first day of menses.
- For 21-pill preparations of Ortho-Novum 1/35 or 1/50, take first tablet on the fifth day of the menstrual cycle, counting the first day of menses as day 1.

Preparations: Available in 21- and 28-tablet preparations.

- The last 7 tablets in 28-tablet preparation usually contain only inert ingredients.
- Quantities of norethindrone (N), ethinyl estradiol (E), and mestranol (N) in the various PO preparations:
  - ▶ Ortho-Novum 7/7/7: first week, 0.5 mg N and 0.035 mg E; second week, 0.75 mg N and 0.035 mg E; third week, 1.0 mg N and 0.035 mg E.
  - ▶ Ortho-Novum 1/35: fixed dose of 1 mg N and 0.035 mg E.
  - ▶ Ortho-Novum 1/50: fixed dose of 1 mg N and 0.050 mg M.
  - ▶ Ortho-Novum 10/11: first 10 days, 0.5 mg N and 0.035 mg E; days 11–21, 1.0 mg N and 0.035 mg E.

Actions: Combination oral contraceptive used to prevent pregnancy.

Selected Side Effects: Serious vascular complications, menstrual changes, hypertension, gallbladder disease, liver tumors, nausea and vomiting, GI distress, breakthrough bleeding, edema, breast changes, weight changes, cervical changes, migraine headache, rash, depression, glucose intolerance, vaginal candidiasis, visual changes from alteration in corneal curvature, intolerance for contact lenses.

Selected Drug Interactions: Contraceptive effectiveness can be decreased by antibiotics (ampicillin, chloramphenicol, isoniazid, nitrofurantoin, penicillin V, rifampin, sulfonamides, tetracycline), analgesics, anxiolytics, antimigraine agents, barbiturates, and phenylbutazone.

Cautions:
- *Contraindicated in patients with thromboembolic or thrombophlebitic disorders, cardiovascular or cerebrovascular disease, vaginal bleeding of unknown cause, endometrial or other estrogen-dependent neoplasms, known or suspected breast cancer, cholestatic jaundice or jaundice with prior pill use, hepatic adenoma or carcinoma, smokers over age 35, or known or suspected pregnancy.*
- Cigarette smoking increases risk of serious cardiovascular complications; patients should be *strongly* advised not to smoke.

Pregnancy Category: X.

Cost: $$$ (≈ $20/month).

Pearls: Patients should undergo complete work-up prior to use with special attention to history of abnormal vaginal bleeding, BP, breast examination, and pelvic examination including cervical cytology.

Ortho Tri-Cyclen contraceptive pills (NORGESTIMATE + ETHINYL ESTRADIOL)

Dose: 1 tablet PO qd; with 21-day regimen, take no pills on days 22–28 then begin a new cycle (3 weeks on, 1 week off).
- For 21-day and 28-day preparations, take first tablet on the first Sunday after onset of menses, or that Sunday if it is first day of menses.

Preparations: Available in 21- and 28-tablet preparations.
- Tablets contain 0.035 mg of ethinyl estradiol and increasing doses of norgestimate (0.180 mg, 0.215 mg, and 0.250 mg); the last seven tablets in the 28-day preparation contain inert ingredients.

Actions: Combination oral contraceptive used to prevent pregnancy.

Selected Side Effects: Serious vascular complications, menstrual changes, hypertension, gallbladder disease, liver tumors, nausea and vomiting, GI distress, breakthrough bleeding, edema, breast changes, weight changes, cervical changes, migraine headache, rash, depression, glucose intolerance, vaginal candidiasis, visual changes from alteration in corneal curvature, intolerance for contact lenses.

Selected Drug Interactions: Contraceptive effectiveness can be decreased by antibiotics (ampicillin, chloramphenicol, isoniazid, nitrofurantoin, penicillin V, rifampin, sulfonamides, tetracycline), analgesics, anxiolytics, antimigraine agents, barbiturates, and phenylbutazone.

Cautions:

- *Contraindicated in patients with thromboembolic or thrombophlebitic disorders, cardiovascular or cerebrovascular disease, vaginal bleeding of unknown cause, endometrial or other estrogen-dependent neoplasms, known or suspected breast cancer, cholestatic jaundice or jaundice with prior pill use, hepatic adenoma or carcinoma, smokers over age 35, or known or suspected pregnancy.*
- Cigarette smoking increases risk of serious cardiovascular complications; patients should be *strongly* advised not to smoke.

Pregnancy Category: X.

Cost: $$$ (≈ $25/month).

Pearls:

- Patients should undergo complete work-up prior to use with special attention to history of abnormal vaginal bleeding, BP, breast examination, and pelvic examination including cervical cytology.
- Contains a newer progestin component; is less androgenic and results in a more favorable lipid profile.

Os-Cal: *see* CALCIUM CARBONATE

OXACILLIN

Dose: 1–2 g IM or IV q4–6h.

Actions: Bactericidal β-lactamase-resistant penicillin that inhibits cell wall synthesis.

- Excellent gram (+) coverage, including staph and strep (but *not* MRSA or enterococci).
- No gram (−) coverage.
- Poor anaerobic coverage.
- *NOTE:* The above-mentioned antimicrobial coverage summary should be used as a guideline only; treatment deci-

sions should take into account not only local epidemiologic patterns of antibiotic susceptibility but also, when available, culture susceptibility results.

Clearance: Metabolized via liver; renally excreted.

- No change in dosage needed in patients with renal insufficiency.
- Avoid in patients with liver disease (because of hepatotoxicity).
- Supplemental dose not required after hemodialysis or peritoneal dialysis.

Selected Side Effects: Rash, occasional elevated LFTs, hepatitis and jaundice, interstitial nephritis, rare neutropenia.

Cautions: *Contraindicated in patients with allergy to any of the penicillins.*

Pregnancy Category: C.

Cost: $$$.

Pearls:

- Monitor LFTs during prolonged therapy.
- Contains high Na^+ load.
- Penicillin provides better coverage than oxacillin for strep.

OXAPROZIN (Daypro)

Dose: 1200 mg PO qd.

Preparations: 600 mg caplets.

Actions: Long-acting NSAID with analgesic and antipyretic activity that may work by inhibiting prostaglandin synthetase; used to treat inflammatory conditions and for pain relief.

OXAZEPAM (Serax)

Dose: 10–30 mg PO tid–qid.

Preparations: 10, 15, and 30 mg tablets or capsules.

Actions: Short-acting benzodiazepine with sedative and anxiolytic effects; used to treat anxiety.

Clearance: Metabolized via liver.

- No change in dosage recommended in patients with renal insufficiency; can cause excess sedation or encephalopathy in patients with end-stage renal disease.

- No change in dosage needed in patients with liver disease.
- Supplemental dose not required after hemodialysis.

Selected Side Effects: Transient mild drowsiness, rare decreased WBCs and liver dysfunction, rare but significant hypotension.

Selected Drug Interactions: Potentiates CNS depressant effects of other CNS depressants.

Cautions: Should probably not be used by pregnant or potentially pregnant patients.

Pregnancy Category: *Oxazepam has not been adequately studied, but other minor anxiolytics are associated with congenital malformations when taken during pregnancy, and therefore should generally not be used by pregnant or potentially pregnant patients.*

Cost: Generic $$, Serax $$$$ ($\approx$ $0.25 each 15 mg generic tablet; $\approx$ $0.85 each 15 mg Serax tablet).

Pearls:
- Abrupt discontinuance after extended use can precipitate barbiturate-like withdrawal reaction.
- Is particularly useful in elderly patients.
- Has relatively short $t_{1/2}$.
- Periodically check CBC and LFTs.

Oxy-5, Oxy-10: *see* BENZOYL PEROXIDE

OXYBUTYNIN (Ditropan)

Dose: 5 mg or 5 mL (1 tsp) PO bid–qid.

Preparations:
- 5 mg tablets.
- 16 oz bottles of syrup containing 5 mg/5 mL (1 tsp).

Actions: Urinary antispasmodic used to treat urinary frequency and incontinence secondary to bladder instability (neurogenic bladder).

Clearance: Metabolized via liver.

Selected Side Effects: Anticholinergic effects (dry mouth, tachycardia, palpitations, constipation and paralytic ileus, urinary hesitancy and retention, impotence, elevated intraocular pressure, decreased sweating and hyperthermia, blurred vision), drowsiness.

Selected Drug Interactions:
- Raises serum level of digoxin.
- Increases anticholinergic blockade.

Cautions:
- *Contraindicated in patients with elevated intraocular pressure associated with angle-closure glaucoma, any disease associated with reduced intestinal motility, or myasthenia gravis.*
- Use with caution in elderly patients and in patients with hepatic disease, renal disease, or autonomic neuropathy.

Pregnancy Category: B.

Cost: Generic $$, Ditropan $$$.

OXYCODONE: *see* Percocet, Percodan

OXYMETAZOLINE (Afrin)

Dose: 2–4 drops (written "gtt") or sprays of 0.05% solution intranasally bid.

Actions: Long-acting α-adrenergic agonist that causes local vasoconstriction; used to treat nasal congestion.

Selected Side Effects: Rebound nasal congestion or irritation with long-term use, hypotension or hypertension, headache, insomnia.

Pregnancy Category: Not established.

Cost: $.

Pearls:
- Prolonged use (> 3–5 days) can lead to "rebound" nasal congestion when treatment is discontinued; therefore, avoid prolonged use.
- Some physicians use intranasal steroids to treat cases of "rebound" nasal congestion.

PACLITAXEL (Taxol)

Dose: Disease dependent.
- *NOTE: Patients need to be pretreated with corticosteroids, diphenhydramine (Benadryl) and an H_2 blocker (such as cimetidine or ranitidine) before treatment (see Pearls section).*
- One regimen is 135 or 175 mg/m^2 administered over 3 h every 3 weeks.

Actions: Naturally occurring antimicrotubule chemotherapeutic agent; used in the treatment of tumors.

- Promotes the assembly of microtubules from tubulin dimers and stabilizes microtubules by preventing depolymerization. This stability results in the inhibition of the normal dynamic reorganization of the microtubule network that is essential for vital interphase and mitotic cellular functions.

Clearance: Predominant clearance is via mechanisms other than renal excretion. Liver metabolism appears to be one such mechanism; biliary excretion may be a second mechanism.

- Information on the effects of renal or hepatic dysfunction on the disposition of paclitaxel is not currently available.

Selected Side Effects: *Severe hypersensitivity reactions (dyspnea, hypotension, angioedema, generalized urticaria), bone marrow suppression (primarily neutropenia),* peripheral neuropathy (usually mild), alopecia, hypotension, nausea and vomiting, diarrhea, mucositis.

Cautions:

- *Because of the risk of hypersensitivity reactions, patients need to be pretreated with corticosteroids, diphenhydramine (Benadryl) and an H_2 blocker (such as cimetidine or ranitidine) before treatment (see Pearls section).*

Pregnancy Category: D.

Pearls:

- Bone marrow suppression (particularly neutropenia) is the dose-limiting side effect.
- Monitor vital signs (particularly blood pressure) frequently during the several hours of infusion.
- Paclitaxel should not be administered if neutrophil count is < 1500 cells/mm^3 or if platelet count is < 100,000 cells/mm^3.
- One suggested premedication regimen consists of the following: (1) dexamethasone (Decadron) 20 mg PO administered 12 and 6 h before paclitaxel, and (2) diphenhydramine (Benadryl) 50 mg IV administered 30–60 min before paclitaxel, and (3) cimetidine (Tagamet) 300 mg IV or ranitidine (Zantac) 50 mg IV administered 30–60 min before paclitaxel.

Pamelor: *see* NORTRIPTYLINE

Pancrease: *see* PANCRELIPASE

PANCRELIPASE (Cotazym, Creon 20, Pancrease, Ultrase, Viokase, Zymase)

Dose: 1–3 capsules (Pancrease) or 1–3 tablets (Viokase) with each meal and 1 capsule with snacks.

Preparations: Capsules containing lipase, protease, and amylase.

Selected Side Effects: GI discomfort, rare allergic-type reactions.

Pregnancy Category: C.

Cost: $$$$ ($\approx$ $2/day).

Pearls:

- Dose may need to be titrated to patients' symptoms.
- For nonenteric-coated preparations, may need to concomitantly give an H_2 blocker so that gastric acid does not destroy the enzymes.

PANCURONIUM (Pavulon)

Dose:

- Initial: Give 0.04–0.10 mg/kg IV push ($\approx$ 6 mg for an average-sized patient).
- Maintenance: 0.01–0.02 mg/kg IV push ($\approx$ 1 mg for an average-sized patient) given q40–60 min as required.

Actions: Neuromuscular blocking agent that relaxes skeletal muscle; used to induce paralysis during intubation, status epilepticus, and mechanical ventilation.

Clearance: Metabolized via liver; renally excreted.

- $t_{1/2}$ is increased in liver dysfunction and in patients with impaired renal function.
- Lengthen dosing interval in patients with renal insufficiency; avoid if GFR < 10 mL/min.

Selected Side Effects: Tachycardia (from acetylcholine block), slight elevation in BP.

Pregnancy Category: C.

Cost: $.

Paraplatin: *see* **CARBOPLATIN**

Parlodel: *see* **BROMOCRIPTINE MESYLATE**

PAROXETINE (Paxil)
Dose:
- Initial: 20 mg PO qd in most patients; 10 mg PO qd in elderly patients and those with severe liver or renal disease.
- Maximum: 50 mg PO qd.

Preparations: 20 and 30 mg tablets.

Actions: Phenylpiperidine derivative serotonin reuptake inhibitor; used to treat depression.

Clearance: Undergoes extensive metabolism.
- Decrease starting dose in patients with severe liver or renal disease.

Selected Side Effects: Rare activation of mania, rare hyponatremia.

Selected Drug Interactions:
- Severe reactions when administered with MAO inhibitors.
- Cimetidine significantly increases its serum level.

Cautions: *Contraindicated in patients who have taken MAO inhibitors within the previous 2 weeks; do not start MAO inhibitor therapy until at least 2 weeks after paroxetine has been discontinued.*

Pregnancy Category: B.

Cost: $$$$ ($\approx$ $2.10 each 20 mg tablet).

Pacvulon: *see* **PANCURONIUM**

Paxil: *see* **PAROXETINE**

PCE 333, 500: *see* **ERYTHROMYCIN**

PENICILLIN (Generic preparations, Pen-Vee K)
Dose: Infection dependent and variable by source. Possible regimens include:
- Strep throat: Penicillin VK 250 mg PO qid for 10 days, taken 30 min before or 2 h after meals.

- Pneumococcal pneumonia: Procaine penicillin G 600,000 units IV q6h; may switch to penicillin VK 250 mg PO qid.
- "Uncomplicated" aspiration pneumonia: Procaine penicillin G 2 million units IV q4h.
- *Streptococcus pneumoniae* or *Neisseria meningitidis* meningitis: Procaine penicillin G 2 million units IV q2h.
- Endocarditis prophylaxis: Penicillin V 2 g PO 1 h before procedure and 1 g PO 6 h later.
- Pediatric dose:
  - ▶ Children < 12 years old, 15–50 mg/kg PO daily in 3 or 4 divided doses.
  - ▶ Children > 12 years, same as adult dose.

Preparations:
- 250, and 500 mg tablets of penicillin V (Pen-Vee K, etc).
- 100 mL bottles containing suspension of penicillin VK, which when reconstituted contains 125 mg/5 mL (1 tsp).
- 100, 150, and 200 mL bottles containing suspension of penicillin VK, which when reconstituted contains 250 mg/5 mL (1 tsp).

Actions: Bactericidal antibiotic that inhibits cell wall synthesis.
- Good gram (+) coverage, including enterococci (but *not* staph).
- Minimal gram (−) coverage (but *not* β-lactamase-producing organisms).
- Good anaerobic coverage (but *not* some *Bacteroides*).
- *NOTE:* The above-mentioned antimicrobial coverage summary should be used as a guideline only; treatment decisions should take into account not only local epidemiologic patterns of antibiotic susceptibility but also, when available, culture susceptibility results.

Clearance: Some liver metabolism; primarily renally excreted.
- Moderately reduce dosage in patients with impaired renal function.
- No change in dosage needed in patients with liver disease.
- Supplemental dose suggested after hemodialysis or peritoneal dialysis.

Selected Side Effects:
- PO: nausea and vomiting, epigastric distress, diarrhea, and black, hairy tongue.

- PO or IV: hypersensitivity reactions (rash, exfoliative dermatitis, urticaria), serum sickness (fever, chills, edema, arthralgia, prostration), anaphylactic reaction, interstitial nephritis, drug fever.
- Rare hemolytic anemia, leukopenia, thrombocytopenia, neuropathy or neurotoxicity, which are usually associated with high doses of parenteral penicillin.

Selected Drug Interactions:
- Possible drug antagonism with chloramphenicol and tetracycline.
- Decreases contraceptive effect of some oral contraceptives.
- Uricosurics (probenecid, indomethacin, etc) can raise its serum level.

Cautions: *Contraindicated in patients with allergy to any of the penicillins.*

Pregnancy Category: Penicillin G is rated as pregnancy category B; penicillin V is not rated.

Cost: $; markedly less expensive than many other IV antibiotics.

Pearls:
- Have patients take PO penicillin 30 min before or 2 h after meals (to ensure maximum absorption); may give penicillin VK with meals.
- Penicillin V (which is administered PO) is the phenoxymethyl analogue of penicillin G (which is administered IV); penicillin V potassium is the potassium salt of penicillin V; the "K" in penicillin VK and Pen Vee K presumably stands for "potassium."

Pentam: *see* **PENTAMIDINE**

PENTAMIDINE (NebuPent, Pentam)
Dose: Use dependent.
- PCP prevention: 300 mg by nebulizer monthly.
- Acute therapy: 4 mg/kg/day IV for 14 days.

Actions: Antiprotozoal agent that interferes with folate transmission; used to treat PCP.

Clearance: Primarily cleared by nonrenal mechanisms.
- Slightly increase dosing interval in patients with impaired renal function.
- Not removed by dialysis.

Selected Side Effects:
- Inhaled: cough and bronchospasm.
- IV: hypotension, hypoglycemia, leukopenia, thrombocytopenia, elevated LFTs or creatinine, pancreatitis; rare deaths have been reported secondary to hypotension, hypoglycemia, or cardiac arrhythmias.

Pregnancy Category: C.

Cost: $$$$ (2-week IV course ≈ $1800 wholesale).

Pearls:
- Patients on PCP prophylaxis can *still* develop PCP.
- Follow CBC, glucose, LFTs, BUN, creatinine, and ECG.
- Preventive therapy is indicated in high-risk patients (T count < 200 or previous PCP infection).

PENTOBARBITAL (Nembutal)

Dose (for induction of coma):
- IV loading dose: 100 mg (for a 70 kg patient).
- Maintenance: 1–3 mg/kg IV given hourly prn.

Actions: Barbiturate used to treat convulsions and to induce coma; also used in certain cases of intracranial hypertension and cerebral edema.

Clearance: Metabolized via liver.
- Reduce dosage in patients with liver disease.

Cautions: Can cause respiratory depression, hypotension, myocardial depression and hypothermia.

Pregnancy Category: D.

Cost: $.

Pearls:
- Avoid perivascular extravasation.
- The weaning of certain patients from pentobarbital who have been on maintenance IV therapy should be performed slowly (over several days) to prevent intracranial hypertension.

PENTOXIFYLLINE (Trental)

Dose:
- Usual: 400 mg PO tid with meals.
- May reduce dosage to 400 mg PO bid if GI or CNS side effects occur.

Preparations: 400 mg controlled-release tablets.
Actions: Methylxanthine analogue that may act by reducing blood viscosity, improving RBC flexibility, reducing RBC and platelet aggregation, and decreasing elevated plasma fibrinogen; used to treat intermittent claudication from peripheral vascular disease.
Clearance: Metabolized via liver.
- No change in dosage needed in patients with renal insufficiency.

Selected Side Effects: Generally well tolerated; rare side effects include nausea and vomiting and CNS symptoms.
Pregnancy Category: C.
Cost: $$$ (≈ $0.60/tablet); no generic form available.
Pearls:
- Can cause a further small reduction in BP in patients taking antihypertensive agents.
- Bleeding and increased PT have been reported in patients both taking and not taking warfarin or antiplatelet agents, but a causal relationship has not been clearly shown; consider more frequent PT monitoring in patients taking warfarin.

Pen-Vee K: *see* PENICILLIN

Pepcid: *see* FAMOTIDINE

Percocet (OXYCODONE + ACETAMINOPHEN)
Dose: 1 tablet PO q6h prn.
Preparations: Each tablet contains 5 mg oxycodone and 325 mg acetaminophen.
Actions: Narcotic analgesic with antipyretic actions used to treat moderate to moderately severe pain.
Clearance: Little information available; probably metabolized via liver with some renal excretion of active metabolites.
- Dosing interval should probably be increased in patients with liver disease.
Selected Side Effects: Lightheadedness, dizziness, sedation, nausea and vomiting, constipation, elevated CSF pres-

sure, euphoria; at high doses can, like morphine, cause respiratory depression.

Cautions:
- *Contraindicated in patients with CNS injury or lesions.*
- Use with caution in elderly or debilitated patients and in patients with severely impaired hepatic or renal function, hypothyroidism, Addison's disease, prostate hypertrophy, or urethral stricture.

Cost: Generic $$, Percocet $$$ (generic ≈ $0.35/tablet, Percocet ≈ $0.80/tablet).

Pregnancy Category: C.

Pearls:
- Raises serum levels of amylase and lipase.
- Can produce drug dependency.
- Remember that Percocet contains acetaminophen, and all the dosing precautions that apply to acetaminophen apply to Percocet.

Percodan (OXYCODONE HCl + OXYCODONE TEREPHTHALATE + ASA)

Dose: 1 tablet PO q6h prn.

Preparations: Each tablet contains 4.5 mg oxycodone HCl, 0.38 mg oxycodone terephthalate, and 325 mg ASA (aspirin).

Actions: Narcotic analgesic with salicylate antipyretic action; used to treat moderate to moderately severe pain.

Clearance: Little information available; oxycodone is probably metabolized in the liver with some renal excretion of active metabolites.
- Dosing interval should probably be increased in patients with liver disease.

Selected Side Effects: Lightheadedness, dizziness, sedation, nausea and vomiting, gastric irritation, upper GI bleeding, constipation, rash, pruritus, elevated CSF pressure; at high doses can, like morphine, cause respiratory depression.

Cautions:
- *Contraindicated in patients with CNS injury or lesions or with ASA allergy.*
- Use with caution in elderly or debilitated patients and in patients with severely impaired hepatic or renal function, hy-

pothyroidism, Addison's disease, prostate hypertrophy, urethral stricture, or history of peptic ulcer disease or upper GI bleeding.

Cost: Generic $$, Percodan $$$ (generic ≈ $0.35/tablet, Percodan ≈ $0.75/tablet).

Pregnancy Category: Not established.

Pearls:

- Can produce drug dependency.
- Remember that Percodan contains ASA, and all the precautions that apply to ASA apply to Percocet.

PERGOLIDE MESYLATE (Permax)

Dose: 0.05 and 0.25 mg tablets.

Preparations: 0.05 and 0.25 mg tablets.

Actions: Ergot derivative dopamine receptor agonist; used as an adjunctive treatment to levodopa/carbidopa (Sinemet) in the treatment of Parkinson's disease.

Clearance: Renally excreted.

Selected Side Effects: Dyskinesia (62% vs 25% in placebo patients), hallucinations, orthostatic hypotension, various body pains, GI effects (nausea, constipation, diarrhea), rhinitis.

Selected Drug Interactions: Dopamine antagonists (phenothiazines, metoclopramide, etc) may diminish its effectiveness.

Cautions: May exacerbate cardiac arrhythmias.

Pregnancy Category: B.

Pearls: Abrupt discontinuation in patients taking levodopa/carbidopa (Sinemet) may precipitate the onset of hallucinations and confusion; discontinuation of pergolide should be done gradually when possible.

Peri-Colace (CASANTHRANOL + DOCUSATE)

Dose: 1 or 2 capsules prn–bid, depending on need and use.

Preparations: Each capsule contains 30 mg casanthranol and 100 mg docusate (Colace).

Actions: Combination mild stimulant laxative and stool soft-ener that provides gently peristaltic stimulation and helps to keep stools softer for easier passage.

Selected Side Effects: Rare GI discomfort.

Cost: Generic $, Peri-Colace $$.

Pearls:

- Usually induces bowel movement overnight or in 8–12 h.
- Should be taken with generous amount of fluid.

Pepto-Bismol: *see* BISMUTH SUBSALICYLATE

Permax: *see* PERGOLIDE MESYLATE

PERPHENAZINE (Trilafon, etc)

Dose: Disease and delivery dependent.

- Nausea and vomiting:
    - ▶ PO: 6–16 mg daily in divided doses (suggestions for each dose range from 2–8 mg).
    - ▶ IV: 5 mg q6h prn.
    - ▶ IM: 5–10 mg.
- Acute psychosis: 5–10 mg IM or IV.

Preparations:

- 2, 4, 8, and 16 mg tablets.
- 4 oz bottle with graduated dropper containing 16 mg/5 mL (1 tsp).

Actions: Phenothiazine that acts at all levels of the nervous system; used to treat severe nausea and vomiting and psychotic disorders.

Clearance: Primary mechanism of clearance is most likely liver metabolism.

- Manufacturer suggests using with caution in renal disease.
- Supplemental dose not required after dialysis.

Selected Side Effects: Extrapyramidal reactions, *tardive dyskinesia, neuroleptic malignant syndrome,* anticholinergic effects (dry mouth, blurred vision, urinary retention, ileus, etc), orthostatic hypotension, quinidine-like ECG changes, drowsiness.

Selected Drug Interactions:

- Antacids reduce its absorption.
- Barbiturates can decrease its effectiveness.

- Potentiates CNS depressant effects of other CNS depressants.
- Can raise serum levels of antidepressants.

Cautions:

- *Contraindicated in patients with liver damage, blood dyscrasias, bone marrow depression, subcortical brain damage, or depressed consciousness and in patients taking large doses of other CNS depressants.*
- Use with caution in elderly patients.

Pregnancy Category: Not established.

Cost: Generic $$, Trilafon $$$ ($\approx$ $0.40 each 8 mg generic tablet; $\approx$ $1 each 8 mg Trilafon tablet).

Pearls:

- Follow CBC, LFTs, and renal function.
- Signs of neuroleptic malignant syndrome include extreme rise in temperature, muscle rigidity and "lead-pipe" syndrome, mental status changes, autonomic instability including irregular pulse or BP, greatly increased HR, diaphoresis, arrhythmias, rhabdomyolysis (with increased CPK, myoglobinuria, and acute renal failure).

Persantine: *see* DIPYRIDAMOLE

Phazyme: *see* SIMETHICONE

PHENAZOPYRIDINE (Pyridium)

Dose: 200 mg PO tid (one source notes 100 mg PO tid to be efficacious).

Preparations: 100 and 200 mg tablets.

Actions: Excreted in urine, where its analgesic action relieves urinary pain, burning, urgency, and frequency.

Selected Side Effects: Rash, GI disturbances, staining of contact lenses, renal and hepatic toxicity (usually at overdose levels), hemolytic anemia, methemoglobinemia.

Pregnancy Category: B.

Cost: Generic $$, Pyridium $$$ ($\approx$ $0.35 each 200 mg generic tablet; $\approx$ $1.05 each 200 mg Pyridium tablet).

Pearls:

- Should be taken after meals.

- Warn patients that phenazopyridine colors the urine deep red-orange (which may be mistaken by the patient for hematuria) and may permanently stain clothing.

Phenergan: *see* PROMETHAZINE

PHENIRAMINE: *see* Naphcon-A ophthalmic solution

PHENOBARBITAL
Dose: Situation and disease dependent:
- Initial therapy for status epilepticus:
  ▶ Recommendations for loading rate and initial IV dose vary significantly.
  ▶ Initial dosage recommendations vary from 200–320 mg to 10 mg/kg IV.
  ▶ Because suggested regimens vary so widely among sources, it is difficult to make any definitive recommendation for dosing. A possible initial regimen for status epilepticus that conforms with many sources would be 5 mg/kg IV given over 10 min. This dose may be repeated, if needed, after 30–60 min.
  ▶ Maximum dose is usually listed as 20 mg/kg (patients can get respiratory depression and require intubation at this point).
  ▶ Some sources recommend an injection rate of 60–100 mg/min; other sources note that injection at rates 360 mg/min can cause hypotension, severely reduced respirations and apnea, and laryngospasm.
- Chronic therapy for seizures: 100–300 mg PO qd.
- Sedation: 30–120 mg daily given in 2 or 3 divided doses.

Preparations:
- 8, 15, 16, 30, 32, 60, 65, and 100 mg tablets.
- 16 ounce bottles of elixir containing 20 mg/5 mL (1 tsp).

Actions: Anticonvulsant, sedative.

Clearance: 50–75% liver metabolized; 25–50% renally excreted.
- Slightly increase dosing interval in patients with end-stage renal disease; no change needed for milder renal impairment.

- Reduce dosage in liver dysfunction.
- Renal excretion is increased with alkaline diuresis.
- Supplemental dose suggested after hemodialysis or peritoneal dialysis.

Selected Side Effects: Somnolence, severe allergic reactions, numerous CNS effects, respiratory depression, rare agranulocytosis, thrombocytopenic purpura or megaloblastic anemia.

Selected Drug Interactions:
- Decreases PT in patients taking warfarin.
- Reduces effectiveness of digoxin and steroids.

Cautions: *Contraindicated in patients with severe pulmonary insufficiency, sensitivity to barbiturates, or history of porphyria.*

Pregnancy Category: D.

Cost: $$ (≈ $0.10 each 100 mg tablet).

Pearls:
- Therapeutic level varies depending on source and institution but is usually in the range of 10–40 mg/mL.
- After IV dose, can take 15–30 min for peak level to be attained in the brain.
- Withdrawal reactions can occur.
- Intermittently check CBC in patients on chronic therapy.
- Signs and symptoms of overdose include CNS depression, Cheyne–Stokes respiration, absent reflexes, hypotension, tachycardia, and hypothermia.

PHENYLEPHRINE (Neo-Synephrine)

Dose: 1 or 2 drops (written "gtt") or sprays into each nostril q4h.

Actions: Topical decongestant that causes vasoconstriction through its α-agonist activity; used to treat nasal congestion.

Selected Side Effects: Local irritation, rebound congestion.

Cautions:
- *May be contraindicated in patients taking MAOI or tricyclics if systemically absorbed.*
- Relatively contraindicated in hypertension, hyperthyroidism, diabetes, and benign prostatic hypertrophy.

Pearls:
- Can antagonize antihypertensive agents if absorbed.
- Prolonged use can lead to "rebound" nasal congestion when treatment is discontinued; therefore, avoid prolonged use.

PHENYLEPHRINE Intravenous (Neo-Synephrine)
Dose:
- Hypotensive crisis: Initial bolus of 200 μg IV; can increase subsequent doses up to a maximum of 500 μg IV.
- Intravenous drip: Initial rate of 100–200 μg/min; maximum dose not well defined—one source suggests can increase dose up to a maximum of 500 μg/min.
- *NOTE:* Dosage is in micrograms, *not* milligrams.

Actions: Potent α-receptor agonist, resulting in vasoconstriction, used to treat hypotension.

Cautions:
- Can decrease cardiac output (due to increased systemic vascular resistance) and can precipitate angina in patients with coronary artery disease.

Pearls:
- Administration through a central IV preferred.

PHENYLPROPANOLAMINE (Acutrim; *see also* Contac, Robitussin-CF)
Dose (for appetite suppression): 75 mg PO after breakfast.

Preparations: 75 mg tablets.

Actions: α-receptor agonist sympathomimetic used as appetite suppressant, for stress incontinence in women, and in many over-the-counter cold products.

Clearance: Primarily excreted unchanged in urine.
- Avoid in renal dysfunction.

Selected Side Effects: Worsening of hypertension, restlessness, insomnia, agitation.

Selected Drug Interactions: *Concomitant use with MAOI, guanethidine, or indomethacin can precipitate hypertensive crisis.*

Cautions: *Contraindicated in significant cardiovascular disease or hypertension, hyperthyroidism, significant renal disease, and acute narrow-angle glaucoma.*

Pearls: Used as decongestant in many cold preparations, including Allerest, Contac, and many others not listed in this guide.

PHENYTOIN (Dilantin)

Dose: Delivery dependent.

- IV loading dose: 15–20 mg/kg (maximum loading rate is 50 mg/min; monitor ECG and BP).
- PO loading dose: 1 g over 4 h, given as 400 mg initially, then 300 mg 2 h later, then another 300 mg 2 h later.
- Usual maintenance: 100 mg PO tid–qid or 300–400 mg PO qd.

Preparations:

- 30, 50, and 100 mg tablets.
- 50 mg chewable tablets.
- 8 oz bottles of orange–vanilla-flavored suspension containing 125 mg/5 mL (1 tsp).

Actions: Medication used primarily as an anticonvulsant.

- Also has some antiarrhythmic properties and can be (although rarely is) used to treat ventricular arrhythmias and certain atrial arrhythmias (particularly those secondary to digoxin toxicity); rarely is used for treatment of trigeminal neuralgia.

Clearance: Metabolized via liver.

- No change in dosage needed in patients with renal insufficiency.
- Dosage may need to be reduced in patients with severe liver disease, but dosing is probably best done by following serum drug levels.
- Supplemental dose not required after hemodialysis or peritoneal dialysis.

Selected Side Effects:

- Acute: Allergic reactions (rash, Stevens–Johnson syndrome, toxic epidermal necrosis, lupus erythematosus), CNS toxicity (confusional states, delirium, psychosis, slurred speech, nystagmus, cerebellar dysfunction, including ataxia), sensory peripheral neuropathy with long-term use, gingival hyperplasia, hirsutism, elevated glucose level or LFTs, rare myelosuppression.

Selected Drug Interactions:
- Reduces efficacy of steroids, warfarin, quinidine, digoxin, and furosemide.
- Acute alcohol ingestion, ASA, cimetidine, and isoniazid raise its serum level.
- Chronic alcohol ingestion and antacids containing calcium reduce its serum level.
- Sucralfate reduces its intestinal absorption.
- In different patients, phenobarbital and valproic acid can either elevate or depress phenytoin levels, and phenytoin can either elevate or depress phenobarbital and valproic acid levels.

Pregnancy Category: Not established; is associated with increased congenital defects, which must be weighed against risk of seizing during pregnancy.

Cost: $$ (≈ $0.20 each 250 mg tablet).

Pearls:
- Usual therapeutic level is 10–20 µg/mL.
- In patients with significant renal failure, follow level of *free Dilantin* secondary to reduced protein binding (therapeutic level of free Dilantin is 1–2 mg/mL).
- Abrupt withdrawal can precipitate seizure.
- Acute alcohol ingestion can raise its serum level and chronic ingestion can reduce it.
- Signs and symptoms of toxicity include delirium, psychosis, encephalopathy, cerebellar dysfunction, nystagmus, lethargy, and tremor.

Phosphaljel: *see* **ALUMINUM PHOSPHATE**

PHOSPHORUS (K-Phos, Neutra-Phos)
Dose: Brand dependent:
- K-Phos: 1–2 tablets PO qid with full glass of water.
- Neutra-Phos: 2 tablets PO bid–qid.

Preparations: 250 mg tablets.
Actions: Phosphorous supplement.
Selected Side Effects: Diarrhea, GI distress, hypocalcemia.

Cautions: Use with caution in patients with renal insufficiency, cirrhosis, or CHF.
Pregnancy Category: C.
Cost: $$.
Pearls:
- IV phosphorus should be used cautiously and only for severe hypophosphatemia (serum phosphorus < 1.0).
- Signs and symptoms of severe hypophosphatemia include neuromuscular effects (weakness, paresthesias, rhabdomyolysis, etc), hematologic abnormalities (hemolysis, platelet dysfunction), and cardiac failure.

PINDOLOL (Visken)
Dose:
- Initial: 5 mg PO bid.
- Maximum: 60 mg PO daily.

Preparations: 5 and 10 mg tablets.
Actions: Nonselective β-receptor blocker with intrinsic sympathomimetic activity used to treat hypertension and CAD.
Clearance: Metabolized via liver; renally excreted.
- No change in dosage needed for patients with impaired renal function but normal liver function.
- Reduce dosage in patients with liver disease, especially in patients with both liver and renal disease.

Selected Side Effects: Elevated LFTs, (rare) anxiety, lethargy, visual changes, bradycardia, claudication, hypotension, syncope.
Cautions: *Contraindicated in bronchial asthma, second- or third-degree heart block, severe bradycardia, or cardiogenic shock.*
Pregnancy Category: B.
Cost: $$$ (≈ $0.90 each 10 mg tablet).
Pearls:
- Can get rebound effect with abrupt discontinuance.
- May be a better β-blocking agent to use in patients with resting bradycardia or borderline CHF (because of its intrinsic sympathomimetic activity).
- Has less cardioprotective effect than other β-blockers.
- Taper when discontinuing (to avoid rebound reactions).

PIPERACILLIN
Dose:
- 3–4 g IV q4–6h.
- Usual maximum dose is 24 g/day.

Actions: Bactericidal semisynthetic antipseudomonal penicillin that inhibits cell wall synthesis.
- Good gram (+) coverage, including enterococci and strep (but *not* staph).
- Excellent gram (−) coverage, including *Pseudomonas aeruginosa.*
- Good anaerobic coverage, including *Bacteroides fragilis.*
- *NOTE:* The above-mentioned antimicrobial coverage summary should be used as a guideline only; treatment decisions should take into account not only local epidemiologic patterns of antibiotic susceptibility but also, when available, culture susceptibility results.

Clearance: Renally excreted.
- Slightly increase dosing interval in patients with impaired renal function.
- Sources differ on whether dosage should be reduced in liver dysfunction.
- Supplemental dose suggested after hemodialysis.

Selected Side Effects: Local thrombophlebitis, hypersensitivity, and rare anaphylactoid reaction.

Cautions: *Contraindicated in patients with allergy to any of the penicillins.*

Pregnancy Category: B.

Cost: $$$.

Pearls:
- (+) CSF penetration in meningeal inflammation.
- Can increase bleeding tendency in patients with renal failure.

PIROXICAM (Feldene)
Dose: 20 mg PO qd or 10 mg PO bid.

Preparations: 10 and 20 mg tablets.

Actions: Nonsteroidal antiinflammatory agent with analgesic and antipyretic actions; used to treat pain and inflammation.

Clearance: Metabolized via liver.
- No change in dosage needed in patients with renal insufficiency.

Selected Side Effects: GI bleeding and ulceration, fluid retention and edema, elevated LFTs, interstitial nephritis and exacerbation of "prerenal" renal failure, rash, prolonged bleeding time (from reversible platelet inhibition).

Cautions:
- *Contraindicated in patients with salicylate sensitivity or history of upper GI bleeding.*
- Should not be used in pregnant or potentially pregnant patients.

Pregnancy Category: Not recommended for use during pregnancy.

Cost: Generic $$$, Feldene $$$$ (generic ≈ $1 each 10 mg tablet, Feldene ≈ $2 each 10 mg tablet).

Pearls:
- Has longest $t_{1/2}$ of the NSAIDs.
- Should be taken with food or antacids (to possibly decrease GI irritation and ulceration).

Pitressin; *see* VASOPRESSIN

Plendil: *see* FELODIPINE

POLYETHYLENE GLYCOL; *see* GoLYTELY

POLYMYXIN B: *see* Cortisporin, Neosporin

POTASSIUM CHLORIDE (K-Dur, K-Tab, Micro-K, Slow-K)
Dose:
- 20–100 mEq PO daily.
- Usually no more than 20–40 mEq is given in a single dose.

Preparations:
- 10 mEq tablets of K-Dur 10.
- 20 mEq tablets of K-Dur 20.
- 10 mEq tablets of K-Tab.

- 10 mEq tablets of Micro K.
- 8 mEq tablets of Slow-K.

Actions: Potassium supplement.

Selected Side Effects: GI irritation, hyperkalemia.

Cautions: Use with caution in renal failure and in patients taking K^+-sparing diuretics or ACE inhibitors.

Pregnancy Category: C.

Cost: $$$.

Pearls:

- K^+ depletion sufficient to cause hypokalemia usually requires loss of > 200 mEq of K^+ from total body stores; however, when treating low blood values, common practice is to administer approximately 40 mEq and then recheck blood value.
- Although the lower limit of "normal" serum potassium level is often listed as approximately 3.5 mEq/L, in patients with active cardiac conditions (especially acute MI or ventricular arrhythmias), many physicians strive to obtain a serum level of ≥ 4.0 mEq/L in the belief that this may reduce ventricular ectopy and arrhythmias (particularly in patients on digoxin).

Pravachol: *see* PRAVASTATIN

PRAVASTATIN (Pravachol)

Dose:

- Initial: 10–20 mg PO qhs.
- Maintenance: 10–40 mg PO qhs.

Preparations: 10 and 20 mg tablets.

Actions: HMG-CoA reductase inhibitor that reduces total cholesterol and LDL and triglyceride levels, and increases HDL cholesterol; used to treat hyperlipidemia.

Clearance: Significant first-pass metabolism and elimination in feces; minor urinary excretion.

- Dosage should be adjusted in patients with liver disease or renal dysfunction.

Selected Side Effects: Rare headache, weakness or fatigue, elevated LFTs, rare increased CPK, myositis, rhabdomyolysis.

Selected Drug Interactions:

- Cholestyramine and colestipol can inhibit its absorption (give pravastatin at least 1 h before or 4 h after these drugs).
- Cyclosporine, gemfibrozil, niacin, or erythromycin may increase the risk of myopathy in patients receiving HMG-CoA reductase inhibitors.

Cautions:

- *Contraindicated in pregnant or potentially pregnant patients.*
- Contraindicated in patients with active liver disease or unexplained transaminase elevations.
- Use with caution in patients with history of liver disease or heavy alcohol use.

Pregnancy Category: X.

Cost: $$$$ ($\approx$ $1.70 each 20 mg tablet).

Pearls:

- Check LFTs and CPK level prior to initiating therapy, every 6 weeks for first 6 months, every 8 weeks during remainder of first year, and then at 6-month intervals.
- Discontinue if persistent LFT increases > 3 times normal, substantial rise in CPK, or myositis occurs.
- Primary effects are reductions in total and LDL cholesterol; usually leads to only modest elevations of HDL cholesterol.

PRAZOSIN (Minipress)

Dose:

- First dose: 1 mg PO given at night (because it might cause hypotension and syncope if the patient is very sensitive to its effects).
- Then begin 1 mg PO bid–tid.
- Usual: 3–5 mg PO bid–tid.
- Maximum: 20 mg PO daily.

Preparations: 1, 2, and 5 mg capsule.

Actions: α-receptor blocker that causes peripheral dilatation; used to treat hypertension.

Clearance: Metabolized via liver.

- No change in dosage needed in patients with renal insufficiency.

- Initial and maintenance doses should probably be reduced in patients with liver disease.
- Supplemental dose not required after hemodialysis or peritoneal dialysis.

Selected Side Effects: Dizziness, orthostatic hypotension, syncope.

Pregnancy Category: C.

Cost: Generic $$, Minipress $$$ ($\approx$ $0.30 each 5 mg generic capsule; $\approx$ $0.95 each 5 mg Minipress capsule).

Pearls:
- Increase dosage *slowly*.
- Patients usually do *not* get reflex tachycardia.
- Is especially good for lowering diastolic BP.
- Diuretic therapy should be held for 1–2 days before beginning therapy with prazosin (volume-depleted patients may have an exaggerated hypotensive response).

PREDNISOLONE (Delta-Cortef, Hydeltrasol, Hydeltra-T.B.A.)

Dose: Preparation dependent.
- Delta-Cortef: 5–60 mg PO daily in 2–4 divided doses.
- Hydeltrasol: Variable dose IM, IV, or directly into lesion or joint (large joint 10–20 mg, small joint 4–5 mg, bursae 10–15 mg, tendon sheath 2–5 mg, ganglia 5–10 mg).
- Hydeltra-T.B.A.: Variable dose given every 2–3 weeks prn IM or into lesion or joint (large joint 20–60 mg, small joint 8–10 mg, bursae 20–30 mg, ganglia 10–20 mg).

Preparations: 5 mg tablets of Delta-Cortef.

Actions: Synthetic corticosteroid with little mineralocorticoid activity; used primarily to treat inflammation and allergic conditions.

Clearance: Metabolized via liver.
- No change in dosage needed in patients with renal insufficiency or liver disease.
- Supplemental dose not required after hemodialysis.

Pregnancy Category: Not established.

Pearls: Is the liver-reduced active metabolite of prednisone.

PREDNISONE
Dose: Highly variable.
- COPD exacerbation: In-patients are often first started on IV methylprednisolone for several days.
- Initial PO doses of prednisone are often 40–60 mg qd. The dose is gradually tapered.

Preparations:
- 2.5, 5, 10, 20, and 50 mg tablets.
- 4 and 8 oz bottles containing 5 mg/5 mL (1 tsp).

Actions: Corticosteroid used to treat inflammation or allergic reactions.

Clearance: Metabolized via liver to active metabolite prednisolone.
- No change in dosage needed in patients with renal insufficiency.
- Supplemental dose suggested after hemodialysis.

Selected Side Effects:
- Elevated serum glucose, Na^+ and water retention (which increases hypertension, edema, and CHF), heightened catabolism, worsening azotemia, psychic derangements ("steroid psychosis").
- Can aggravate peptic ulcer disease, insomnia, and night terrors.
- Myopathy, osteoporosis, vertebral compression fractures, aseptic necrosis, hirsutism, moon facies, and glucose intolerance can develop with chronic therapy.

Selected Drug Interactions:
- Decreases hypoglycemic effect of insulin and OHAs.
- Increases risk of hypokalemia with K^+-depleting diuretics.
- May either prolong or shorten PT in patients taking warfarin.

Pregnancy Category: Not established; watch newborns for signs of hypoadrenalism.

Cost: $.

Pearls:
- Follow serum glucose levels in patients receiving acute steroid therapy.
- When switching from IV Solu-Medrol to PO prednisone during treatment of reactive airway disease, a somewhat ar-

bitrary but commonly used initial dose is 40 mg PO qd with gradual tapering. Usually taper over weeks in patients who have worse airway disease or are more steroid-dependent; in patients with milder disease, taper by 5 mg daily or every several days.

- Even with significant liver disease, enough prednisolone should be produced to achieve therapeutic effects.
- Relative activity comparison of commonly used steroids:

Steroid	Relative Antiinflammatory and Glucocorticoid Activity	Relative Mineralocorticoid Activity
Cortisone	0.8	0.8
Hydrocortisone	1.0	1.0
Prednisone	4.0	0.8
Methylprednisolone	5.0	0.5
Dexamethasone	25–30	0.0

Premarin (oral conjugated estrogens)

Dose: Disease dependent:

- *NOTE:* In the past, Premarin was given in 4-week cycles, with the administration regimen being—drug for 3 weeks and then no drug for 1 week (due to a concern of increased risk of endometrial cancer with unopposed estrogen treatment); more recently, Premarin is usually proscribed to be taken with the progesterone agent Provera. When so prescribed, Premarin is to be taken every day (ie, *not* 3 weeks on—1 week off). The following dosing schedules are those that are recommended when Premarin is prescribed with Provera. *NOTE*: Prescription information from the manufacturer and that listed in the 1995 *PDR* still suggest the 3 weeks on—1 week off schedule.
- Menopausal vasomotor symptoms: 1.25 mg PO qd (with Provera).
- Osteoporosis: 0.625 mg PO qd (with Provera).

Preparations: 0.3, 0.625, 0.9, 1.25, and 2.5 mg tablets.

Actions: Estrogen supplement used to treat various hormone-responsive conditions.

Clearance: Metabolized and inactivated primarily in the liver.

Selected Side Effects: Changes in vaginal bleeding pattern, breast tenderness and engorgement, increased risk of cardiovascular events, elevated calcium level in patients with breast cancer metastatic to bone, increased risk of gallbladder disease, GI distress, headache, depression, changes in libido.

Cautions:

- *Contraindicated in pregnant or potentially pregnant patients.*
- Use with caution in cardiovascular or circulatory disease.

Pregnancy Category: X.

Cost: $$.

Pearls:

- Estrogen increases risk of endometrial cancer when administered without progestin.
- In patients whose uterus has been removed, there is obviously no concern about the risk of endometrial cancer, and thus no need to prescribe Provera with Premarin.
- Provera itself, when prescribed with Premarin, is taken in one of two regimens: (1) 2.5 mg qd taken every day or (2) 10 mg qd for 2 weeks, and then no Provera for 2 weeks.

Preparation H ointment, cream, and suppositories

Dose: Manufacturer suggests applying to anal region or inserting a suppository whenever symptoms occur or 3–5 times daily, especially at night, in the morning, and after each bowel movement.

Preparations:

- 1 and 2 oz containers of ointment.
- 0.9 and 1.8 oz containers of cream.
- Packages of 12, 24, 36, and 48 suppositories.

Actions: Preparation containing live yeast cell derivative that (manufacturer states) acts by increasing oxygen uptake of dermal tissues and facilitating collagen formation, and shark liver oil that acts as a protectant, softening and sooth-

ing tissues; used to help shrink swelling of hemorrhoidal tissue and to relieve pain and itching.
Pearls: Actual clinical efficacy is controversial.

Prevacid: *see* LANSOPRAZOLE

Prilosec: *see* OMEPRAZOLE

Primaxin (IMIPENEM + CILASTATIN)
Dose: Delivery dependent.
- IV: 250–500 mg q6h.
- IM: 500–750 mg q12h.

Actions: Bactericidal antibiotic that inhibits cell wall synthesis.
- Good gram (+) coverage, including strep, staph, and enterococci (but *not* MRSA).
- Excellent gram (−) coverage, including *Pseudomonas aeruginosa* and β-lactamase-producing organisms.
- Good anaerobic coverage, including *Bacteroides fragilis.*
- *NOTE:* The above-mentioned antimicrobial coverage summary should be used as a guideline only; treatment decisions should take into account not only local epidemiologic patterns of antibiotic susceptibility but also, when available, culture susceptibility results.

Clearance: Imipenem undergoes some liver metabolism but is predominantly metabolized in kidneys and renally excreted; cilastatin inhibits renal metabolism of imipenem.
- Slightly reduce dosage or increase dosing interval in patients with impaired renal function.
- No change in dosage needed in patients with liver disease.
- Supplemental dose suggested after hemodialysis.

Selected Side Effects:
- Generally well tolerated.
- Rare elevation of LFTs, (+) Coombs' reaction, or yeast overgrowth.
- Can cause seizures when used at high doses, in renal failure, in elderly patients, or in patients with history of head trauma, seizures, or CNS pathology.
- Rapid infusion can cause nausea and vomiting.

Cautions: Patients allergic to β-lactams *may* have cross-sensitivity allergic reactions to imipenem.
Pregnancy Category: C.
Cost: $$$.

Primidone (Mysoline)
Dose: Disease dependent:
- Seizures: Usual maintenance dose is 250 mg PO tid–qid.
- Action ("essential") tremor: 50 mg PO bid–tid.

Preparations:
- 50 and 250 mg tablets.
- 8 oz bottles of suspension containing 250 mg/5 mL (1 tsp).

Actions: Anticonvulsant similar in structure to the barbiturates; used to treat tonic–clonic seizures and complex partial seizures.

Clearance: Metabolized via liver to phenobarbital; 40% excreted unchanged in urine
- Reduce dose or increase dosing interval in patients with renal insufficiency.

Selected Side Effects: Somnolence, gait ataxia, bone marrow depression.
Cautions: *Contraindicated in patients with porphyria.*
Cost: $.
Pearls: Monitor CBC due to possible bone marrow depression.

Prinivil: *see* LISINOPRIL

Prinzide 12.5, Prinzide 25 (LISINOPRIL + HYDROCHLOROTHIAZIDE)
Dose (Usual): 1 or 2 tablets of Prinzide 12.5 or Prinzide 25 PO qd.
Preparations: Each tablet contains 20 mg lisinopril with 12.5 mg hydrochlorothiazide (Prinzide 12.5) or 25 mg hydrochlorothiazide (Prinzide 25).
Actions: Combination medication containing an ACE inhibitor (lisinopril) and a diuretic (hydrochlorothiazide); used to treat hypertension.

Selected Side Effects: Dizziness, orthostatic effects, non-productive cough, impairment of renal function, angio-edema, rare neutropenia

Cautions:

- Do not use as initial therapy for hypertension (must first determine whether the patient needs more than one type of anti-hypertensive medication and determine that the combination of ACE inhibitor and diuretic will not cause hypertension).
- Patients should already be taking lisinopril before this medication is begun.
- *Contraindicated in second and third trimesters of pregnancy* (because of lisinopril component).

Pregnancy Category: D.

Cost: $$$ (≈ $1 each Prinzide-25 tablet).

PROBUCOL (Lorelco)

Dose: 500 mg PO bid.

Preparations: 250 and 500 mg tablets.

Actions:

- Cholesterol-lowering agent that reduces both LDL and HDL; used to treat hypercholesterolemia.
- Also is a potent antioxidant.

Selected Side Effects:

- *QT interval prolongation and ventricular arrhythmias.*
- Multiple GI, CNS, hematologic, and dermatologic adverse reactions have also been reported; however, the exact incidence of these reactions and whether they occurmore frequently with probucol than with a placebo is unclear.

Cautions: *Contraindicated in patients with prolonged QT interval, recent myocardial damage, or history of ventricular arrhythmias or unexplained syncope.*

Pregnancy Category: B.

Cost: $$$$ (≈ $1.15 each 500 mg tablet).

Pearls:

- Obtain baseline and periodic ECGs to follow QT interval; discontinue therapy if prolongation of the corrected QT interval occurs with therapy.
- Benefits of lowering LDL levels must be weighed against possible detrimental effects of lowering HDL levels.

- It is recommended that probucol be taken with morning and evening meals.

PROCAINAMIDE (Procan SR, Pronestyl)

Dose: Route and brand dependent.
- IV: Several regimens for loading dose exist:
  - ▶ 100 mg procainamide q3–5min to maximum of approximately 1–1.5 g (17 mg/kg) *or* if therapy is limited by hypotension or the QRS complex widening by 50% of its original width.
  - ▶ IV infusion at maximum rate of 20–30 mg/min (some sources recommend administering at a maximum rate of 20 mg/min to avoid hypotension; the AHA 1994 ACLS guidelines suggest an administration rate of 20–30 mg/min) up to a maximum of 1–1.5 mg/kg (17 mg/kg) or if therapy is limited by hypotension or the QRS complex widening by 50% of its original width.
- IV maintenance: 2–4 mg/min.
- PO maintenance:
  - ▶ Pronestyl: 500–1000 mg q4–6h.
  - ▶ Procan SR: 500–1000 mg q8h.

Preparations:
- 250, 375, and 500 mg tablets of Pronestyl.
- 500, 750, and 1000 mg tablets of Procan SR.

Actions: Type Ia antiarrhythmic used to treat ventricular and supraventricular arrhythmias.

Clearance: Metabolized via liver; renally excreted.
- Metabolite (NAPA) is active.
- Moderately to markedly increase dosing interval in patients with impaired renal function.
- Sources differ on whether to reduce dosage in patients with liver disease, so at minimum monitor serum levels carefully.
- Reduce dosage in elderly patients.
- Supplemental dose suggested after hemodialysis.

Selected Side Effects: Hypotension (with IV administration), *QT prolongation, ventricular arrhythmias (particularly torsade de pointes),* frequent SLE-like syndrome (with prolonged therapy), nausea and vomiting, agranulocytosis.

Cautions: *Contraindicated in patients with the ventricular arrhythmia torsade de pointes, SLE, or severe conduction abnormalities.*

Pregnancy Category: C.

Cost: Generic $$, Procan SR $$$.

Pearls:

- Give an AV blocker prior to use in atrial flutter (not atrial fibrillation) because procaine can slow the atrial flutter rate and increase effective AV conduction, resulting in an increased ventricular response rate.
- Some physicians follow procainamide (PA) and NAPA levels. Usual therapeutic levels differ among sources and among hospital laboratories. "Therapeutic" levels usually are given as approximately from 4–8 to 4–10 mg/L.
- *Follow QRS complex width and corrected QT intervals during loading and initial therapy. Increases of > 50% in the QRS complex width or of > 25% in the corrected QT interval are associated with increased risk of torsade de pointes and necessitate dose reductions.*
- Observe patients for hypotension during IV load.

Procan SR: *see* **PROCAINAMIDE**

Procardia, Procardia XL: *see* **NIFEDIPINE**

PROCHLORPERAZINE (Compazine)

Dose: Route dependent:

- PO: 5–10 mg tid–qid prn.
- Long-acting PO (Spansule): Initially try 15 mg every morning or 10 mg bid; maximum 20 mg bid.
- IM: 5–10 mg q4–6h prn; maximum 40 mg in 24 h.
- PR: 25 mg bid prn.

Preparations:

- 5, 10, and 25 mg tablets.
- 10 and 15 mg long-acting Compazine Spansules.
- 4 oz bottle of syrup containing 5 mg/mL.
- 2.5, 5, and 25 mg suppositories.

Actions: Phenothiazine that suppresses the chemoreceptor trigger zone; used to treat nausea.

Clearance: Metabolized primarily via liver.

Selected Side Effects: Extrapyramidal symptoms, drowsiness, dizziness, blurred vision, dry mouth, hypotension, increased risk of convulsions, neuroleptic malignant syndrome.

Pregnancy Category: Not established, but use during pregnancy is generally not recommended.

Cost: $$$$ (≈ $1 each 10 mg tablet).

Proleukin: *see* INTERLEUKIN-2

PROMETHAZINE (Phenergan)

Dose: Use dependent.
- Nausea and vomiting: 12.5–25 mg PO, PR, IM, or IV.
- Sedation: 25–50 mg PO, PR, IM, or IV.

Preparations:
- 12.5, 25, and 50 mg tablets.
- 4 oz and 1 pint bottles of syrup containing 6.25 mg/5 mL (1 tsp).
- 12.5, 25, and 50 mg suppositories.

Actions: Phenothiazine derivative with antihistaminic, sedative, antiemetic, and anticholinergic effects; used to treat nausea and vomiting, motion sickness, allergic reactions, and for sedation.

Clearance: Metabolized via liver.
- No change in dosage needed in patients with renal insufficiency.
- Dosage may need to be reduced in patients with end-stage renal disease (because of excessive drowsiness).

Selected Side Effects: Drowsiness, extrapyramidal reactions, anticholinergic effects.

Selected Drug Interactions:
- Potentiates CNS depressant effects of other CNS depressants.
- Can increase extrapyramidal reactions in patients taking MAOI.

Cautions: Use with caution in patients with bone marrow depression, asthma, narrow-angle glaucoma, prostate hypertrophy, stenosing peptic ulcer, or bladder neck obstruction.
Pregnancy Category: C.
Cost: $$ ($\approx$ $0.10 each 25 mg tablet).

Pronestyl: *see* PROCAINAMIDE

PROPAFENONE (Rythmol)
Dose:
- Initial: 150 mg PO q8h for 3–4 days.
- Usual maintenance: 150–300 mg PO tid.

Preparations: 150, 225, and 300 mg tablets.
Actions: Type Ic antiarrhythmic (blocks sodium channels and slows impulse conduction); used to treat ventricular arrhythmias; also used to treat supraventricular arrhythmias (though not FDA approved).
- Is structurally similar to propranolol and has β-blocking properties.

Clearance: Metabolized via liver with two patterns of metabolism: (1) $t_{1/2}$ of 2–10 h in > 90% of patients and (2) 10–32 h in the remainder; metabolites may be active.
- Reduce dosage in patients with impaired renal function.
- Decrease dosage to 150 mg PO q8–12h in patients with liver disease.

Selected Side Effects: Proarrhythmic effects, conduction abnormalities (first-degree AV block, intraventricular conduction delay), CHF, unusual taste sensation, constipation, (+) ANA titer.
Selected Drug Interactions:
- Raises serum levels of propranolol and metoprolol.
- Increases serum level of digoxin by 35%–85%.
- Cimetidine raises its serum level by 20%.
- Quinidine causes the slow pattern of metabolism ($t_{1/2}$ 10–32 h).
- Prolongs PT in patients taking warfarin.

Cautions: Use with caution in patients with CHF, conduction abnormalities, or bronchospasm.
Pregnancy Category: C.
Cost: $$$$ ($\approx$ $1.05 each 150 mg tablet).

Propofol: *see* DIPRIVAN

PROPOXYPHENE (Darvon, Darvon-N; see also Darvocet)
Dose: 65–100 mg PO q4h prn.
Preparations:
- 32 and 65 mg capsules of Darvon.
- 100 mg capsules of Darvon-N.

Actions: Narcotic analgesic used to treat mild to moderate pain.

Clearance: Metabolized primarily via liver.
- Reduce dosage or avoid in patients with end-stage renal disease (active metabolites accumulate that have dysrhythmic activity).
- Decrease dosage in patients with liver disease.
- Supplemental dose not required after hemodialysis or peritoneal dialysis.

Pregnancy Category: Not established.

Cost: Generic $$, Darvon $$$$ (generic ≈ $0.10 each 65 mg tablet, Darvon ≈ $0.40 each 65 mg tablet).

Pearls: Subject to abuse and addiction.

PROPRANOLOL (Inderal, Inderal LA)
Dose: Delivery dependent:
- Regular-strength PO: Usual dose is 20–40 mg bid–qid (usually given bid for hypertension).
- Long-acting PO (Inderal LA): 80–160 mg qd.
- IV: 1–3 mg (at an injection rate of no more than 1 mg/min); a second dose may be repeated after 2 min if necessary; most commonly is administered 1 mg at a time.

Preparations:
- 10, 20, 40, 60, 80, and 90 mg tablets.
- 60, 80, 120, and 160 mg tablets of Inderal LA.

Actions: Nonselective β-blocker used to treat ischemic heart disease and hypertension.

Clearance: Metabolized via liver.
- No change in dosage needed in patients with renal insufficiency.
- Reduce dosage in patients with liver disease.
- Supplemental dose not required after hemodialysis.

Selected Side Effects: Hypotension, bradycardia, AV block, Raynaud-like symptoms, depression, fatigue, bronchospasm, impotence.
Selected Drug Interactions:
• Decreases clearance of lidocaine and theophylline.
Pregnancy Category: C.
Cost: Generic $, Inderal $$$ (≈ $0.10 each 30 mg generic tablet; ≈ $0.40 each 30 mg Inderal tablet; ≈ $0.90 each 60 mg Inderal LA tablet).
Pearls: Taper dose when discontinuing (to avoid rebound reactions).

Propulsid: *see* CISAPRIDE

PROPYLTHIOURACIL (PTU)
Dose:
• Initial: 100–150 mg PO tid–qid.
• Maintenance: 50–300 mg daily (usually given in divided doses tid).
Preparations: 50 mg tablets.
Actions: Medication that inhibits synthesis of thyroid hormone and conversion of T_4 to T_3; used to treat hyperthyroidism.
Clearance: Metabolized via liver; renally excreted.
• Slightly reduce dosage in patients with impaired renal function.
Selected Side Effects: Rash, pruritus, occasional GI discomfort, headache, arthralgia, paresthesias, rare leukopenia (usually during first 2 months of therapy), elevated LFTs and hepatitis.
Pregnancy Category: D.
Cost: $$.

ProSom: *see* ESTAZOLAM

ProStep: *see* NICOTINE transdermal patch

Proventil: *see* ALBUTEROL

Provera: *see* MEDROXYPROGESTERONE

Prozac: *see* FLUOXETINE

PSEUDOEPHEDRINE (Sudafed; *see also* Actifed, Robitussin-PE, Seldane-D)
Dose: 60–120 mg PO tid–qid.
Preparations: 30 and 60 mg tablets.
Actions: Oral decongestant that stimulates release of endogenous catecholamines, leading to both α- and β-receptor stimulation; used to treat nasal, sinus, or eustachian tube congestion.
Cautions:
- *Contraindicated in patients taking MAOI or tricyclics.*
- Use with caution in patients with hypertension.

PSYLLIUM: *see* Metamucil

PTU: *see* PROPYLTHIOURACIL

Purinethol: *see* MERCAPTOPURINE

PYRAZINAMIDE (PZA)
Dose: 25 mg/kg PO qd.
Preparations: 500 mg tablets.
Actions: Bactericidal nicotinamide analogue used to treat mycobacterial infections (in combination with other antimycobacterial agents).
Clearance: Metabolized via liver; renally excreted.
- Reduce dosage in patients with impaired renal function.
Selected Side Effects: Dose-related hepatotoxicity, frequent hyperuricemia, arthralgias, gastric irritation.
Cautions: Use with caution, if at all, in patients with liver disease or gout.
Cost: $$$$ (≈ $3/day).
Pearls:
- Check LFTs before beginning treatment.
- Follow LFTs and uric acid levels.

Pyridium: *see* **PHENAZOPYRIDINE**

PYRIDOXINE (VITAMIN B$_6$)
Dose: Use dependent.
- B$_6$ deficiency: 10–250 mg PO qd.
- Prophylactic therapy for patients taking isoniazid who are at risk for developing neuropathy: 25–50 mg PO qd (*Washington Manual* recommends 50 mg PO qd for prophylactic therapy when isoniazid [INH] is administered).

Preparations: 10, 25, 50, 100, 200, 250, and 500 mg tablets.

PZA: *see* **PYRAZINAMIDE**

Questran: *see* **CHOLESTYRAMINE**

Quinaglute: *see* **QUINIDINE**

Quinamm: *see* **QUININE**

Quinidex: *see* **QUINIDINE**

QUINAPRIL (Accupril)
Dose:
- Initial: 10 mg PO qd (5 mg PO qd for patients taking diuretics).
- Maintenance: 10–80 mg PO daily in 1 or 2 divided doses.

Preparations: 10, 20, and 40 mg tablets.

Actions: ACE inhibitor used to treat hypertension.

Clearance: Deesterified in the liver to active metabolite quinaprilat, which is eliminated primarily by renal excretion.
- In patients with impaired renal function, reduce initial dose to 2.5–5.0 mg, and titrate subsequent dose to BP response.

Selected Side Effects: Hypotension and dizziness, hyperkalemia (especially in patients with impaired renal function or taking K$^+$-sparing drugs or K$^+$ supplements), nonproductive cough, impairment of renal function, angioedema, rare neutropenia.

Cautions:

- *Contraindicated during second and third trimesters of pregnancy and in patients with significant aortic stenosis or hyperkalemia.*
- Patients should almost never be given both an ACE inhibitor and a K^+ supplement, unless clearly indicated by serial serum K^+ testing.

Pregnancy Category: D.

Cost: $$$ ($\approx$ $0.95 each 20 mg tablet).

Pearls:

- Diuretics potentiate its antihypertensive effects; the risk of hypotension is increased in volume-depleted and elderly patients.
- Follow BUN, creatinine, and K when beginning therapy.
- Patients should be instructed not to use potassium supplements or salt substitutes containing potassium.
- Patients should be made aware of the possibility of developing a nonproductive cough and of developing angioedema.
- The frequently seen nonproductive cough with ACE inhibitors is presumed to be due to the inhibition of the degradation of endogenous bradykinin.
- Patients who develop a cough with one ACE inhibitor usually also develop such a cough with other ACE inhibitors.

QUINIDINE (QUINIDINE SULFATE, Quinaglute, Quinidex Extentabs)

Dose: Preparation dependent.

- Quinidine sulfate: 200–400 mg q6h.
- Quinaglute: 324–648 mg q8–12h.
- Quinidex Extentabs: 300–600 PO q8–12h.
- "Loading dose" for converting atrial arrhythmias: 600 mg of quinidine sulfate once PO.

Preparations:

- 100, 200, and 300 mg tablets of quinidine sulfate.
- 324 mg long-acting Quinaglute.
- 300 mg extended release tablets of Quinidex Extentabs.

Actions: Type Ia antiarrhythmic (blocks sodium channels leading to slowed impulse conduction); used to treat ventricular and supraventricular arrhythmias.

- Also prolongs repolarization, leading to QT interval prolongation.

Clearance: Metabolized primarily via liver.

- No change in dosage needed in patients with renal insufficiency.
- Reduce dosage in elderly patients and in patients with liver dysfunction or decreased liver perfusion.
- Supplemental dose suggested after hemodialysis or peritoneal dialysis.

Selected Side Effects: Diarrhea (common and often dose-limiting), nausea, *QT interval prolongation, proarrhythmic effects (especially the ventricular arrhythmia torsade de pointes),* cinchonism (tinnitus, headache, nausea and vomiting, visual changes, etc), thrombocytopenia, fever, hepatitis.

Selected Drug Interactions:

- Prolongs PT in patients taking warfarin.
- *Greatly increases serum level of digoxin (up to 100%).*

Cautions: *Contraindicated in patients with the ventricular arrhythmia torsade de pointes, severe conduction abnormalities, or a prolonged QT interval.*

Cautions: Use with caution in AV nodal disease.

Pregnancy Category: C.

Cost: Generic $, brands $$$ (≈ $0.10 each 200 mg generic tablet; ≈ $0.25 each 200 mg brand-name tablet; ≈ $0.25 each 324 mg Quinaglute tablet).

Pearls:

- Follow QRS and corrected QT intervals; discontinue for an increase of ≥ 50% in the QRS interval or an increase of ≥ 25% in the corrected QT interval.
- For toxicity (ie, greatly increased QT and QRS, torsade de pointes), may treat with lactate, bicarbonate, isoproterenol, or overdrive pacing.
- Give an AV blocker prior to use in atrial flutter (not fibrillation) because quinidine can slow the atrial flutter rate and increase effective AV conduction, resulting in an increased ventricular response rate.

QUININE (QUININE SULFATE, Quinamm)
Dose: 260–520 mg PO qhs.
Preparations: 260 mg tablets.

Actions: Medication used to prevent and treat nocturnal leg cramps.

Clearance: Metabolized via liver; renally excreted.

- Moderately reduce dosage or increase dosing interval in patients with impaired renal function.
- Supplemental dose suggested after hemodialysis but not after peritoneal dialysis.

Selected Side Effects: Cinchonism (tinnitus, headache, nausea and vomiting, visual changes, etc), hemolysis, ITP.

Selected Drug Interactions:

- Raises serum level of digoxin.
- Potentiates effects of neuromuscular blocking agents.

Cautions: *Contraindicated in G6PD deficiency, optic neuritis, ITP, tinnitus, and in pregnant or potentially pregnant patients.*

Pregnancy Category: X.

Cost: $.

Pearls: Has cardiac effects similar to those of quinidine.

RAMIPRIL (Altace)

Dose:

- Initial: 2.5 mg PO qd (1.25 mg PO qd in patients taking diuretics to avoid possible hypotension).
- Maintenance: 2.5–20 mg daily given qd–bid.

Preparations: 1.25, 2.5, 5, and 10 mg capsules.

Actions: ACE inhibitor used to treat hypertension.

Clearance: Metabolized via liver to more active metabolite, ramiprilat; drug and metabolite are excreted in urine and feces.

- Reduce dosage in renal failure.

Selected Side Effects: Hypotension and dizziness, hyperkalemia (especially in patients with impaired renal function or taking K^+-sparing drugs or K^+ supplements), nonproductive cough, impairment of renal function, angioedema, rare neutropenia.

Cautions:

- *Contraindicated during second and third trimesters of pregnancy and in patients with significant aortic stenosis or hyperkalemia.*
- Patients should almost never be given both an ACE inhibitor and a K^+ supplement, unless clearly indicated by serial serum K^+ testing.

Pregnancy Category: D.
Cost: $$$ (≈ $0.80 each 5 mg tablet).
Pearls:
- Diuretics potentiate its antihypertensive effects; the risk of hypotension is increased in volume-depleted and elderly patients.
- Follow BUN, creatinine, and K when beginning therapy.
- Patients should be instructed not to use potassium supplements or salt substitutes containing potassium.
- Patients should be made aware of the possibility of developing a nonproductive cough and of developing angioedema.
- The frequently seen nonproductive cough with ACE inhibitors is presumed to be due to the inhibition of the degradation of endogenous bradykinin.
- Patients who develop a cough with one ACE inhibitor usually also develop such a cough with other ACE inhibitors.

RANITIDINE (Zantac)
Dose:
- Regimens for acute therapy include: (1) 150 mg PO bid, (2) 300 mg PO qhs, or (3) 50 mg IV q8h.
- Maintenance: 150 mg PO qhs.
Preparations:
- 150 and 300 mg tablets.
- 1 pint bottle of flavored syrup containing 75 mg/5 mL (1 tsp).
Actions: H_2 blocker used to treat peptic ulcer disease.
Clearance: Renally excreted.
- Slightly reduce dosage in patients with impaired renal function.
- No change in dosage required in patients with liver disease.
- Supplemental dose suggested after hemodialysis.
Selected Side Effects: Rare confusion and agitation in elderly patients, rare decrease in platelets, occasional elevated LFTs and rare hepatitis, rare severe headache, rare conduction abnormalities or arrhythmias.
Selected Drug Interactions: Magnesium- and aluminum-containing antacids, such as Maalox and Mylanta, reduce its bioavailability (give at least 2 h apart from ranitidine).
Cost: $$$$ (≈ $2.60 each 300 mg tablet).
Pearls: Gives false (+) protein results on urinalysis.

Reglan: *see* METOCLOPRAMIDE

Relafen: *see* NABUMETONE

RESERPINE (Serpasil)
Dose (for hypertension therapy):
- Initial: 0.5 mg PO qd for 1–2 weeks.
- If satisfactory decrease in BP is achieved, may decrease dosage to 0.1–0.25 mg PO qd.

Preparations: 0.1 and 0.25 mg tablets.

Actions: Central-acting agent that decreases HR and lowers BP by depleting catecholamine stores, thereby depressing sympathetic nerve function; used to treat hypertension.
- Is also occasionally used to treat psychosis refractory to traditional antipsychotics.

Clearance: Metabolized via liver.
- No change in dosage needed for mild or moderate renal failure; avoid in patients with end-stage renal disease (GFR < 10 mL/min).
- Supplemental dose not required after hemodialysis or peritoneal dialysis.

Selected Side Effects: Dose-related depression, drowsiness, weakness, activation of peptic ulcer disease (increases secretion of hydrochloric acid) and ulcerative colitis, GI distress, nasal congestion, sexual dysfunction, bradycardia and arrhythmias, weight gain, edema.

Selected Drug Interactions:
- Tricyclics can increase its antihypertensive effect.
- Can prolong effect of direct-acting amines (epinephrine, isoproterenol, phenylephrine, metaraminol). Inhibits action of indirect-acting amines (ephedrine, tyramine, amphetamines).
- Decreases effect of levodopa.

Cautions:
- *Avoid concomitant use with MAOI.*
- *Contraindicated in active peptic ulcer disease, ulcerative colitis, and pheochromocytoma and in patients with depression or undergoing ECT.*

- Use with caution in patients with history of previous peptic ulcer disease, ulcerative colitis, or gallstones (can cause biliary colic).

Pregnancy Category: C.

Cost: $.

Pearls:

- Dose-related depression is a common and important side effect.
- Some sources suggest a maximum dose of 0.5 mg PO qd, though, as noted, depression is dose related.
- Is more effective when used with a diuretic or vasodilator, and several fixed-combination preparations are available.

Restoril: *see* TEMAZEPAM

Retin-A: *see* TRETINOIN topical cream, gel, and liquid

Retrovir: *see* ZIDOVUDINE

Rhinocort: *see* BUDESONIDE

Rifadin: *see* RIFAMPIN

RIFAMPIN (Rifadin, Rimactane)

Dose: Disease dependent:

- Tuberculosis: 600 mg PO or IV qd.
- Meningococcal carrier: 600 mg PO bid for 2 days.

Preparations: 150 and 300 mg tablets.

Actions: Semisynthetic antibiotic that binds to DNA-dependent RNA polymerase and inhibits RNA synthesis; used as an antitubercular agent and in asymptomatic *Neisseria meningitidis* infection (and potential *N meningitidis* carriers).

Clearance: Metabolized to active metabolites; undergoes enterohepatic circulation.

- No change in dosage needed in patients with renal insufficiency.
- Reduce dosage in hepatic or biliary disease.
- Supplemental dose not required after hemodialysis.

Selected Side Effects:
- Elevated LFTs, *hepatitis and liver damage* (with toxic effects potentiated by isoniazid), rare severe hypersensitivity reactions (including hemolytic anemia, interstitial nephritis, etc), rare thrombocytopenia.

Selected Drug Interactions:
- Can diminish effects of methadone, barbiturates, diazepam, verapamil, β-blockers, digoxin, quinidine, disopyramide, mexiletine, theophylline, anticonvulsants, OHAs, and warfarin.
- Substantially reduces effectiveness of oral contraceptives.

Pregnancy Category: C.

Cost: $$$$ (≈ $4/day); no generic form is available.

Pearls:
- Liver toxicity is the major side effect; check LFTs before starting therapy and periodically during treatment.
- Warn patients that it colors urine, saliva, feces, sputum, nasal discharge, sweat, and tears orange-red, and that it can permanently stain soft contact lenses.
- Interferes with laboratory assays of vitamin B and folate.
- Should be taken at least 1 h before or 2 h after meals.

Rimactane: *see* RIFAMPIN

Robitussin: *see* GUAIFENESIN and the following Robitussin preparations

Robitussin A-C (GUAIFENESIN + CODEINE + ALCOHOL)

Dose: 10 mL (2 tsp) PO q4h prn.

Preparations:
- Available in 2 oz, 4 oz, 1 pint, and 1 gallon bottles.
- Each 5 mL (1 tsp) contains 100 mg guaifenesin, 10 mg codeine, and 3.5% alcohol.

Actions: Combines expectorant with centrally acting narcotic that elevates the threshold for cough; used to treat persistent cough.

Cautions: *Contraindicated in patients who have taken MAOI within 2 weeks.*

Pearls: Warn patients of somnolent effects of codeine and that they should not drive or operate potentially dangerous machinery while taking codeine.

Robitussin-CF (GUAIFENESIN + PHENYLPROPANOLAMINE + DEXTROMETHORPHAN + ALCOHOL)

Dose: 10 mL (2 tsp) PO q4h prn.

Preparations:
- Available in 4, 8, and 16 oz bottles.
- Each 5 mL (1 tsp) contains 100 mg guaifenesin, 12.5 mg phenylpropanolamine, 10 mg dextromethorphan, and 4.75% alcohol.

Actions: Combines expectorant, decongestant, and centrally acting cough suppressants; used to treat persistent cough.

Robitussin-DM (GUAIFENESIN + DEXTROMETHORPHAN + ALCOHOL)

Dose: 10 mL (2 tsp) PO q4–6h prn.

Preparations:
- Available in 4, 8, and 12 oz bottles.
- Each 5 mL (1 tsp) contains 100 mg guaifenesin, 15 mg dextromethorphan, and 1.4% alcohol.

Actions: Combines expectorant and centrally acting cough suppressant; used to treat persistent cough.

Robitussin-PE (GUAIFENESIN + PSEUDOEPHEDRINE + ALCOHOL)

Dose: 10 mL (2 tsp) PO q4h prn.

Preparations:
- Available in 4, 8, and 16 oz bottles.
- Each 5 mL (1 tsp) contains 100 mg guaifenesin, 30 mg pseudoephedrine, and 1.4% alcohol.

Actions: Combines expectorant and decongestant; used to treat persistent cough and nasal congestion.

Rocephin: *see* CEFTRIAXONE

Roferon-A: *see* INTERFERON

Rogaine: *see* MINOXIDIL

Rolaids (DIHYDROXYALUMINUM SODIUM CARBONATE)
Dose:
- 1 or 2 tablets hourly prn.
- Maximum: 24 tablets in 24 h.

Preparations: Each tablet contains 334 mg dihydroxyaluminum sodium carbonate.

Rolaids (CALCIUM CARBONATE)
Dose:
- 1–2 tablets hourly prn.
- Maximum: 14 tablets in 24 h.

Preparations: Each tablet contains 550 mg calcium carbonate.

Rolaids, Extra Strength (CALCIUM CARBONATE)
Dose:
- 1 or 2 tablets hourly prn.
- Maximum: 8 tablets in 24 h.

Preparations: Each extra-strength tablet contains 1000 mg calcium carbonate.

Rolaids, Sodium-Free (CALCIUM CARBONATE + MAGNESIUM HYDROXIDE)
Dose: 1 or 2 tablets hourly prn; maximum 18 tablets in 24 h.

Preparations: Each tablet contains 317 mg calcium carbonate and 64 mg magnesium hydroxide.

Romazicon: *see* FLUMAZENIL

Rufen: *see* IBUPROFEN

Rythmol: *see* PROPAFENONE

SALBUTAMOL: *see* ALBUTEROL

SALMETEROL (Serevent)
Dose:
- Maintenance treatment of asthma: 2 puffs bid, taken approximately 12 h apart.
- Prophylactic treatment before exercise: 2 puffs at least 30–60 min before exercise.

Preparations: 13 g canisters provided 120 metered actuations.

Actions: Long-acting β_2-selective β-receptor agonist bronchodilator; used as maintenance therapy in select patients with asthma who require regular treatment with inhaled, short-acting β_2 agonists, and to prevent exercise-induced asthma (*is* not *used for the acute treatment of asthma exacerbation or nocturnal asthma*).

Cautions:
- *Should not be used for the acute treatment of asthma symptoms or asthma exacerbation.*
- Salmeterol should not *be used in patients with asthma who can be treated with occasional use of short-acting inhaled bronchodilators.*
- Should be used with extreme caution in patients being treated with MAO inhibitors or tricyclic antidepressants.

Pregnancy Category: C.

Cost: $$$$ (≈ $55 each inhaler).

Pearls: All patients requiring salmeterol should also be prescribed a short-acting β-receptor agonist to be used for exacerbations between salmeterol doses.

SALSALATE (Disalcid)
Dose: 1 g PO tid or 1.5 g PO bid
- Titrate according to individual response (full benefits may not be evident for 3–4 days).

Preparations:
- 500 and 750 mg tablets.
- 500 mg capsules.

Actions: Nonsteroidal antiinflammatory agent with antipyretic and analgesic properties; used to treat inflammatory conditions.

Clearance: Undergoes esterase hydrolysis in the body and renal excretion.

Selected Side Effects: Tinnitus, hearing impairment, nausea, rash, vertigo.

Selected Drug Interactions:
- Can enhance hypoglycemic effect of OHAs.
- Is antagonistic to uricosuric agents.

Cautions: Use with caution in renal insufficiency or peptic ulcer disease.

Pregnancy Category: C.

Cost: Generic $, Disalcid $$$ ($\approx$ $0.10 each 500 mg generic tablet; $\approx$ $0.50 each 500 mg Disalcid tablet).

Pearls:
- Patients with ASA sensitivity rarely show cross-sensitivity.
- Causes less upper GI bleeding than other NSAIDs.
- Monitor plasma salicylate levels.
- Therapeutic level is 10–30 mg/dayL.
- Signs and symptoms of overdose include tinnitus, vertigo, headache, confusion, drowsiness, sweating, hyperventilation, diarrhea, and vomiting.
- Can lower measured T_4 level.
- Acidification of urine can markedly increase its plasma level.

SCOPOLAMINE (Transderm Scop)

Dose:
- Apply 1 disk to an area of intact skin behind the ear.
- Apply approximately 3 h prior to travel to attain adequate blood levels.

Preparations: Each disk delivers 0.5 mg of scopolamine over 3 days.

Actions: Belladonna alkaloid with antiemetic and antinauseant actions; used to treat motion sickness.

Selected Side Effects: Dry mouth (extremely frequent), drowsiness, confusion, disorientation.
Cautions: Use with caution in elderly patients, patients with obstruction of the pylorus or urinary bladder neck, patients with metabolic, liver, or renal failure, and patients taking drugs that have CNS effects or anticholinergic activity.
Pregnancy Category: C.
Cost: $$$ (≈ $4 each disk).

SECOBARBITAL (Seconal)
Dose: Delivery dependent.
- PO (as hypnotic): 100 mg PO qhs.
- IV: Up to 250 mg, given at maximum rate of 50 mg over 15 s; usually given in divided doses (50–100 mg is usually adequate).

Preparations: 50 and 100 mg Seconal Pulvules.
Actions: Rapidly acting barbiturate used to induce sleep.
Clearance: Metabolized via liver; eliminated in urine and feces.
- Reduced dosage recommended in patients with impaired renal function or liver disease.

Pregnancy Category: D.
Cost: $.
Pearls:
- As noted, give IV push *slowly*.
- Is addictive and can be habit-forming.
- Can cause skin ulceration if extravasated.

Seconal: *see* SECOBARBITAL

Sectral: *see* ACEBUTOLOL

Seldane: *see* TERFENADINE

Seldane-D (PSEUDOEPHEDRINE + TERFENADINE)
Dose: 1 tablet PO bid.
Preparations: Each tablet contains 120 mg pseudoephedrine and 60 mg terfenadine.

Actions: Combination antihistamine and decongestant; used to treat rhinorrhea.

Cautions: *Concurrent use of terfenadine with erythromycin or ketoconazole, and use in patients with hepatic dysfunction that interferes with terfenadine metabolism, have been associated with ventricular arrhythmias and death. Terfenadine should, therefore, not be prescribed under these conditions.*

Pregnancy Category: C.

Cost: $$$$ (≈ $1/tablet).

SELEGILINE (Eldepryl)

Dose: 5 mg PO bid, taken at breakfast and at lunch.

Preparations: 5 mg tablets.

Actions: MAO inhibitor; used as an adjunct treatment for Parkinson's disease in patients taking levodopa/carbidopa (Sinemet) who exhibit deterioration in the quality of their response to this therapy.

Clearance: Partially renally excreted.

Selected Side Effects: Exacerbation of levodopa-associated side effects; nausea; confusion; dizziness, lightheadedness, fainting; dry mouth.

Cautions:

- *Contraindicated in patients taking meperidine (Demerol) and, probably, other opioids.*
- Tricyclic antidepressants and fluoxetine (Prozac) should not be prescribed until at least 14 days after discontinuation of MAO inhibitors.

Pregnancy Category: C.

Pearls: After 2–3 days of therapy, consider attempting to reduce the dose of levodopa/carbidopa (Sinemet).

Septra: *see* Bactrim

Serax: *see* OXAZEPAM

Serevent: *see* SALMETEROL

Serpasil: *see* RESERPINE

SERTRALINE (Zoloft)
Dose:
- Initial: 50 mg PO qd (one source notes an initial dose of 25 mg can be used in some patients).
- Can titrate dose upward at 1 week interval up to a maximum of 200 mg PO qd.

Preparations: 50 and 100 mg scored tablets.

Actions: Serotonin reuptake inhibitor used to treat depression.

Clearance: Liver metabolized.
- Decrease dose or increase dosing interval in patients with liver disease.

Selected Side Effects: GI distress, tremor, insomnia or somnolence, male sexual dysfunction, dry mouth, increased sweating, rare activation of mania, rare hyponatremia.

Selected Drug Interactions:
- Severe reactions when administered with MAO inhibitors.
- Cimetidine significantly increases its serum level.

Cautions: *Contraindicated in patients who have taken MAO inhibitors within the previous 2 weeks; do not start MAO inhibitor therapy until at least 2 weeks after paroxetine has been discontinued.*

Pregnancy Category: B.

Cost: $$$$ ($\approx$ $1.90 each 50 mg tablet).

Silvadene: *see* SILVER SULFADIAZINE cream

SILVER SULFADIAZINE cream (Silvadene)
Dose: Apply thin layer to affected area qd–bid.

Preparations: 20, 50, 85, 400, and 1000 mg containers of 1% cream.

Actions: Topical sulfonamide antibiotic used to prevent and treat burn wound infections.

Selected Side Effects: Hypersensitivity reaction, skin discoloration, transient decrease in neutrophil levels.

Cautions:
- Some systemic absorption of sulfonamide can occur.
- Some hemolysis can occur in G6PD-deficient patients.

- Its use over an extensive body surface area can result in significant serum levels.
- Use with caution in sulfa allergy.

Pregnancy Category: B.
Cost: $$.

SIMETHICONE (Gas-X, Mylicon, Phazyme; *see also* Mylanta)

Dose: 40–125 mg PO after each meal and qhs.
Preparations: 40, 80, and 125 mg tablets and 125 mg capsules.
Actions: Medication that disperses or prevents formation of mucus-surrounded gas pockets; used to treat flatulence and functional gastric bloating.
Pregnancy Category: C.
Pearls: Actual clinical efficacy, if any, unclear.

SIMVASTATIN (Zocor)

Dose:
- Initial: 5–10 mg PO qhs.
- Maximum: 40 mg PO Qhs.
- Preparations: 5, 10, 20, and 40 mg tablets

Actions: HMG-CoA inhibitor that lowers total and LDL cholesterol and triglyceride levels, and increases HDL cholesterol; used to treat hypercholesterolemia.
Clearance: Hydrolyzed to its active form; primarily cleared by the liver.
Selected Side Effects: Elevated LFTs, increased CPK (MM), and myopathy (especially when given with immunosuppressants, gemfibrozil, niacin, or erythromycin).
Selected Drug Interactions:
- Can prolong PT in patients taking warfarin.
- Cyclosporine, gemfibrozil, niacin, or erythromycin may increase the risk of myopathy.

Cautions:
- *Contraindicated in pregnant or potentially pregnant patients.*
- Contraindicated in patients with active liver disease or unexplained transaminase elevations.

- Use with caution in patients with history of liver disease or heavy alcohol use.

Pregnancy Category: X.

Cost: $$$–$$$$.

Pearls:

- Should be taken in the evening.
- Obtain LFTs and CPK level before starting therapy.
- Recommended frequency for checking liver function during treatment has been liberalized to every 6 weeks for first 3 months, then every 8 weeks for remainder of first year and approximately every 6 months thereafter.
- Discontinue if persistent LFTs > 3 times normal, substantial rise in CPK, or myositis occurs.
- Primary effects are reductions in total and LDL cholesterol; usually leads to only modest elevations of HDL cholesterol.

Sinemet, Sinemet CR (CARBIDOPA + LEVODOPA)

Dose: Highly variable.

- Initial dose often 1 tablet PO tid of Sinemet 25/100; optimal daily dose is determined by careful titration.
- Sinemet CR (controlled release) can be substituted for regular-duration Sinemet once the ideal daily dose of medication is determined. The conversion guidelines from Sinemet to Sinemet CR are complex; therefore, consult *PDR* for conversion guidelines.

Preparations:

- Each tablet of Sinemet 10/100, Sinemet 25/100, and Sinemet 25/250 contains 10, 25, and 25 mg carbidopa and 100, 100, and 250 mg levodopa, respectively.
- Each tablet of controlled-release Sinemet CR 25/100 and Sinemet CR 50/200 contains 25 and 50 mg carbidopa and 100 and 200 mg levodopa, respectively.

Actions: Antiparkinsonian medication; used to treat Parkinson's disease and parkinsonian syndrome.

- Levodopa crosses the blood–brain barrier and is converted to dopamine, which has antiparkinsonian effects.

- Carbidopa prevents non-CNS conversion of levodopa to dopamine.

Clearance: Metabolized via liver.

- No change in dosage needed in patients with renal insufficiency.

Selected Side Effects: Involuntary dyskinetic movements, rare CNS effects.

Selected Drug Interactions:

- *Can cause hypertensive crisis in patients taking MAOI.*
- Concomitant use with sympathomimetics increases risk of arrhythmias.
- Concomitant use with antihypertensive agents increases risk of postural hypotension.

Cautions:

- *Contraindicated in patients with narrow-angle glaucoma, history of melanoma, or taking MAOI.*
- May precipitate neuroleptic malignant syndrome-like complex if abruptly discontinued.
- Should not be given to patients currently taking single-agent levodopa.
- Use with caution in patients with history of MI, arrhythmias, or peptic ulcer disease (can cause upper GI bleeding).

Pregnancy Category: Not established.

Cost: $$$ ($\approx$ $0.40 each generic 25/100 tablet; $\approx$ $0.60 each 25/100 Sinemet tablet).

Pearls: Can cause (+) Coombs' test.

Slo-bid: *see* THEOPHYLLINE

Slo-Niacin: *see* NICOTINIC ACID

Slo-Phyllin: *see* THEOPHYLLINE

Slow-K: *see* POTASSIUM CHLORIDE

SODIUM BICARBONATE: *see* BICARBONATE

SODIUM POLYSTYRENE SULFONATE (Kayexalate)

Dose: Route dependent:
- PO:
  - ▶ 15–30 g in 50–100 mL of 20% sorbitol.
  - ▶ This dose may repeat q3–4h up to 4 or 5 doses in 24 h until hyperkalemia resolves.
- PR:
  - ▶ 50 g in 200 mL of 20% sorbitol; should be retained 30–60 min.
  - ▶ This dose may be repeated q4–6h up to 4 doses in 24 h.

Actions:
- Cation exchange resin that binds K^+ in exchange for other cations (usually Na^+) in the intestinal tract, thereby removing K^+ from the body; used to treat hyperkalemia.
- Sorbitol serves as an osmotic laxative to decrease constipation.

Selected Side Effects: Constipation, fecal impaction, gastric irritation, exacerbation of CHF or peripheral edema (due to its large Na^+ load).

Selected Drug Interactions: May cause concretions if given with aluminum hydroxide.

Cautions: Use with caution in patients who may not tolerate the Na^+ load.

Pregnancy Category: C.

Cost: $.

Pearls: Removes approximately 1 mEq of K^+ for each gram of resin administered and can lower serum K^+ 0.5–1.0 mEq/L for each 50 g of resin administered.

Solu-Cortef: *see* HYDROCORTISONE

Solu-Medrol: *see* METHYLPREDNISOLONE

SOTALOL (Betapace)
Dose:
- Initial: 80 mg PO bid.
- Total daily dose can be titrated upward every 2–3 days, up to a usual maximum daily dose of 240–320 mg, administered in divided doses bid.

Preparations: 80, 160, and 240 mg scored tablets.

Actions: Antiarrhythmic with actions of both class II (β-receptor blocker) and class III (prolongation of cardiac action potentiation duration by potassium channel blockade, similar to lidocaine) antiarrhythmics; used to treat arrhythmias.
- The class II actions lead to slowed heart rate, decreased AV node conduction, and increased AV node refractoriness; the class III actions include prolongation of the atrial and ventricular myocardial refractory periods and repolarization time (increased repolarization time reflected as a prolongation of the QT interval).
- Also prolongs refractoriness of AV node and of bypass tracts.

Clearance: Renally excreted; undergoes no metabolism prior to excretion.
- Moderate increase in dosing interval required in patients with renal insufficiency (administer qd).

Side Effects: Proarrhythmic effects, QT prolongation and torsade de pointes, bradycardia, CHF, and other side effects similar to those caused by β-blockers.

Drug Interactions:
- *Should not be used simultaneously with class Ia antiarrhythmics (quinidine, procainamide, disopyramide) because these agents also prolong the QT interval; should not be used simultaneously with β-blockers.*
- Should be used with caution with other medications that may prolong the QT interval, including phenothiazines, tricyclic antidepressants, and the antihistamines terfenadine (Seldane) and astemizole (Hismanal).

Cautions:
- *Contraindicated in patients with bronchial asthma, sinus bradycardia, second- or third-degree heart block (unless a*

*functioning pacemaker is present), QT prolongation, or un-
controlled CHF or cardiogenic shock.*
Pregnancy Category: B.
Cost: $$$$ (≈ $1.50 each 80 mg tablet).
Pearls:
- Therapy should be begun in a monitored setting, and the corrected QT interval should be followed.
- Cautions regarding the use of β-receptor blockers also apply to sotalol.

SPIRONOLACTONE (Aldactone; *see also* Aldactazide)

Dose: 25–50 mg PO tid–qid.
Preparations: 25, 50, and 100 mg tablets.
Actions: K^+-sparing diuretic that competitively inhibits aldosterone; usually used to treat ascites.
Clearance: Metabolized via liver; renally excreted.
- Markedly increase dosing interval in patients with impaired renal function; avoid in patients with end-stage renal disease.
- No change in dosage needed in patients with liver disease.
Selected Side Effects: Hyperkalemia, dehydration, hyponatremia, gynecomastia, hyperchloremic metabolic acidosis.
Selected Drug Interactions: Can increase risk of digoxin toxicity.
Pregnancy Category: Not established.
Cost: $.
Pearls: Follow serum electrolytes.

Sporanox: *see* ITRACONAZOLE

Stelazine: *see* TRIFLUOPERAZINE

Streptase: *see* STREPTOKINASE

STREPTOKINASE (Kabikinase, Streptase)

Dose: Acute MI: 1.5 million units IV over 1 h.
Actions: Thrombolytic agent that acts with plasminogen to produce an "activator complex" that converts plasminogen

to proteolytic enzyme plasmin, leading to thrombolysis; used to treat acute MI and certain other thrombotic conditions.

Clearance: Partially cleared by formation of an antigen–antibody complex; the reticuloendothelial system may also play a role in clearance.

- Dosage adjustment in patients with impaired renal function is not explicitly recommended.

Selected Side Effects: *Bleeding,* reperfusion arrhythmias, hypotension (1–10%), hypersensitivity, anaphylactoid reactions, fever (0–21%).

Pregnancy Category: C.

Cost: $$ (≈ $200 wholesale); markedly less expensive than TPA and anistreplase (Eminase, APSAC).

Pearls:

- In certain specific cases, consider its use in treatment of pulmonary embolism, deep vein thrombosis, arterial thrombus, or embolism.
- May not be effective if administered 5 days–6 months after previous use or after streptococcal infection, due to possible development of antibodies; the use of TPA should instead be considered.
- Some authorities believe that adjunctive heparin therapy may not be necessary (as long as the patient has received aspirin). When heparin is to be used as adjunctive therapy, one regimen for administering the heparin is to begin therapy (without a bolus) when the PTT falls to < 2 times control (this is in contrast to heparin therapy in the setting of TPA use, in which immediate heparinization is required).
- *The lists of what constitutes absolute contraindications to thrombolytic therapy and what other factors should be considered as increasing the risks of adverse events have been evolving and are being updated as new data become available.* The following should serve as guidelines only; *in decisions regarding thrombolytic therapy, the risks of administering thrombolytic agents must be weighed against the potential benefit.*
- Generally accepted absolute contraindications:
  ▶ History of hemorrhagic strokes (regardless of when the bleed occurred); thromboembolic stroke within the past 1 year.

- ► Active or recent (within 2 weeks) internal bleeding (*not* including menses).
- ► Recent CNS surgery or trauma; known CNS (or spinal cord) tumor, or AV malformation.
- ► Severe hypertension on presentation (> 180/110), which increases the risk for hemorrhagic stroke.
- ► Major recent (within 2 weeks) surgery.
- ► CPR that is prolonged (> 10 min) or suspected to have been traumatic (ie, suspected multiple rib fractures).
- ► Suspected aortic dissection.
- ► Pregnancy.
- Other factors that should be considered when the potential risks and benefits of thrombolytic therapy are considered:
  - ► Thromboembolic strokes greater than 1-year old; TIA within the prior 6 months *may* increase the risk of CNS adverse events.
  - ► Known bleeding diathesis or significantly elevated INR (≥ 2–3) from warfarin therapy.
  - ► Active peptic ulcer disease or recent significant GI bleeding (a distant history of a GI bleed may not be a significant risk factor with thrombolytic therapy).
  - ► Hemorrhagic retinopathy was in the past regarded as a relative contraindication to therapy; some sources no longer regard it as a contraindication; vitreous hemorrhage may, however, be a contraindication to treatment.
  - ► Older age was in the past considered a relative contraindication to therapy; however, although the risk of CNS bleeding in elderly patients is greater, the benefits in terms of mortality reduction are also greater, thus age per se is now not generally regarded as a contraindication to thrombolytic therapy. The greater risks and benefits with thrombolytic therapy in elderly patients should be weighed when considering such therapy in these patients.
  - ► Patients with cardiogenic shock on presentation do not generally derive significant benefit from thrombolytic therapy, and primary angioplasty, when available, should be considered.

STREPTOMYCIN
Dose:
- 1 g IM qd (for tuberculosis).
- With prolonged treatment, some sources suggest that frequency can eventually be reduced to 1 or 2 times weekly.

Preparations: 1 and 5 g vials.

Actions: Bactericidal antibiotic that inhibits protein synthesis; used to treat tuberculosis and other infections.

Clearance: Renally excreted via glomerular filtration.
- Significantly reduce dosage in patients with impaired renal function.

Selected Side Effects: Neurotoxic reactions (including peripheral neuritis, encephalopathy, vestibular dysfunction and vertigo, and paresthesias of the face), auditory dysfunction (from damage to cranial nerve VIII), rash, fever, urticaria, angioedema, eosinophilia, neuromuscular blockade.

Cautions:
- Risk of severe neurotoxic reactions is sharply increased in patients with impaired renal function or prerenal azotemia.
- Should not be given to pregnant or potentially pregnant patients.

Pregnancy Category: D.

Cost: $.

Pearls:
- Contains sulfite.
- Sanford's antimicrobial guide suggests obtaining monthly audiograms.
- Is known to cause fetal cranial nerve damage.

SUCCINYLCHOLINE
Dose: 1 mg/kg IV.

Actions: Short-acting neuromuscular blocker; used to obtain temporary neuromuscular paralysis.

Clearance: Rapidly hydrolyzed by plasma pseudocholinesterase.

Selected Side Effects: Bradycardia or tachycardia, myalgias.

SUCRALFATE (Carafate)
Dose: Use dependent.
- Acute therapy: 1 g PO qid.
- Maintenance: 1 g PO bid.

Preparations:
- 1 g tablets.
- 14 oz bottles of suspension containing 1g/10 mL.

Actions: Nonsystemic medication that works locally; used to treat duodenal ulcers.

Clearance: Poorly absorbed.
- Use with caution in patients with end-stage renal disease (small amounts of aluminum are absorbed and can accumulate).

Selected Side Effects: Constipation.

Selected Drug Interactions: Can decrease absorption of cimetidine, ciprofloxacin, digoxin, norfloxacin, phenytoin, ranitidine, tetracycline, or theophylline when administered simultaneously.

Pregnancy Category: B.

Cost: $$$ (acute therapy ≈ $2.40/day, maintenance ≈ $1.20/day).

Pearls:
- Administer at a separate time from other drugs when alterations in absorption are a concern.
- Not approved to treat gastric ulcers.

Sudafed: *see* PSEUDOEPHEDRINE

SULBACTAM: *see* Unasyn

SULFAMETHOXAZOLE: *see* Bactrim

SULFASALAZINE (Azulfidine)
Dose: 3–4 g daily, given in divided doses bid–qid.

Preparations:
- 500 mg tablets.
- 1 pint oral suspension containing 250 mg/5 mL (1 tsp).

Actions: Combines 5-ASA and sulfapyridine; used to treat ulcerative colitis.

- Sulfasalazine's effectiveness was discovered accidentally and its mechanism of action is still not completely understood; action may be related to inhibition of arachidonic acid metabolism and production of prostaglandins and leukotrienes, which mediate inflammation in ulcerative colitis; 5-ASA is believed to be the more active and important component.

Clearance: Intestinal flora split most of the parent compound into its two components in the bowel; most of 5-ASA is eliminated in feces; most of sulfapyridine is absorbed, then metabolized in liver and excreted in urine.

Selected Side Effects: Nausea and vomiting, anorexia, gastric distress, headache, orange-yellow discoloration of urine.

Cautions:
- *Contraindicated in patients with sulfa allergy.*
- Use with caution in patients with G6PD deficiency.

Pregnancy Category: B.

Cost: Generic $, Azulfidine $$ (≈ $0.15 each generic tablet; ≈ $0.25 each Azulfidine tablet).

Pearls: Warn patients of possible urine discoloration.

SULINDAC (Clinoril)
Dose: 150–200 mg PO bid.

Preparations: 150 and 200 mg tablets.

Actions: Nonsteroidal antiinflammatory agent with analgesic and antipyretic actions; used to treat pain and inflammation.

Clearance: Metabolized via liver.
- No change in dosage needed in patients with impaired renal function.
- Reduce dosage in patients with liver disease.

Selected Side Effects: Upper GI ulceration and bleeding, fluid retention and edema, elevated LFTs, interstitial nephritis and exacerbation of "prerenal" renal failure, rash, prolonged bleeding time (from reversible platelet inhibition).

Cautions:
- *Contraindicated in patients with salicylate sensitivity or history of peptic ulcer or upper GI bleeding.*

- Use with caution in elderly patients.
- Can cause premature closure of the ductus arteriosus when used during last trimester of pregnancy.

Pregnancy Category: *Should not be used during last trimester of pregnancy.*

Cost: $$$ (≈ $0.60 each 150 mg tablet).

Pearls: Should be taken with food or antacids (to possibly decrease GI irritation and ulceration).

Suprax: *see* CEFIXIME

Symmetrel: *see* AMANTADINE

Synthroid: *see* L-THYROXINE

T₄: *see* L-THYROXINE

Tagamet: *see* CIMETIDINE

Tambocor: *see* FLECAINIDE

TAMOXIFEN

Dose: 10–20 mg PO bid.

Preparations: 10 mg tablets.

Actions: Synthetic nonsteroidal agent with antiestrogenic properties that competes for estrogen-binding sites; usually used to treat breast cancer.

Clearance: Extensively metabolized and excreted in bile and feces.

- No change in dosage needed in patients with impaired renal function.

Selected Side Effects: Hot flashes, vaginal bleeding, menstrual irregularities, nausea and vomiting, thromboembolic disorders, rare myelosuppression, priapism, possible hypercalcemia, possible endometrial cancer.

Selected Drug Interactions: Can increase PT in patients taking warfarin.

Cautions: Use with caution in patients with decreased WBCs or platelets.

Pregnancy Category: D.
Cost: $$$ (≈ $1.25/day).
Pearls: Periodically check CBC.

Tapazole: *see* METHIMAZOLE

Taxol: *see* PACLITAXEL

Tazicef: *see* CEFTAZIDIME

Tazidime: *see* CEFTAZIDIME

Tegretol: *see* CARBAMAZEPINE

TEMAZEPAM (Restoril)
Dose: 15–30 mg PO qhs prn.
Preparations: 15 and 30 mg capsules.
Actions: Benzodiazepine used to treat insomnia.
Clearance: Metabolized via liver.
• No change in dosage needed in patients with renal insufficiency or liver disease.
Cautions: *Contraindicated in pregnant or potentially pregnant patients.*
• Avoid in elderly patients.
Pregnancy Category: X.
Cost: Generic $, Restoril $$$ (≈ $0.15 each 15 mg generic tablet; ≈ $0.70 each 15 mg Restoril tablet).

Tenormin: *see* ATENOLOL

Terazol: *see* TERCONAZOLE
vaginal cream and suppositories

TERAZOSIN (Hytrin)
Dose (for hypertension):
• Initial: 1 mg PO qhs (first dose or first several doses given at night in case patient develops orthostatic hypotension or frank hypotension).

- If tolerated, can then gradually increase dosage and have patient take dose in the morning.
- Usual: 1–5 mg PO qd.
- Maximum: 20 mg PO daily.
- If response is substantially diminished at 24 h, consider increasing dosage or giving bid.

Preparations: 1, 2, 5, and 10 mg tablets.

Actions: α-receptor blocker that causes peripheral dilatation; used to treat hypertension.

- Also now used for the treatment of benign prostatic hypertrophy (BPH).

Selected Side Effects: *Hypotension, orthostatic hypotension,* dizziness, syncope, asthenia, nasal congestion.

Pregnancy Category: C.

Cost: $$$ (≈ $1.20 each 5 mg tablet).

Pearls: Caution patients about possible hypotensive effects, especially with first several doses.

TERBUTALINE inhaler, injection, and tablets (Brethaire, Brethine, Bricanyl)

Dose:

- Inhaler: 2 inhalations, 1 min apart, q4–6h.
- PO: 5 mg of Brethine or Bricanyl PO tid (with doses taken 6 h apart); if significant side effects dose can be decreased to 2.5 mg tid.
- SQ: 0.25 mg of Brethine injected subcutaneously into the lateral deltoid area; if no significant clinical improvement within 15–30 min, a second 0.25 mg dose may be administered.

Preparations:

- 75 mg canister of Brethaire, either with mouthpiece or as refill without mouthpiece, delivering at least 300 inhalations.
- 2.5 and 5 mg tablets of Brethine and Bricanyl.

Actions: β-adrenergic agonist bronchodilator used to treat reversible obstructive airway disease.

Selected Side Effects (most are related to systemic actions): Tremor, nervousness, palpitations, dyspnea or wheezing, dysrhythmias.

Cautions: Use with caution in patients taking MAOI or tricyclics, in cardiac disease (especially CAD and arrhythmias), hypertension, or hyperthyroidism, and in diabetes (large IV doses have been associated with worsening of diabetes and diabetic ketoacidosis).
Pregnancy Category: B.
Cost: $$$ (inhaler ≈ $25 retail).

TERCONAZOLE vaginal cream and suppositories (Terazol 3 cream, Terazol 7 cream, Terazol 3 vaginal suppositories)
Dose:
- Terazol cream: Apply full applicator intravaginally qhs for 3 days (Terazol 3) or 7 days (Terazol 7).
- Terazol suppository: Insert 1 suppository intravaginally qhs for 3 days.

Preparations:
- Terazol 7 cream contains 0.4% terconazole and is available as 45 g tube with measured applicator. Terazol 3 cream contains 0.8% terconazole and is available as 20 g tube with measured applicator.
- Each 2.5 g Terazol 3 vaginal suppository contains 80 mg terconazole.

Actions: Topical antifungal used to treat candidiasis.
Selected Side Effects: Headache, body pain, dysmenorrhea, abdominal or genital pain.
Pregnancy Category: C.
Cost: $$$ (≈ $30 for Terazol 7 cream).

TERFENADINE (Seldane; *see also* Seldane-D)
Dose: 60 mg PO bid.
Preparations: 60 mg tablets.
Actions: Antihistamine used to treat allergy symptoms.
Clearance: Metabolized via liver.
- No change in dosage needed in patients with renal insufficiency.

Selected Side Effects: Minimal side effects compared with those in patients receiving placebo, QT interval prolongation and rare ventricular arrhythmias.

Selected Drug Interactions: *Concurrent use of terfenadine with erythromycin or ketoconazole has been associated with ventricular arrhythmias and death (see Cautions).*

Cautions:

- *Concurrent use of terfenadine with erythromycin and ketoconazole, and use in patients with hepatic dysfunction that interferes with terfenadine metabolism, have been associated with ventricular arrhythmias and death. Terfenadine should, therefore,* not *be prescribed in patients taking erythromycin and the related drugs clarithromycin and troleandomycin, ketoconazole and the related drugs troleandomycin, itraconazole, fluconazole, metronidazole and miconazole, and in patients with hepatic dysfunction.*
- Avoid in patients taking medications that can prolong the QT interval, in patients with congenital QT prolongation, patients with electrolyte abnormalities or those on diuretics with the potential to induce electrolyte abnormalities (secondary to concerns about ventricular arrhythmias).

Pregnancy Category: C.

Cost: $$$ (≈ $0.90/tablet); similar to daily cost of astemizole (Hismanal).

Pearls:

- *Warn patients that if they experience syncope they should discontinue the medicine and consult their physician.*
- Does not generally have the sedative and drowsiness effects of many other antihistamines.

TETRACYCLINE (Achromycin)

Dose: Route or disease dependent:

- PO: 250–500 mg qid.
- IV: 500–1000 mg q12h.
- *Chlamydia trachomatis* infection: 500 mg PO qid for 7 days or longer.

Preparations:
- 250 and 500 mg capsules.
- 16 oz bottle of flavored suspension containing 250 mg/5 mL (1 tsp).

Actions: Bacteriostatic antibiotic that inhibits protein synthesis.
- Some gram (+) coverage, including some strep and staph (but *not* enterococci).
- Some gram (−) coverage (but frequent resistance).
- Some anaerobic coverage (but many *Bacteroides fragilis* are resistant).
- Good coverage of *Mycoplasma, Rickettsia, Chlamydia,* and *Borrelia burgdorferi* (Lyme disease).
- *NOTE:* The above-mentioned antimicrobial coverage summary should be used as a guideline only; treatment decisions should take into account not only local epidemiologic patterns of antibiotic susceptibility but also, when available, culture susceptibility results.

Clearance: Metabolized via liver; renally excreted.
- Moderately decrease dosage in patients with impaired renal function.
- Reduce dosage in liver dysfunction.
- Supplemental dose not required after hemodialysis or PT.

Selected Side Effects:
- *Yellowing of developing teeth,* photosensitivity, GI distress, elevated BUN, hepatotoxicity, hypersensitivity reactions.
- Can lead to azotemia, hyperphosphatemia, or acidosis in patients with impaired renal function.
- IV administration is associated with frequent phlebitis.

Selected Drug Interactions:
- Can interfere with bactericidal actions of penicillins.
- Can prolong PT in patients taking warfarin.
- All antacids, calcium products, iron products, $NaHCO_3$, and sucralfate decrease its absorption.

Cautions: *Contraindicated in patients* < 8 years old and during second half of pregnancy (animal studies show embryo and fetal toxicity).

Pregnancy Category: D. *Should not be used during second half of pregnancy; hepatic failure may occur in preg-*

nant and postpartum women treated with IV tetracycline for pyelonephritis.
Cost: $ (≈ $5 for 250 qid for 10 days).
Pearls:
- Doxycycline is generally better tolerated.
- Caution patients to avoid intense sun exposure while taking tetracycline.
- PO dose should be given 1 h before or 2 h after meals.

Theo-24: *see* THEOPHYLLINE

Theo-Dur: *see* THEOPHYLLINE

Theolair: *see* THEOPHYLLINE

THEOPHYLLINE (Slo-bid, Slo-Phyllin, Theo-24, Theo-Dur, Theolair: *see also* AMINOPHYLLINE for IV administration)

Dose: Highly variable.
- Initial: 300–400 mg PO or 5 mg/kg PO daily.
- May increase 25% q3d to maximum of 900 mg daily.

Preparations:
- Slo-Phyllin: 60, 125, and 250 mg tablets given bid–tid.
- Slo-bid: 50, 100, 200, and 300 mg capsules given bid–tid.
- Theo-Dur: 100, 200, 300, and 450 mg tablets given bid.
- Theo-24: 100, 200, 300, and 400 mg capsules given qd.
- Theolair: 125 and 250 mg tablets given tid–qid.
- 16 oz bottles of Slo-Phyllin syrup or Theolair liquid, each containing 80 mg/15mL (1 Tbsp) given tid–qid.

Actions: Xanthine derivative that may act by directly relaxing smooth muscles of the bronchial airways, increasing diaphragmatic contractility, and by other mechanisms; used to treat reactive airway disease.

Clearance: Metabolized via liver.
- No change in dosage needed in patients with renal insuffciency.
- Reduce dosage by at least 50% in liver dysfunction.

Selected Side Effects: Tachycardia, palpitations, arrhythmias, nausea and vomiting, reflux secondary to decreased lower esophageal sphincter pressure, seizures.

Selected Drug Interactions:

- Drugs that lead to elevated theophylline levels: cimetidine, propranolol, fluoroquinolones (Cipro, Floxin, etc), macrolide antibiotics (erythromycin, Biaxin, etc), isoniazid (INH), oral contraceptives.
- Drugs that lead to lower theophylline levels: phenytoin (Dilantin), phenobarbital, rifampin, carbamazepine, furosemide.

Pregnancy Category: C.

Cost: Generic \$\$, brands \$\$\$ ($\approx$ \$0.15 each 300 mg generic tablet; $\approx$ \$0.40 each 300 mg Theo-24 tablet).

Pearls:

- $t_{1/2}$ is increased in COPD, cor pulmonale, CHF, liver disease, viral infections and high fevers, and in elderly patients.
- $t_{1/2}$ is decreased in smokers.
- To calculate the PO dose, when converting from IV drip, multiply the hourly IV dose by 10, and give that amount bid (eg, for a patient on an IV drip of 30 mg/h, the PO dose is 300 mg PO bid).
- Suggested dosage adjustments:

Serum Level (μg/mL)	Dose Adjustment
10 <	Increase dosage 25% at 3-day intervals until "therapeutic level" or symptomatic relief is achieved.
20–25	Decrease dosage 10% and recheck after 3 days.
25–30	Omit next dose and decrease subsequent doses 25%; recheck level after 3 days.
>30	Omit next 2 doses and decrease subsequent doses 50%; recheck level after 3 days.

THIAMINE (VITAMIN B$_1$)

Dose: 100 mg PO, IM, or IV daily (usually given for 3 days to prevent Wernicke's encephalopathy).

Preparations: 10, 25, 50, 100, 250, and 500 mg tablets.

Selected Side Effects: Burning at injection site, anaphylactic reaction.

Pregnancy Category: A.
Cost: $.
Pearls: For IV use, give in dilute solution or at high IV fluid rate (is often added to the liter of IV fluid the patient is already receiving).

THIORIDAZINE (Mellaril, Mellaril-S)
Dose: Disease dependent:
- Psychotic manifestations:
  - ▶ Usual starting dose: 50–100 mg PO tid.
  - ▶ Maintenance: 200–800 mg PO daily given in 2 or 3 divided doses.
- Depression with anxiety:
  - ▶ Usual starting dose: 25 mg PO tid.
  - ▶ Doses can vary widely, from 10 mg PO bid–qid to 50 mg PO tid–qid.
- Use lower doses in elderly patients.

Preparations:
- 10, 15, 25, 50, 100, 150, and 200 mg tablets of Mellaril.
- 1 pint buttermint-flavored oral suspension of Mellaril-S containing 25 mg/5 mL (1 tsp).
- 1 pint buttermint-flavored oral suspension of Mellaril-S containing 100 mg/5 mL (1 tsp).

Actions: Phenothiazine that blocks postsynaptic dopamine receptors in the basal ganglia, hypothalamus, limbic system, brainstem, and medulla; used to treat psychotic disorders and depression with anxiety.

Clearance: Metabolized via liver; metabolites are active; undergoes enterohepatic recirculation and renal excretion.
- Reduce dosage in patients with impaired renal function.

Selected Side Effects: Sedation and drowsiness, anticholinergic effects (dry mouth, blurred vision, etc), extrapyramidal reactions, *tardive dyskinesia, neuroleptic malignant syndrome,* ECG changes (corrected QT is prolonged, T wave changes), inhibition of ejaculation.

Selected Drug Interactions: Potentiates CNS depressant effects of other CNS depressants.

Cautions:
- *Contraindicated in severe CNS depression or coma and in severe hypertensive or hypotensive heart disease.*
- Reduces the convulsive threshold.

Pregnancy Category: C.
Cost: Generic $$, Mellaril $$$$ (≈ $0.15 each 50 mg generic tablet; ≈ $0.55 each 50 mg Mellaril tablet).
Pearls: Signs of neuroleptic malignant syndrome include extreme rise in temperature; muscle rigidity and "lead-pipe" syndrome; mental status changes; autonomic instability, including irregular pulse or BP; greatly increased HR; diaphoresis; arrhythmias; rhabdomyolysis (with increased CPK, myoglobinuria, and acute renal failure).

Thorazine: *see* CHLORPROMAZINE

L-THYROXINE (LEVOTHYROXINE, T_4, Levoxine, Synthroid)
Dose:
- Initial: 25–50 μg PO qd.
- May increase in 25 μg doses every 2–3 weeks.
- Usual: < 200 μg qd.
- *NOTE:* Dose is in micrograms, not milligrams.

Preparations: 25, 50, 75, 88, 100, 112, 125, 150, 175, 200, and 300 μg tablets.
Actions: Synthetic thyroxine supplement used to treat hypothyroidism.
Clearance: Deiodinated to T_3, an active metabolite, in liver, kidney, and other tissues.
Selected Side Effects: Signs and symptoms of hyperthyroidism if overrepeated.
Selected Drug Interactions:
- Thyroid replacement increases sensitivity to warfarin (warfarin dose may need to be reduced). Cholestyramine binds T_4 and T_3 in the intestine (give Synthroid > 5 h after cholestyramine).

Cautions:
- *Contraindicated in uncorrected adrenocortical insufficiency.*
- Use with caution in patients with history of angina or MI and in elderly patients.

Pregnancy Category: May be used during pregnancy.
Cost: Generic $, Synthroid $$ (≈ $0.10 each 50 mg generic tablet; ≈ $0.20 each 50 mg Synthroid tablet).

Pearls:
- Symptoms of thyroid hormone toxicity include chest pain, tachycardia, palpitations, excess sweating, heat intolerance, weight loss, nervousness.
- Adequate therapy usually results in normal levels of thyroid-stimulating hormone and T_4 after 2–3 weeks of the maintenance dose.
- Follow PT in patients taking warfarin.
- Onset of action is 6–8 h for IV therapy and 3–5 days for PO therapy.
- Aggravates diabetes (dosage of insulin or OHA may need to be increased).

TICARCILLIN (Ticar; *see also* Timentin)
Dose: 3 g IV q4h; may be given IM.
Actions: Bactericidal semisynthetic penicillin that inhibits cell wall synthesis.
- Some gram (+) coverage, including strep (some coverage for enterococci but less than with ampicillin, and *not* MRSA).
- Some gram (−) coverage (acts synergistically with aminoglycosides against *Pseudomonas aeruginosa*).
- Good anaerobic coverage, including some *Bacteroides fragilis.*
- *NOTE:* The above-mentioned antimicrobial coverage summary should be used as a guideline only; treatment decisions should take into account not only local epidemiologic patterns of antibiotic susceptibility but also, when available, culture susceptibility results.
Clearance: Renally excreted.
- Markedly increase dosing interval in patients with impaired renal function.
- No change in dosage needed in patients with liver disease.
- Supplemental dose suggested after hemodialysis or peritoneal dialysis.
Selected Side Effects: Hypersensitivity reactions and rare anaphylaxis, rare cases of coagulation abnormalities and bleeding at high doses, elevated LFTs, rare hematologic abnormalities.

COMMONLY USED DRUGS **363**

Cautions: *Contraindicated in patients with allergy to any of the penicillins.*
Pregnancy Category: B.
Cost: $$$.
Pearls:
- (+) CSF penetration with meningeal inflammation.
- Carries high Na^+ load.

Ticlid: *see* TICLOPIDINE

TICLOPIDINE (Ticlid)
Dose: 250 mg PO bid.
Preparations: 250 mg tablets.
Actions:
- Antiplatelet agent that causes time- and dose-dependent inhibition of both platelet aggregation and release of platelet granule constituents.
- Used to decrease the incidence of future stroke in patients who have had transient ischemic attacks, prior thrombotic strokes, or unstable angina, or who are allergic to aspirin, and in some patients in whom coronary stents are placed.
Clearance: Extensively metabolized in the liver.
- Patients with moderate renal failure may have greater prolongation of bleeding time.
- Should not be given in advanced liver disease (in part because of increased risk of bleeding).
Selected Side Effects: GI effects (diarrhea, nausea, dyspepsia), *neutropenia,* elevated cholesterol, prolonged bleeding time, rare elevation of LFTs, rare thrombocytopenia.
Selected Drug Interactions:
- Antacids reduce its absorption.
- Cimetidine decreases clearance and increases risk of toxicity.
Cautions:
- *Contraindicated in patients with neutropenia, thrombocytopenia, hemostatic disorders, active bleeding, or severe liver disease.*
- Cimetidine should not be given to patients taking ticlopidine.

- Use with caution in patients with lesions (such as ulcers) that are predisposed to bleeding.

Pregnancy Category: B.

Cost: $$$$ (≈ $1.40/tablet).

Pearls:

- Giving with food increases its absorption.
- Should be reserved only for patients allergic to aspirin (because of potential for drug-induced neutropenia) or selected patients receiving coronary stents.
- Neutropenia occurs in 2.4% of patients and is usually reversible after cessation of therapy.
- *Monitor WBC and neutrophil count every 2 weeks for first 3 months of therapy, more frequently if absolute neutrophil counts are consistently declining or are 30% less than pretreatment values.*
- Platelet inhibition is irreversible for the life of the platelet.
- Prolongs bleeding time; this can be normalized within 2 h by methylprednisolone 20 mg IV; platelet transfusions can also be used to reverse its effects on bleeding.
- Should be taken with food to increase its absorption.

Tigan: *see* TRIMETHOBENZAMIDE

Timentin (TICARCILLIN + CLAVULANATE)

Dose: 3.1 g IV q4–6h.

Preparations: Each 3.1 g contains 3 g ticarcillin and 100 mg clavulanate.

Actions: Antibacterial agent consisting of semisynthetic penicillin and β-lactamase inhibitor (clavulanate).

- Good gram (+) coverage, including *Staphylococcus aureus, S epidermidis,* and enterococci (but *not* MRSA).
- Good gram (−) coverage (but *not* ticarcillin-resistant *Pseudomonas aeruginosa*).
- Good anaerobic coverage, including some *Bacteroides fragilis.*
- *NOTE:* The above-mentioned antimicrobial coverage summary should be used as a guideline only; treatment decisions should take into account not only local epidemiologic patterns of antibiotic susceptibility but also, when available, culture susceptibility results.

Clearance: Primarily renally excreted.
- Moderately to markedly increase dosing interval in patients with impaired renal function.
- No change in dosage needed in patients with liver disease.
- Supplemental dose suggested after hemodialysis.

Selected Side Effects: Hypersensitivity reactions and rare anaphylaxis, rare cases of coagulation abnormalities and bleeding at high doses, elevated LFTs, rare hematologic abnormalities.

Cautions: *Contraindicated in patients with allergy to any of the penicillins.*

Pregnancy Category: B.

Cost: $$$.

Pearls:
- (+) CSF penetration with meningeal inflammation.
- Causes false (+) Coombs' test and false (+) test for proteinuria.

TIMOLOL (Blocadren)

Dose: Disease dependent:
- Hypertension:
  - ► Initial: 10 mg PO bid.
  - ► Usual: 10–30 mg PO bid.
- Post-MI prophylaxis: 10 mg PO bid.

Preparations: 5, 10, and 20 mg tablets.

Actions: Nonselective β-blocker; used to treat hypertension and as post-MI prophylaxis.

Clearance: Metabolized primarily via liver; some renal excretion.
- One source states dosage adjustment is not needed in patients with impaired renal function; another source recommends using with caution in renal disease.
- Reduce dosage in patients with liver disease.

Selected Side Effects: Fatigue, bradycardia, hypotension, conduction abnormalities, worsening of systolic ejection fraction.

Cautions: *Contraindicated in second- or third-degree heart block, bronchial asthma or COPD, severe bradycardia, and overt heart failure.*

Pregnancy Category: C.
Cost: $$ (≈ $0.40 each 10 mg tablet).
Pearls: Taper when discontinuing (to avoid rebound reactions).

TISSUE PLASMINOGEN ACTIVATOR (ALTEPLASE, t-PA, Activase)
Dose:
- Nonweight-adjusted for acute MI: 15 mg IV bolus, then 50 mg infusion over 30 min, then 35 mg over 1 h.
- Weight-adjusted for acute MI: 15 mg IV bolus, then 0.75 mg/kg (up to a maximum of 50 mg) IV over 30 min, then 0.5 mg/kg (up to a maximum of 35 mg) over 1 h.
- Life-threatening pulmonary embolus: 100 mg IV administered over 2 h.

Actions: Thrombolytic agent that produces thrombus-specific conversion of plasminogen to plasmin, causing local fibrinolysis; used to treat acute MI with ST segment elevations or left bundle branch block (LBBB) not known to be old.

Selected Side Effects: Bleeding (intracranial bleeding, 1%), reperfusion arrhythmias.

Pregnancy Category: C.

Cost: $$$$ ($2600 wholesale); streptokinase is markedly less expensive.

Pearls:
- Begin ASA and IV heparin simultaneously with administration.
- Protocols for reocclusion therapy may vary by institution. Suggested guidelines:
  - ▶ Early reocclusion (< 48 h): 6 mg IV bolus, then 20 mg/h IV infusion to total dose of 50 mg.
  - ▶ Late reocclusion (> 48 h): 15 mg IV bolus, then 50 mg IV infusion over first 30 min, then 35 mg IV over 1 h for total dose of 100 mg (or use weight-adjusted regimen as above).
  - ▶ *The lists of what constitute absolute contraindications to thrombolytic therapy and what other factors should be*

considered as increasing the risks of adverse events have been evolving and are being updated as new data become available. The following should serve as guidelines only; *in decisions regarding thrombolytic therapy, the risks of administering thrombolytic agents must be weighed against the potential benefit.*

- Generally accepted absolute contraindications:
  - ► History of hemorrhagic strokes (regardless of when the bleed occurred); thromboembolic stroke within the past 1 year.
  - ► Active or recent (within 2 weeks) internal bleeding (*not* including menses).
  - ► Recent CNS surgery or trauma; known CNS (or spinal cord) tumor, or AV malformation.
  - ► Severe hypertension on presentation (> 180/110), which increases the risk for hemorrhagic stroke.
  - ► Major recent (within 2 weeks) surgery.
  - ► CPR that is prolonged (> 10 min) or suspected to have been traumatic (ie, suspected multiple rib fractures).
  - ► Suspected aortic dissection.
  - ► Pregnancy.
- Other factors that should be considered when the potential risks and benefits of thrombolytic therapy are considered:
  - ► Thromboembolic strokes greater than 1-year old; TIA within the prior 6 months *may* increase the risk of CNS adverse events.
  - ► Known bleeding diathesis or significantly elevated INR (≥ 2–3) from warfarin therapy.
  - ► Active peptic ulcer disease or recent significant GI bleeding (a distant history of a GI bleed may not be a significant risk factor with thrombolytic therapy).
  - ► Hemorrhagic retinopathy was in the past regarded as a relative contraindication to therapy; some sources no longer regard it as a contraindication; vitreous hemorrhage may, however, be a contraindication to treatment.
  - ► Older age was in the past considered a relative contraindication to therapy; however, although the risk of CNS bleeding in elderly patients is greater, the benefits in

terms of mortality reduction are also greater, thus age per se is now not generally regarded as a contraindication to thrombolytic therapy. The greater risks and benefits with thrombolytic therapy in elderly patients should be weighed when considering such therapy in these patients.

▶ Patients with cardiogenic shock on presentation do not generally derive significant benefit from thrombolytic therapy, and primary angioplasty, when available, should be considered.

TOBRAMYCIN
Dose:
- Loading: 2 mg/kg.
- Maintenance: 1–1.67 mg/kg q8h IM or IV.

Actions: Bactericidal aminoglycoside antibiotic that irreversibly inhibits protein synthesis.

- Excellent aerobic gram (–) coverage with variable, hospital-dependent coverage for *Pseudomonas aeruginosa* (better *P aeruginosa* coverage than with gentamicin but some nosocomial strains are resistant).
- *NOTE:* The above-mentioned antimicrobial coverage summary should be used as a guideline only; treatment decisions should take into account not only local epidemiologic patterns of antibiotic susceptibility but also, when available, culture susceptibility results.

Clearance: Renally excreted.
- Markedly decrease dosage or increase dosing interval in patients with impaired renal function.
- No change in dosage needed in patients with liver disease.
- Supplemental dose suggested after hemodialysis or peritoneal dialysis.

Selected Side Effects: *Nephrotoxicity,* ototoxicity, increased neuromuscular blockade.

Selected Drug Interactions:
- Concomitant use with cephalothin, cisplatin, cyclosporine, loop diuretics, or vancomycin increases its nephrotoxicity and ototoxicity.

- Prolongs PT in patients taking warfarin.
- Penicillins can decrease its effectiveness in renal failure.

Pregnancy Category: D.

Cost: $$.

Pearls:

- No significant CSF penetration.
- Follow serum peak and trough levels.
- Gentamicin is often a less expensive alternative.

TOCAINIDE (Tonocard)

Dose:

- Initial: 400 mg PO q8h.
- Usual maintenance: 400–600 mg PO q8h or tid.
- Maximum: 2400 mg PO daily.
- Manufacturer notes that patients who have a therapeutic response with the tid regimen may be tried on a bid regimen if carefully monitored.

Preparations: 400 and 600 mg tablets.

Actions: Class Ib antiarrhythmic (blocks sodium channels and slows impulse conduction) similar to lidocaine and mexiletine; used to treat ventricular arrhythmias.

Clearance: Metabolized via liver; renally excreted.

- Slightly reduce dosage in patients with impaired renal function.
- Dosage may need to be lowered in patients with hepatic dysfunction (one source suggests up to 50% reduction in patients with severe liver disease).
- Supplemental dose suggested after hemodialysis.

Selected Side Effects: Proarrhythmic effects, CNS effects (including tremor, ataxia, dizziness, vertigo, paresthesias), nausea, rare but important blood dyscrasias (leukopenia, thrombocytopenia, anemia), very rare pulmonary fibrosis.

Selected Drug Interactions: May have additive side effects if administered with lidocaine.

Pregnancy Category: C.

Cost: $$$$ (≈ $0.85 each 400 mg tablet).

Pearls: Follow CBC, especially during first 12 weeks.

Tofranil: *see* IMIPRAMINE

TOLAZAMIDE (Tolinase)
Dose:
- Initial: 100–250 mg PO qd.
- Maintenance: 100–1000 mg PO daily.
- If total daily dose > 500 mg, should be given in divided doses bid.

Preparations: 100, 250, and 500 mg tablets.

Actions: Oral hypoglycemic agent used to treat noninsulin-dependent diabetes.

Clearance: Metabolized via liver.
- No change in dosage needed in patients with impaired renal function.

Selected Side Effects: *Hypoglycemia,* skin reactions, rare hyponatremia (second-degree increased ADH secretion), rare disulfiram-like (Antabuse) reactions.

Cost: $$ (≈ $0.55 each 250 mg tablet).

TOLBUTAMIDE (Orinase)
Dose: 500–3000 mg daily, given in 1 or 2 divided doses.

Preparations: 250 and 500 mg tablets.

Actions: Oral hypoglycemic agent used to treat noninsulin-dependent diabetes.

Clearance: Metabolized via liver; renally excreted.
- No change in dosage needed in patients with renal insufficiency.
- Supplemental dose not required after hemodialysis.

Selected Side Effects: Hypoglycemia, skin reactions, rare hyponatremia (second-degree increased ADH secretion), rare disulfiram-like (Antabuse) reactions.

Cost: Generic $, Orinase $$ (≈ $0.10 each 500 mg tablet; ≈ $0.25 each 500 mg tablet).

Tolinase: *see* TOLAZAMIDE

Tonocard: *see* TOCAINIDE

Toprol XL: *see* METOPROLOL

Toradol: *see* KETOROLAC

TORSEMIDE (Demadex)

Dose: Disease dependent:

- Congestive heart failure or chronic renal failure: Initial dose of 10–20 mg PO or IV qd; titrate dose upward as clinically indicated (usually by doubling the previous dose) up to a maximum of approximately 200 mg.
- Hepatic cirrhosis: Initial dose of 5–10 mg PO or IV qd, administered concurrently with either an aldosterone antagonist or a K$^+$-sparing diuretic; titrate dose upward as clinically indicated (usually by doubling the previous dose) up to a maximum of approximately 200 mg.
- Hypertension: Initial dose of 5 mg PO qd; if after 4–6 weeks antihypertensive response not adequate, can increase dose to 10 mg PO qd; if antihypertensive response still inadequate, an additional agent should be added to the regimen (or another agent should be tried as monotherapy).

Preparations: 5, 10, 20, and 100 mg scored tablets.

Actions: Diuretic that acts in the thick ascending portion of the loop of Henle, inhibiting the Na$^+$/K$^+$//Cl$^-$/carrier system; used in the treatment of hypertension or in the treatment of edema due to congestive heart failure, liver disease, or renal insufficiency.

Selected Side Effects: Possible ototoxicity (tinnitus and hearing loss), hypokalemia (more in patients with CHF or renal or hepatic disease and less in patients with hypertension), modest increases in total cholesterol and glucose levels.

Drug Interactions:

- Indomethacin (Indocin) decreases its effectiveness.
- Decreases renal excretion of salicylates and may lead to salicylate toxicity in patients receiving high dose salicylates.
- Other diuretics are associated with increased risk of lithium toxicity and may increase the ototoxicity of aminoglycosides.

Cautions:

- *Contraindicated in patients who are anuric or have sulfonylurea allergies.*
- Use with caution in cirrhosis and ascites (rapid fluid shifts may precipitate hepatic coma).

Pregnancy Category: B.

Pearls:
- May be taken without regard to meals.
- PO and IV preparations provide comparable efficacy per milligram administered.
- With IV administration, onset of diuresis occurs within 10 min and the peak effect occurs within first hour; with PO administration, onset of diuresis occurs within onset and peak effect occurs in 1–2 hours.

TPA: *see* TISSUE PLASMINOGEN ACTIVATOR

Trandate: *see* LABETALOL

Transderm-Nitro: *see* NITROGLYCERIN patch

Transderm-Scop: *see* SCOPOLAMINE

TRAZODONE (Desyrel)
Dose:
- Initial: 150 mg PO daily in divided doses.
- May increase total daily dose by 50 mg every 3–4 days.
- Maximum: 400–600 mg PO daily in divided doses.
- Should be taken with food.

Preparations: 50, 100, 150, and 300 mg tablets.

Actions: Nontricyclic antidepressant, associated with down-regulation of β-receptors, that can inhibit serotonin uptake or potentiate behavioral changes induced by 5-hydroxytryptophan (5-HT), a serotonin precursor; used to treat depression.

Clearance: Metabolized in the liver to a 5-HT agonist metabolite.

Selected Side Effects: Dizziness, lightheadedness, drowsiness (frequent); hypotension; anticholinergic effects (dry mouth, blurred vision, constipation); fatigue; incoordination; priapism.

Selected Drug Interactions:
- Can raise serum levels of digoxin or phenytoin.
- Dosage of concurrently administered antihypertensives may need to be reduced.

- Fluoxetine (Prozac) increases its serum level and toxicity if the two are administered within weeks of each other.
- Augments effects of warfarin.

Cautions:
- Can cause priapism that requires surgical intervention.
- Can aggravate preexisting ventricular arrhythmias.

Pregnancy Category: C.

Cost: Generic $$$, Desyrel $$$$ ($\approx$ $0.85 each 150 mg generic tablet; $\approx$ $2.40 each 150 mg Desyrel tablet).

Pearls:
- Warn patients to stop the drug and seek medical advice if priapism occurs (one third of patients who develop priapism require surgery).
- Warn patients of possible CNS effects and to avoid potentially hazardous tasks when taking the drug, at least initially.
- How it reacts with MAOI is not well known.
- Most patients respond during first week of therapy and achieve optimal response within 2 weeks; 25% of patients require 2–4 weeks for optimal response.

Trental: *see* PENTOXIFYLLINE

TRETINOIN topical cream, gel, and solution (Retin-A)

Dose: Initially, apply to dry cleansed skin qhs; may adjust dosage as needed.

Preparations: Multiple different strengths and sized containers of cream and gel (see *PDR*).

Actions: Topical medication that decreases comedone formation; used to treat acne vulgaris.

Selected Side Effects: Stinging on application, skin irritation, photosensitivity.

Pregnancy Category: C.

Cost: $$$ (tube $\approx$ $30 retail).

Pearls:
- Acne can appear worsened during first 4–6 weeks of therapy.
- Avoid contact with mucous membranes.
- Patients should be advised to use sun screen (at least SPF-15) when significant sun exposure is anticipated.

TRIAMCINOLONE (Azmacort)
Dose: 2 inhalations tid–qid.
Preparations: 20 g package containing 60 mg triamcinolone that delivers at least 240 oral inhalations.
Actions: Antiinflammatory aerosolized steroid used for *chronic* treatment of bronchial asthma in patients with disease severe enough to require steroid therapy.
Selected Side Effects:
- Localized *Candida* infections, hoarseness, dry or irritated throat, dry mouth.
- Possible systemic absorption leading to steroid-like effects and hypothalamic–pituitary–adrenal suppression.

Pregnancy Category: D.
Cost: $$$$ (≈ $46 each inhaler).

TRIAMCINOLONE nasal inhaler (Nasacort)
Dose:
- Usual starting dose: 2 sprays in each nostril qd.
- If needed, may increase to a total dose of 4 sprays in each nostril daily, administered qd, bid, or qid.
- Some patients may be maintained on 1 spray in each nostril qd.

Preparations: 15 mg canister that delivers at least 100 sprays.
Actions: Topical steroid used to treat allergic rhinitis.
Selected Side Effects: Headache, sneezing, epistaxis, dry mucous membranes, nasosinus congestion, systemic absorption with resultant steroid side effects, rare candidiasis.
Pregnancy Category: C.
Cost: $$$.

TRIAMCINOLONE ACETONIDE cream, lotion, and ointment (Aristocort A, etc)
Dose: Apply thin film to affected skin bid–qid.
Preparations:
- 15 and 60 g tubes of 0.025% cream.
- 15, 60, and 240 g tubes of 0.1% cream.

- 15 and 240 g tubes of 0.5% cream.
- 15, 60, and 240 g tubes of 0.1% ointment.

Actions: Topical steroid used to treat steroid-responsive dermatologic conditions.

Selected Side Effects: Local irritation, folliculitis, hypertrichosis, dermatitis, epidermal and dermal atrophy, adrenal axis suppression.

Cautions: *Contraindicated in varicella or vaccinia.*

Cost: $$.

Pearls:

- Occlusive dressings enhance its systemic absorption.
- Prolonged use of this midpotency steroid may cause skin atrophy, telangiectasias, and pigmentary changes.

TRIAMTERENE (Dyrenium; *see also* Dyazide, Maxzide)

Dose: 100 mg PO bid.

Preparations: 50 and 100 mg capsules.

Actions: K^+-sparing diuretic used to treat hypertension.

Clearance: Metabolized via liver; metabolites are active; some renal and biliary excretion.

- Avoid in patients with GFR < 10 mL/min and in patients with liver disease.

Selected Side Effects: Hyperkalemia.

Selected Drug Interactions:

- Decreases clearance of lithium.
- Concomitant use with ACE inhibitors, K^+ supplements, salt substitutes, or β-blockers increases risk of hyperkalemia.
- Raises serum level of digoxin.

Pregnancy Category: B.

Cost: $$$ (0.50 each 100 mg Dyrenium tablet).

Pearls:

- Hyperkalemia is especially common in patients with GFR < 30 mL/min.
- Warn patients to avoid potassium-containing salt substitutes during use.
- Interferes with catecholamine and quinidine testing.
- Can aggravate megaloblastic anemia in patients with alcoholic cirrhosis.

TRIAZOLAM (Halcion)

Dose: 0.125–0.250 mg PO qhs.

Preparations: 0.125 and 0.250 mg tablets.

Actions: Benzodiazepine hypnotic that decreases sleep latency, increases sleep duration, and reduces the number of nocturnal awakenings; used for short-term management of insomnia.

Clearance: Metabolized via liver.

- No change in dosage needed in patients with renal insufficiency or liver disease.

Selected Side Effects: Drowsiness, dizziness and lightheadedness, rare amnesia, abnormal thinking and behavior changes, mood changes.

Selected Drug Interactions:

- Potentiates CNS depressant effects of other CNS depressants.
- Cimetidine and erythromycin double its $t_{1/2}$ and serum level.

Cautions:

- *Contraindicated in pregnant and potentially pregnant patients.*
- Avoid in elderly patients.

Pregnancy Category: X.

Cost: Generic \$\$, Halcion \$\$\$ (≈ \$0.50 each 0.25 mg generic tablet; ≈ \$0.70 each 0.25 mg Halcion tablet).

Pearls: Patients can get rebound insomnia after discontinuance.

TRIETHANOLAMINE otic solution (Cerumenex)

Dose and usage:

- (1) Tilt head at 45° angle; (2) fill ear canal with Cerumenex; (3) insert cotton plug; (4) allow to remain in ear 15–30 min; (5) gently flush ear with lukewarm water.
- Repeat this procedure if necessary.

Preparations: 6 and 12 mL bottles with dropper.

Actions: Ceruminolytic agent that emulsifies and disperses excess or impacted ear wax used to treat excessive, symptomatic cerumen build-up in the ear.

Selected Side Effects: Rare local dermatitis reactions.

Cautions: Contraindicated in patients with perforated tympanic membrane or otitis media. Discontinue if sensitization or irritation occurs.
Cost: $$$ (6 mL≈ $17, 12 mL ≈ $26).
Pregnancy Category: C.

TRIFLUOPERAZINE (Stelazine)
Dose: Disease dependent:
- Nonpsychotic anxiety: 1–2 mg PO bid.
- Acute therapy for psychotic disorder: 1–2 mg IM q4–6h prn.
- Chronic therapy for psychotic disorder: Usual starting dose is 2–5 mg PO bid; some patients may require higher doses.

Preparations: 1, 2, 5, and 10 mg tablets.
Actions: Phenothiazine derivative used to treat psychotic disorders and nonpsychotic anxiety.
Clearance: Extensively metabolized in the liver; metabolites are active.
Selected Side Effects: Drowsiness, dizziness, extrapyramidal reactions, fatigue and muscle weakness, dry mouth, blurred vision, *neuroleptic malignant syndrome, tardive dyskinesia,* ECG changes (especially Q wave and T wave changes), cholestasis.
Selected Drug Interactions:
- Concomitant use with methyldopa increases BP.
- Phenothiazines can decrease effect of warfarin, counteract antihypertensive effects of guanethidine and related compounds, and lower the convulsive threshold.
- Concomitant administration of propranolol and a phenothiazine can raise serum levels of both drugs.

Cautions:
- *Contraindicated in patients with depressed CNS state, existing blood dyscrasias, or bone marrow depression, or preexisting liver disease.*
- Lowers the seizure threshold and can increase risk of seizures in patients taking anticonvulsants.
- Can exacerbate anginal pain and orthostatic hypotension.

Pregnancy Category: Not established.
Cost: Generic $$, Stelazine $$$$ (≈ $0.35 each 2 mg tablet; ≈ $0.95 each 2 mg Stelazine tablet).

Pearls:
- Should only be used short term (< 12 weeks) for treatment of nonpsychotic anxiety.
- Concentrate preparation contains bisulfite and should be given diluted in juice, milk, carbonated beverages, coffee, soup, or pudding.
- Signs of neuroleptic malignant syndrome include extreme rise in temperature, muscle rigidity and "lead-pipe" syndrome, mental status changes, autonomic instability, including irregular pulse or BP, greatly increased HR, diaphoresis, arrhythmias, rhabdomyolysis (with increased CPK, myoglobinuria, and acute renal failure).

TRIHEXYPHENIDYL (Artane)
Dose: Disease and preparation dependent:
- Idiopathic parkinsonism:
  ▶ Give 1 mg PO the first day.
  ▶ May then increase daily dose by 2 mg increments every 3–5 days up to total of 6–10 mg PO given in 3 divided doses (ie, 2–3 mg PO tid).
- Drug-induced parkinsonism:
  ▶ Initially give 1 mg PO; may give subsequent higher doses after several hours if needed.
  ▶ Total daily dose required is usually 5–15 mg PO, given in divided doses.
- Concomitant use of Artane and levodopa: 3–6 mg PO daily, given in divided doses (such as 1–2 mg PO tid).
- Artane Sequels: Long-acting tablets that can be given qd–bid; once the total daily dose of trihexyphenidyl is established, Artane Sequels may be substituted on a mg per mg basis to achieve total daily dose.

Preparations:
- 2 and 5 mg scored tablets.
- 16 oz elixir containing 2 mg/5 mL (1 tsp).
- 5 mg sustained-action Artane Sequels.

Actions: Synthetic antispasmodic used to treat parkinsonian symptoms, particularly tremor and rigidity.

Selected Side Effects: Common side effects that often decrease with time include dry mouth, blurred vision, dizziness, nausea, and nervousness.

Cautions: Use with caution in patients with cardiovascular, renal, or liver disease, hypertension, acute angle-closure glaucoma, benign prostatic hypertrophy, or obstructive GI disease.

Pregnancy Category: C.

Cost: $$ (≈ $0.50/day).

Pearls:

- Patients should have gonioscopic examination and intraocular pressure monitoring at regular intervals (can raise intraocular pressure).
- Do not discontinue abruptly.
- Doses should be given around mealtime (some patients tolerate it better before meals and some afterward, depending on which side effects most affect them).

Trilafon: *see* PERPHENAZINE

Tri-Levlen (LEVONORGESTREL + ETHINYL ESTRADIOL)

Dose:

- 1 tablet PO qd, preferably after dinner or qhs; with 21-day preparation, take no pills on days 22–28 then begin a new cycle.
- For both 21- and 28-day preparations, take first tablet on the first day of menses. (*Note:* Other sources recommend different protocols for beginning therapy.)

Preparations: Available in 21- and 28-pill preparations.

- Days 1–6: 0.050 mg levonorgestrel and 0.030 mg ethinyl estradiol; days 7–11: 0.075 mg levonorgestrel and 0.040 mg ethinyl estradiol; days 12–21: 0.125 mg levonorgestrel and 0.030 mg ethinyl estradiol.
- Days 22–28 (with 28-day preparation): inert tablets.

Actions: Oral contraceptive with varying dose combintions; used to prevent pregnancy.

Selected Side Effects:

- Serious vascular complications, menstrual changes, cervical changes, breast changes, vaginal candidiasis, hypertension, edema, weight changes, gallbladder disease, GI distress, nausea and vomiting, liver tumors, migraine headache, rash, depression, glucose intolerance, visual changes from alteration in corneal curvature, intolerance for contact lenses.

• Breakthrough bleeding can occur during first several months of use.

Selected Drug Interactions: Concomitant use with antibiotics (ampicillin, chloramphenicol, isoniazid, nitrofurantoin, penicillin VK, phenytoin, rifampin, sulfonamides, tetracycline), analgesics, anxiolytics, antihistamines, migraine preparations, phenylbutazone, phenytoin, or tranquilizers can decrease its contraceptive effectiveness.

Cautions:

• *Contraindicated in patients with thromboembolic or thrombophlebitic disorders, cardiovascular or cerebrovascular disease, vaginal bleeding of unknown cause, endometrial or other estrogen-dependent tumors, known or suspected breast cancer, jaundice, hepatic tumors, smokers over age 35, or possible pregnancy.*

• Cigarette smoking increases risk of serious cardiovascular complications; patients should be *strongly* advised not to smoke.

Pregnancy Category: X.

Cost: $$$ (≈ $20/month).

Pearls: Patients should undergo complete work-up prior to use with special attention to history of abnormal vaginal bleeding, BP, breast examination, and pelvic examination including cervical cytology.

TRIMETHOBENZAMIDE (Tigan)

Dose: Delivery dependent.

• PO: 250 mg tid–qid.

• Suppository: 200 mg tid–qid.

• IM: 200 mg (2 mL) tid–qid.

Preparations:

• 100 and 250 mg tablets.

• 200 mg suppositories.

Actions: Anticholinergic agent used to treat nausea and vomiting.

• Mechanism of action may be related to central effects of the chemoreceptor trigger zone.

Selected Side Effects: Drowsiness, CNS reactions, including parkinsonian symptoms.
Cost: $$$ (~ $0.50 each 250 mg tablet).

TRIMETHOPRIM: *see* Bactrim

Tri-Norinyl (NORETHINDRONE + ETHINYL ESTRADIOL)
Dose: 1 pill PO qd, preferably qhs.
- With 21-day preparation, take no pills on days 22–28 then begin a new cycle.
- Take first pill on first Sunday after onset of menses, or that Sunday if it is first day of menses.

Preparations: Available in 21- and 28-pill preparations.
- Days 1–12: 0.5 mg norethindrone and 0.035 mg ethinyl estradiol; days 13–21: 1.0 mg norethindrone and 0.035 mg ethinyl estradiol.
- Days 22–28 (with 28-pill preparations): inert ingredients.

Actions: Oral contraceptive with varying dose combinations; used to prevent pregnancy.

Selected Side Effects:
- Serious vascular complications, menstrual changes, cervical changes, breast changes, vaginal candidiasis, hypertension, edema, weight changes, gallbladder disease, GI distress, nausea and vomiting, liver tumors, migraine headache, rash, depression, glucose intolerance, visual changes from alteration in corneal curvature, intolerance for contact lenses.
- Breakthrough bleeding can occur during first several months of use.

Selected Drug Interactions: Concomitant use with antibiotics (ampicillin, chloramphenicol, isoniazid, nitrofurantoin, penicillin V, phenytoin, rifampin, sulfonamides, tetracycline), analgesics, anxiolytics, antihistamines, migraine preparations, phenylbutazone, phenytoin, or tranquilizers can decrease its contraceptive effectiveness.

Cautions:
- *Contraindicated in patients with thromboembolic or thrombophlebitic disorders, cardiovascular or cerebrovascular*

382 POCKET GUIDE TO COMMONLY PRESCRIBED DRUGS

disease, vaginal bleeding of unknown cause, endometrial or other estrogen-dependent tumors, known or suspected breast cancer, jaundice, hepatic tumors, smokers over age 35, or possible pregnancy.

- Cigarette smoking increases risk of serious cardiovascular complications; patients should be *strongly* advised not to smoke.

Pregnancy Category: X.

Cost: $$$ (≈ $21/month retail).

Pearls: Patients should undergo complete work-up prior to use with special attention to history of abnormal vaginal bleeding, BP, breast examination, and pelvic examination including cervical cytology.

Triphasil (LEVONORGESTREL + ETHINYL ESTRADIOL)

Dose: 1 tablet PO qd, preferably after dinner or qhs.

- With 21-day preparation, take no pills on days 22–28 then begin a new cycle.
- For both 21- and 28-day preparations, take first tablet on the first day of menses. If begun after discontinuance of another oral contraceptive, take first pill on first day of withdrawal bleeding.
- If tablets are begun later than first day of menstruation, use an additional form of contraception for the first week.

Preparations: Available in 21- and 28-pill preparations.

- Days 1–6: 0.050 mg levonorgestrel and 0.030 mg ethinyl estradiol; days 7–11: 0.075 mg levonorgestrel and 0.040 mg ethinyl estradiol; days 12–21: 0.125 mg levonorgestrel and 0.030 mg ethinyl estradiol.
- Days 22–28 (with 28-pill preparations): inert ingredients.

Actions: Oral contraceptive with varying dose combintions; used to prevent pregnancy.

Selected Side Effects: Serious vascular complications, menstrual changes, cervical changes, breast changes, vaginal candidiasis, hypertension, edema, weight changes, gallbladder disease, GI distress, nausea and vomiting, liver tumors, migraine headaches, rash, depression, glucose intolerance, visual changes from alteration in corneal curvature, intolerance for contact lenses. Breakthrough bleeding can occur during first several months of use.

Selected Drug Interactions: Concomitant use with antibiotics (ampicillin, chloramphenicol, isoniazid, nitrofurantoin, penicillin VK, phenytoin, rifampin, sulfonamides, tetracycline), analgesics, anxiolytics, antihistamines, migraine preparations, phenylbutazone, phenytoin, or tranquilizers can decrease its contraceptive effectiveness.

Cautions:
- *Contraindicated in patients with thromboembolic or thrombophlebitic disorders, cardiovascular or cerebrovascular disease, vaginal bleeding of unknown cause, endometrial or other estrogen-dependent tumors, known or suspected breast cancer, jaundice, hepatic tumors, smokers over age 35, or possible pregnancy.*
- Cigarette smoking increases risk of serious cardiovascular complications; patients should be *strongly* advised not to smoke.

Pregnancy Category: X.

Cost: $$$ (≈ $22/month).

Pearls: Patients should undergo complete work-up prior to use with special attention to history of abnormal vaginal bleeding, BP, breast examination, and pelvic examination including cervical cytology.

Tums, Tums E-X antacid tablets (CALCIUM CARBONATE)

Dose: Use dependent.
- Antacid: Chew 1 or 2 tablets hourly prn up to a maximum of 16 tablets in 24 h of regular Tums or Tums E-X.
- Calcium supplement: 1 or 2 tablets after meals.

Preparations:
- Each regular-strength Tums contains 500 mg calcium carbonate.
- Each Tums E-X contains 750 mg calcium carbonate.

Actions: Antacid and calcium supplement.

Pearls: Each regular-strength Tums provides 20%, and each Tums E-X 30%, of the adult US RDA for calcium.

Tylenol: *see* ACETAMINOPHEN

Tylenol with Codeine
Dose:
- Tylenol Nos. 1, 2, or 3: 1–2 tablets q4h PO prn.
- Tylenol No. 4: 1 tablet q4h PO prn.

Preparations:
- Each tablet contains 300 mg acetaminophen and the following amount of codeine: No. 1, 7.5 mg; No. 2, 15 mg; No. 3, 30 mg; No. 4, 60 mg.
- Also available as 5 mL, 15 mL, and 1 pint elixir containing 120 mg acetaminophen and 12 mg codeine per 5 mL (1 tsp).

Actions: Combination analgesic used to treat mild to moderately severe pain.

Clearance: Metabolized via liver; codeine metabolites include norcodeine and morphine.
- Slightly decrease dosage in patients with impaired renal function.
- Reduce dosage in patients with liver disease.

Selected Side Effects: Sedation, respiratory depression, nausea and vomiting, constipation, hepatotoxicity (with overdose or chronic therapy).

Cautions:
- *Avoid in patients with liver disease.*
- Use with caution in patients disease.

Pregnancy Category: C.

Cost: $$ ($\approx$ $0.50 for each Tylenol 3 tablet).

Pearls:
- *All the precautions that apply to acetaminophen, particularly regarding hepatotoxicity, also apply to Tylenol with Codeine (see listing under ACETAMINOPHEN).*
- Patients allergic to morphine can have cross-allergy to codeine.
- Urine tests will be positive for morphine.

Ultrase: *see* PANCRELIPASE

Unasyn (AMPICILLIN + SULBACTAM)
Dose: 1.5–3.0 g IM or IV q6h.

Preparations: Each 1.5 g of Unasyn contains 1.0 g ampicillin and 0.5 g sulbactam.

Actions: β-Lactamase-resistant (from sulbactam) bactericidal semisynthetic penicillin antibiotic that inhibits cell wall biosynthesis.
- Good gram (+) coverage, including strep, staph, and enterococci (but *not* MRSA).
- Good gram (−) coverage, including β-lactamase-producing organisms (but *not Pseudomonas aeruginosa* and some resistant nosocomial organisms).
- Good anaerobic coverage, including *Bacteroides fragilis.*
- *NOTE:* The above-mentioned antimicrobial coverage summary should be used as a guideline only; treatment decisions should take into account not only local epidemiologic patterns of antibiotic susceptibility but also, when available, culture susceptibility results.

Clearance: Predominantly renally excreted.
- Moderately increase dosing interval in patients with impaired renal function.
- No change in dosage needed in patients with liver disease.

Selected Side Effects: Thrombophlebitis, pain at IM injection site, hypersensitivity and rare anaphylactic reactions.

Cautions: *Contraindicated in patients with allergy to any of the penicillins.*

Pregnancy Category: B.

Cost: $$.

Pearls:
- Can give false (+) urine glucose test.
- Risk of rash is increased in patients with mononucleosis or who are taking allopurinol.

Urecholine: *see* BETHANECHOL

UROKINASE (Abbokinase Open-Cath)
for catheter clearance
Dose and administration:
- After reconstituting as directed, inject urokinase in an amount equal to catheter volume; attempt aspiration after 35 min.
- May repeat aspiration attempts q5min for 30 min.
- If catheter is not opened in 30 min, retry after additional 30–60 min.
- A second injection may be necessary in resistant cases.

Actions: Thrombolytic agent produced by the kidney and found in urine; used to treat clotted IV catheters.
Clearance: Rapidly cleared by the liver.
Cautions: Contraindicated in patients with active internal bleeding, recent CVA, intracranial or intraspinal surgery, or CNS neoplasm (theoretically, can enter the systemic circulation).
Pregnancy Category: B.
Cost: $.

Valium: *see* DIAZEPAM

VALPROIC ACID (DIVALPROEX SODIUM, VPA, Depakene, Depakote)
Dose:
- Initial: 15 mg/kg PO in 3 divided doses (5 mg/kg PO tid).
- May increase daily (not tid) dose by 5–10 mg/kg at 1-week intervals.
- Maximum: 60 mg/kg PO daily (20 mg/kg PO tid).

Preparations:
- Depakene: 250 mg capsules; 16 oz bottles containing 250 mg/5 mL (1 tsp).
- Divalproex sodium: 125, 250, and 500 mg enteric-coated tablets.

Actions: Antiepileptic agent that may increase CNS levels of γ-aminobutyric acid; used to treat absence and tonic-clonic seizures
Clearance: Metabolized primarily via liver.
- No change in dosage needed in patients with renal insufficiency.
- Reduce dosage in patients with liver disease.
- Supplemental dose not required after hemodialysis or peritoneal dialysis.

Selected Side Effects: *Liver toxicity and hepatic failure,* decreased platelets or increased coagulation profile (or both), drowsiness, ataxia, transient GI side effects that usually resolve.
Selected Drug Interactions:
- Raises serum level of phenobarbital and can cause severe CNS depression.

- May decrease or increase serum level of phenytoin.
- Phenytoin and phenobarbital can alter its serum level.
- Concomitant use with carbamazepine can alter serum levels of both drugs.

Pregnancy Category: D.

Cost: $$$$ (≈ $5 each 250 mg tablet).

Pearls:

- Depakote (divalproex sodium) is a compound containing equal amounts of sodium valproate and valproic acid, formed by partial neutralization of valproic acid with NaOH; divalproex sodium dissociates to valproate in the GI tract.
- Follow LFTs, especially for first 6 months.
- Follow platelets and coagulation profile, especially in patients undergoing surgery.
- Usual therapeutic level is 50–100 mg/mL.
- Divalproex sodium is enteric-coated and has fewer GI side effects than other preparations.
- Alters urine ketone test.

Vancenase, Vancenase AQ:
see **BECLOMETHASONE**
nasal inhaler and spray

Vanceril: *see* **BECLOMETHASONE**
oral inhaler

VANCOMYCIN

Dose:

- 1 g IV q12h.
- Pseudomembranous colitis: 125–500 PO mg q6h (Sanford's antimicrobial booklet recommends 125 mg q6h).

Preparations: 125 and 250 mg capsules.

Actions: Bactericidal antibiotic that inhibits cell wall synthesis.

- Excellent gram (+) coverage, including *Staphylococcus aureus, S epidermidis,* MRSA, and enterococci, as well as gram (+) anaerobes.
- No gram (–) coverage.

- *NOTE:* The above-mentioned antimicrobial coverage summary should be used as a guideline only; treatment decisions should take into account not only local epidemiologic patterns of antibiotic susceptibility but also, when available, culture susceptibility results.

Clearance: Renally excreted.
- Markedly increase dosing interval in patients with impaired renal function.
- Dosage adjustment probably not needed in patients with liver disease.
- Supplemental dose not required after hemodialysis or peritoneal dialysis.

Selected Side Effects: *Nephrotoxicity,* ototoxicity, local phlebitis, decreased WBCs, "red man" syndrome.

Pregnancy Category: C.

Cost: $$$.

Pearls:
- Administer over > 60 min to avoid hypotension and anaphylactoid reactions.
- Follow serum peak and trough levels.

Vascor: *see* BEPRIDIL

VASOPRESSIN (Pitressin)

Dose (for bleeding esophageal varices):
- Initial: 0.2–0.4 units/min.
- Maintenance: 0.2–0.6 units/min.
- An initial bolus is *not* recommended.

Actions: Dose dependent:
- Low dose has antidiuretic effect; higher doses stimulate smooth muscle contractions, leading to decreased blood flow to splanchnic, coronary, pancreatic, GI, skin, and muscular systems; used to treat bleeding esophageal varices.

Selected Side Effects: Hypertension, angina, MI, arrhythmias, decreased urine output, finger necrosis, hypersensitivity reactions.

Pregnancy Category: C.

Cost: $$.

Pearls:
- After variceal bleeding is controlled, may taper by 0.1 unit q6–12h.

- Consider giving with nitrates to reduce systemic side effects (can decrease peripheral and coronary vasoconstriction).

Vasotec: *see* ENALAPRIL

VECURONIUM (Norcuron)
Dose:
- Initial intubating dose: 0.08–0.10 mg/kg IV.
- Subsequent maintenance doses of 0.010–0.015 mg/kg IV may be given as needed (the first maintenance dose may be required 25–40 min after initial dose; subsequent maintenance doses may be required every 12–15 minutes thereafter).
- Continuous infusion: Begin with 0.001 mg/kg/min IV; adjust as clinically indicated; usually maintenance dose is 0.0008–0.0012 mg/kg/min.

Actions: Nondepolarizing neuromuscular blocking agent that competes for cholinergic receptors at the motor endplate; used during endotracheal intubation and to provide skeletal muscle relaxation during surgery or mechanical ventilation.

Clearance: Recovery time is not significantly increased by impaired renal function but may be prolonged in patients with liver disease.

Selected Drug Interactions:
- Concomitant use with succinylcholine, aminoglycosides, lidocaine, quinidine, or tetracycline can prolong duration of neuromuscular blockade.
- Patients taking quinidine can experience recurrent paralysis.

Pregnancy Category: C.

Pearls:
- Is one third more potent than pancuronium and has shorter duration of action.
- Good intubation conditions are usually achieved 2.5–3.0 min after administration.
- Maximum neuromuscular blockade occurs within 3–5 min after administration.
- Time to 95% recovery is 45–60 min.
- Its action is reversed by acetylcholinesterase inhibitors (neostigmine, edrophonium, pyridostigmine, etc).

VENLAFAXINE (Effexor)
Dose:
- Initial: 75 mg daily, administered in 2–3 divided doses.
- The total daily dose can be increased to 150 and then 225 mg, allowing at least 4 days between any dose changes.

Preparations: 25, 37.5, 50, 75, and 100 mg tablets.

Actions: Structurally novel antidepressant that inhibits serotonin and norepinephrine reuptake.

Clearance: Metabolized via liver; renally excreted.
- Daily dose should be reduced by 50% in patients with moderate liver disease; those with even more limited liver function may require even greater reductions in dose.
- Daily dose should be reduced 25% in patients with mild to moderate renal impairment; in patients undergoing dialysis the total daily dose should be reduced by 50%, and the dose should be withheld until dialysis treatment is finished.

Selected Side Effects: Sustained elevation of blood pressure, nausea, constipation, somnolence or insomnia, anorexia and dose-dependent weight loss, nervousness, abnormal ejaculation/orgasm or impotence, seizures (rare).

Selected Drug Interactions: *Administration with MAO inhibitors associated with multiple serious adverse reactions.*

Cautions: *Should not be administered concurrent with or within 14 days of MAO inhibitor use; at least 7 days should be allowed between the discontinuation of venlafaxine and the initiation of MAO inhibitor treatment.*

Pregnancy Category: C.

Pearls:
- Venlafaxine should be taken with food.
- Blood pressure should be checked prior to initiating and during therapy.

Ventolin: *see* ALBUTEROL

VePesid: *see* ETOPOSIDE

VERAPAMIL (Calan, Calan SR, Isoptin, Isoptin SR, Verelan)

Dose: Delivery dependent.
- Regular-acting PO: 40–160 mg tid.
- Long-acting Calan SR and Isoptin SR: 120–240 mg qd–bid.
- Long-acting Verelan: 120–480 mg PO qd.
- IV: 2.5–5 mg over 2 min (3 min in elderly patients); may repeat dose if indicated.

Preparations:
- 40, 80, and 120 mg tablets of Calan and Isoptin.
- 120, 180, and 240 mg long-acting tablets of Calan SR and Isoptin SR.
- 120 and 240 mg long-acting tablets of Verelan.

Actions: Calcium channel blocker predominantly causing (−) cardiac inotropy, (−) cardiac chronotropy, and decreased cardiac conduction; used to treat angina and supraventricular arrhythmias and for diastolic dysfunction.

Clearance: Metabolized via liver; metabolites are active.
- Slightly reduce dosage in patients with end-stage renal disease; no change needed for milder renal dysfunction.
- Markedly decrease dosage in patients with liver disease.
- $t_{1/2}$ is prolonged in elderly patients.
- Supplemental dose not required after hemodialysis.

Selected Side Effects: Hypotension, bradycardia, CHF, constipation, AV node block.

Selected Drug Interactions: *Significantly raises serum level of digoxin (by 50–75%).*

Cautions: *Contraindicated in patients with decreased ejection fraction, substantially reduced BP, sick sinus syndrome, or second- or third-degree AV block (unless a ventricular pacemaker is in place) and in patients with atrial flutter or fibrillation* and *WPW syndrome or Lown-Ganong-Levine syndrome.*

Pregnancy Category: C.

Cost: PO $$$, IV $ (≈ $0.90 each 80 mg verapamil tablet; ≈ $1.30 each 240 mg Verelan tablet).

Verelan: *see* VERAPAMIL

Versed: *see* MIDAZOLAM

Vibramycin: *see* DOXYCYCLINE

Vibra-Tabs: *see* DOXYCYCLINE

Vicodin, Vicodin ES (ACETAMINOPHEN + HYDROCODONE)

Dose:
- Usual: 1–2 Vicodin tablets or 1 Vicodin ES tablet PO q4–6h.
- Maximum: 8 Vicodin or 5 Vicodin ES tablets over 24 h.

Preparations:
- Each Vicodin tablet contains 500 mg acetaminophen and 5.0 mg hydrocodone.
- Each Vicodin ES tablet contains 750 mg acetaminophen and 7.5 mg hydrocodone.

Actions: Schedule III narcotic preparation, in same category as Tylenol with Codeine and Fiorinal with Codeine, used to treat pain.

Clearance: Acetaminophen is metabolized in the liver; hydrocodone is metabolized to hydromorphone in the liver.

Cautions:
- *Contraindicated in patients with liver disease.*
- Use with caution in patients with pulmonary disease.

Pregnancy Category: C.

Cost: $$$ (Generic ≈ $0.30/tablet, Vicodin ≈ $0.55/tablet).

Pearls:
- *All the cautions that apply to acetaminophen, particularly those regarding hepatotoxicity, also apply to Vicodin.*
- As with other schedule III substances, may be prescribed by telephone in most states and may be refilled up to 5 times within 6 months.
- Has fewer GI side effects than codeine.

Videx: *see* DIDANOSINE

VINBLASTINE

Dose: Tumor dependent; often given weekly if WBC count permits. Give IV.

Actions: Antineoplastic agent that can interfere with metabolic pathways or mitosis; used to treat malignancies.

Clearance: Predominantly biliary excreted.

- May need to reduce dosage in patients with hepatobiliary insufficiency (toxicity can be increased).
- No change in dosage required in patients with impaired renal function.

Selected Side Effects:

- *Leukopenia, severe local irritation if extravasated,* acute bronchospasm and shortness of breath (especially when used in combination with mitomycin), constipation, hypertension, pain in tumor-containing organs (possibly from swelling of tumor tissue), reversible alopecia, rare nausea and vomiting.
- Has minimal direct effect on RBC count.

Pregnancy Category: D.

Cost: $$.

Pearls:

- WBC depression is dose-limiting side effect.
- WBC nadir occurs at days 5–10; recovery is complete 7–14 days after nadir.
- Platelets are decreased only in patients who have had previous radiation therapy or other bone marrow suppression.

VINCRISTINE

Dose: Tumor dependent.

- Often 1.4 mg/m^2 IV given weekly.
- Maximum single dose should not exceed 2 mg.

Actions: Antineoplastic alkylating agent that arrests mitosis by interfering with function of intracellular tubules; used to treat neoplasms.

Clearance: Cleared via hepatobiliary system.

- Reduce dosage in patients with hepatobiliary insufficiency.
- No change in dosage needed in patients with renal insufficiency.

Selected Side Effects: *Neurotoxicity, severe local irritation and possible tissue necrosis if extravasated, significant constipation and paralytic ileus,* increased uric acid and uric acid nephropathy, acute bronchospasm and shortness of breath (especially when used with mitomycin-C), common alopecia, occasional decrease in WBCs (especially with pre-existing bone marrow suppression), urine retention (especially in elderly patients), rare SIADH.

Pregnancy Category: D.
Cost: $$$.
Pearls:

- Dose-limiting neurotoxicity can include neuritic pain, sensory loss, paresthesias, difficulty walking, slapping gait, loss of deep tendon reflexes, muscle wasting, and cranial nerve impairment; loss of deep tendon reflex, by itself, is not a reason to withhold treatment.
- Neuromuscular effects frequently develop sequentially: sensory impairment and paresthesias, then neuritic pain, then motor dysfunction.
- Give anticonstipation agents aggressively (severe constipation can develop).
- Serious bone marrow depression is usually *not* a dose-limiting event.

VINORELBINE (Navelbine)

Dose: Usual dose is 30 mg/m², administered over 6–10 minutes, given weekly.
Actions: Vinca alkaloid that interferes with microtubule assembly; used as a chemotherapeutic agent.
Clearance: Metabolized via liver.

- Dose adjustment necessary in patients with liver disease.

Selected Side Effects: *Granulocytopenia,* peripheral neuropathy (usually mild or moderate), nausea, pain at local injection site, rare acute bronchospasm and dyspnea, occasional mild alopecia.
Cautions:
Pregnancy Category: D.
Pearls:

- Granulocyte counter nadir occurs 7–10 days after treatment, with recovery usually within the following 7–14 days.
- Granulocytopenia is the major dose-limiting side effect.
- Follow CBC.

Viokase: *see* **PANCRELIPASE**

Visken: *see* **PINDOLOL**

Vistaril: *see* **HYDROXYZINE**

VITAMIN B: *see* **THIAMINE**

VITAMIN B: *see* **PYRIDOXINE**

VITAMIN B: *see* **COBALAMIN**

Volmax: *see* **ALBUTEROL**

VITAMIN K
Dose: Use dependent:
- Acute therapy (in patients with coagulopathy believed secondary to Vitamin K deficiency): 10 mg SQ for 3 days.
- Chronic therapy: 10 mg SQ or IM monthly or 5–10 mg PO qd (if patient can absorb it orally).

Pearls: The administration of higher dose vitamin K (10 mg doses) to reverse elevated prothrombin times due to warfarin (Coumadin) treatment makes it extremely difficult to quickly reinitiate anticoagulant therapy for these patients with warfarin; therefore, vitamin K should be administered in either low doses (such as suggested in the American College of Chest Physicians' guidelines, which are periodically published in *Chest*) or not at all in patients in whom reinitiating anticoagulant therapy is anticipated (FFP administration may be preferable).

VPA: *see* **VALPROIC ACID**

VP-16: *see* **ETOPOSIDE**

WARFARIN (Coumadin)
Dose: Extremely variable. Some sources suggest 10 mg PO qd for 3 days, then 2–10 mg PO qd. Others do not give this

3-day "load," but begin therapy with the dose they believe
will be therapeutic.

- Consider beginning therapy at a lower dose (2–5 mg) if patient has liver disease, is elderly, chronically malnourished,
or on medication that can significantly potentiate warfarin.

Preparations: 2, 2.5, 5, 7.5, and 10 mg tablets.

Actions: Anticoagulant that inhibits production of vitamin
K-dependent coagulation factors; used to prevent or treat
thrombosis.

Clearance: Metabolized via liver.

- No change in dosage needed in patients with impaired renal
function.
- Although 21% of warfarin is excreted in urine, one source
notes that its $t_{1/2}$ is not increased in patients with liver disease, so no dosage adjustment is necessary.
- Supplemental dose not required after hemodialysis or peritoneal dialysis.

Selected Side Effects: Bleeding, rare necrosis of skin or
tissues (occurs in patients with protein C deficiency).

Selected Drug Interactions: Raises serum levels of OHAs,
phenytoin, and phenobarbital.

Cautions:

- *Contraindicated in pregnant patients and those of child-
bearing age who are likely to become pregnant.*
- Relatively contraindicated in patients with metastasis of
hemorrhagic tumors.

Pregnancy Category: X.

Cost: $$ (no generic form is available).

Pearls:

- *Factors that prolong PT response: Amiodarone, anesthet-
ics, many antibiotics, allopurinol, cancer, cimetidine, colla-
gen vascular diseases, CHF, diarrhea, diuretics, alcohol,
liver dysfunction, methyldopa, MAOI, NSAID, narcotics,
phenytoin, poor nutritional status, quinidine, ranitidine, sal-
icylates, thyroid medications, vitamin K deficiency.*
- Factors that shorten PT response: Antacids, antihistamines,
barbiturates, cholestyramine, diuretics, alcohol, haloperidol,
oral contraceptives, ranitidine, rifampin, vitamin C.
- Recommendations for what is the "ideal" INR for various
conditions are in evolution. The table shown here gives one

possible set of guidelines. These should be used as guidelines only, and the reader should consult other sources of information (particularly the American College of Chest Physicians' Consensus Conference recommendation in *Chest* 1992; 102 (supl): 312S–326S, as well as several articles on atrial fibrillation and mechanical heart valves in *N Eng J Med* 1995, volume 333(1) and hospital specialists before deciding on therapy.

Condition	INR Range
Venous Thrombosis (DVT)	2–3
Nonrheumatic Atrial Fibrillation	2–3
Mechanical Heart Valves	3–4
Ventricular Aneurism With Clot	3–4

Wellbutrin: *see* BUPROPION

Wytensin: *see* GUANABENZ

Xanax: *see* ALPRAZOLAM

Xylocaine: *see* LIDOCAINE

ZALCITABINE (ddc, DIDEOXYCYTIDINE, Hivid)
Dose: 0.75 mg PO q8h (NOT tid)
- When given in combination with zidovudine (AZT), the recommended dose of zidovudine is 200 mg PO q8h.

Preparations: 0.375 and 0.750 mg tablets.

Actions: Synthetic analogue of deoxycytidine that inhibits viral DNA synthesis; used as monotherapy in patients intolerant of zidovudine or with disease progression on zidovudine, or concurrently with zidovudine, for the treatment of advanced HIV infections.

Clearance: Primarily renally excreted; no significant liver metabolism.
- Dosage adjustment is recommended in patients with renal insufficiency.

Selected Side Effects: *Peripheral neuropathy,* rare pancreatitis, rare lactic acidosis, possible rare liver failure.

Selected Drug Interactions:

- Concomitant use of zalcitabine with other drugs known to cause peripheral neuropathy (dapsone, disulfiram, ethionamide, gold, hydralazine, isoniazid, metronidazole, nitrofurantoin, phenytoin (Dilantin), ribavirin, chloramphenicol, cisplatin, vincristine, etc) should be avoided when possible.
- Drugs, including amphotericin, cimetidine, probenecid, and aminoglycosides, may increase the risk of peripheral neuropathy and other toxicities by interfering with the renal clearance of zalcitabine.
- Maalox reduces its absorption.

Cautions:

- *Should be used with extreme caution, if at all, in patients with preexisting peripheral neuropathy.*
- Should be used with caution in patients at risk for or with pancreatitis or liver failure.

Pregnancy Category: C.

Cost: $$$$$.

Pearls:

- Peripheral neuropathy is the major side effect associated with zalcitabine; treatment should be promptly terminated in patients who develop signs or symptoms of peripheral neuropathy.
- Should be taken on an empty stomach.

Zantac: *see* RANITIDINE

Zarontin: *see* ETHOSUXIMIDE

Zaroxolyn: *see* METOLAZONE

ZDV: *see* ZIDOVUDINE

Zestoretic (LISINOPRIL + HYDROCHLOROTHIAZIDE)

Dose: 1 tablet PO qd.

Preparations: Tablets containing 20 mg lisinopril with either 12.5 or 25 mg hydrochlorothiazide.

Actions: Combination ACE inhibitor and diuretic used to treat hypertension.

Cost: $$$ (≈ $1.15/tablet).

Pearls: Should not be prescribed until it is first established that patients can tolerate this combination of medications at lower doses (potential for hypotension is high).

Pregnancy Category: D.

Side Effects, Drug Interactions, and Pearls: *see* LISINOPRIL and HYDROCHLOROTHIAZIDE.

Zestril: *see* LISINOPRIL

Ziac (BISOPROLOL + HYDROCHLOROTHIAZIDE)

Dose: Initial dose is one 2.5/6.25 tablet PO daily; titrate dose upward at 14-day intervals as clinically indicated up to a maximum dose of 20 mg of bisoprolol and 12.5 mg hydrochlorothiazide.

Preparations: Ziac 2.5/6.25, 5/6.25, and 10/6.25 tablets contain 2.5, 5, and 10 mg bisoprolol, respectively, and 6.25 mg of hydrochlorothiazide.

Actions: Combination of a β_1-selective β-receptor blocker (bisoprolol) and thiazide diuretic (hydrochlorothiazide); used for the treatment of hypertension.

ZIDOVUDINE (AZT, Retrovir, ZDV)

Dose: 100–200 mg PO q4h while awake.

• Lower dose is equally effective in many situations and has substantially less toxicity.

Preparations:

• 100 mg capsules.

• 240 mL bottles of syrup containing 50 mg/5 mL (1 tsp).

Actions: Antiretroviral drug that inhibits RNA-dependent DNA polymerase; used to treat HIV infection.

Clearance: Metabolized primarily via liver; some renal excretion.

• Dosage may need to be adjusted in patients with severe renal disease; no change needed for milder renal impairment.

• Requires cautious use and possible dosage adjustment in patients with liver disease.

Selected Side Effects: Leukopenia, anemia (most commonly after 4–6 weeks), headache, insomnia, nausea and vomiting, fatigue, myositis, neurotoxicity.

Selected Drug Interactions:
- Can raise or lower serum level of phenytoin.
- Decreases serum level of theophylline.
- Concomitant use with ganciclovir or dapsone increases risk of myelosuppression.
- Use with acyclovir increases risk of neurotoxicity.
- Acetaminophen can exacerbate its toxicity.

Pregnancy Category: C.

Cost: $$$$$ (≈ $1.50 each 100 mg tablet); cost is a *major,* if not prohibitive factor for many patients.

Pearls:
- Frequently check CBC.
- Has not been shown to decrease infectivity.

Zinacef: *see* CEFUROXIME

Zithromax: *see* AZITHROMYCIN

Zocor: *see* SIMVASTATIN

Zofran: *see* ONDANSETRON

Zoloft: *see* SERTRALINE

ZOLPIDEM (Ambien)

Dose:
- 10 mg PO qhs.
- Use 5 mg PO qhs in elderly and debilitated patients and those with hepatic dysfunction.

Preparations:

Actions: Imidazopyridine hypnotic agent used for the short-term treatment of insomnia.
- Actions are believed to be related to its effects on GABA receptors.

Clearance: Metabolized to inactive metabolites.
- No dose adjustment necessary in patients with renal failure.

Selected Side Effects: Daytime drowsiness requiring discontinuation occurs only rarely (0.5–1.6%); few significant side effects compared with rates in placebo-treated patients.

Pregnancy Category: B.

Pearls:
- Is not structurally related to benzodiazepine hypnotic agents.
- Absorption is decreased by food.

ZORprin: *see* ACETYLSALICYLIC ACID

Zostrix: *see* CAPSAICIN cream

Zovirax: *see* ACYCLOVIR

Zyloprim: *see* ALLOPURINOL

INDEX

Pro-Step. *See* NICOTINE transdermal patch
Proventil. *See* ALBUTEROL
Provera. *See* MEDROXYPROGESTERONE
Prozac. *See* FLUOXETINE
PSEUDOEPHEDRINE (Sudafed), 12, 325. *See also* Actifed; Robitussin-PE; Seldane-D
PSYLLIUM. *See* Metamucil
PTU. *See* PROPYLTHIOURACIL
Purinethol. *See* MERCAPTOPURINE
PYRAZINAMIDE (PZA), 325
Pyridium. *See* PHENAZOPYRIDINE
PYRIDOXINE (VITAMIN B$_6$), 326
PZA. *See* PYRAZINAMIDE

Q

Questran. *See* CHOLESTYRAMINE
Quinaglute. *See* QUINIDINE
Quinamm. *See* QUININE
QUINAPRIL (Accupril), 8, 326–327
Quinidex. *See* QUINIDINE
QUINIDINE (QUINIDINE SULFATE, Quinaglute, Quinidex Extentabs), 3, 327–328
QUININE (QUININE SULFATE, Quinamm), 9, 328–329

R

RAMIPRIL (Altace), 8, 329–330
RANITIDINE (Zantac), 3, 14, 330
Reglan. *See* METOCLOPRAMIDE
Relafen. *See* NABUMETONE
RESERPINE (Seprasil), 8
RESERPINE (Serpasil), 331–332
Restoril. *See* TEMAZEPAM
Retin-A. *See* TRETINOIN topical cream, gel, and liquid
Retrovir. *See* ZIDOVUDINE
Rhinocort. *See* BUDESONIDE
Rifadin. *See* RIFAMPIN
RIFAMPIN (Rifadin, Rimactane), 332–333

Rimactane. *See* RIFAMPIN
Robinul. *See* GLYCOPYRROLATE
Robitussin. *See* GUAIFENESIN; Robitussin preparations
Robitussin A-C (GUAIFENESIN + CODEINE + ALCOHOL), 9, 333–334
Robitussin-CF (GUAIFENESIN + PHENYLPROPANOLAMINE + DEXTROMETHORPHAN + ALCOHOL), 334
Robitussin-DM (GUAIFENESIN + DEXTROMETHORPHAN + ALCOHOL), 9, 334
Robitussin-PE (GUAIFENESIN + PSEUDOEPHEDRINE + ALCOHOL), 334–335
Rocephin. *See* CEFTRIAXONE
Roferon-A. *See* INTERFERON
Rogaine. *See* MINOXIDIL
Rolaids (CALCIUM CARBONATE), 335
Rolaids (DIHYDROXYALUMINUM SODIUM CARBONATE), 3, 335
Rolaids, Extra Strength (CALCIUM CARBONATE), 335
Rolaids, Sodium-Free (CALCIUM CARBONATE + MAGNESIUM HYDROXIDE), 335
Romazicon. *See* FLUMAZENIL
Rufen. *See* IBUPROFEN
Rythmol. *See* PROPAFENONE

S

SALBUTAMOL. *See* ALBUTEROL
SALMETEROL (Serevent), 336
SALSALATE (Disalcid), 2, 336–337
SCOPOLAMINE, 6
SCOPOLAMINE (Transderm Scop), 337–338
SCRALFATE (Carafate), 3
SECOBARBITAL (Seconal), 2, 338
Seconal. *See* SECOBARBITAL
Sectral. *See* ACEBUTOLOL